ADVANCES IN OCULAR IMMUNOLOGY

Acknowledgement

The Sixth International Symposium on the Immunology and Immunopathology of the Eye gratefully acknowledges the generous support of the following organizations:

Alcon Laboratories
Allergan, Inc.
Chiron Vision
Iolab
Kowa Company, Ltd.
Rhein Medical

ADVANCES IN OCULAR IMMUNOLOGY

Proceedings of the 6th International Symposium on the Immunology and Immunopathology of the Eye, Bethesda, USA

Editors:

Robert B. Nussenblatt
Scott M. Whitcup
Rachel R. Caspi
Igal Gery

Laboratory of Immunology
National Eye Institute,
National Institute of Health
Bethesda, MD
USA

1994

ELSEVIER

Amsterdam - Lausanne - New York - Oxford - Shannon - Tokyo

International Congress Series No. 1068
ISBN 0-444-81742-5

This book is printed on acid-free paper.

Published by:
Elsevier Science B.V.
P.O. Box 211
1000 AE Amsterdam
The Netherlands

        Library of Congress Cataloging-in-Publication Data

International Symposium on the Immunology and Immunopathology of the
  Eye (6th : 1994 : Bethesda, Md.)
    Advances in ocular immunology : proceedings of the 6th
  International Symposium on the Immunology and Immunopathology of the
  Eye, Bethesda, USA / editors, Robert B. Nussenblatt ... [et al.].
      p.   cm. -- (International congress series)
    Includes index.
    ISBN 0-444-81742-5 (alk. paper)
    1. Eye--Immunology--Congresses. 2. Eye--Inflammation--Congresses.
  I. Nussenblatt, Robert B. II. Title. III. Series.
    [DNLM: 1. Eye Diseases--immunology--congresses. 2. Eye-
  -immunology--congresses. 3. Inflammation--immunology--congresses.
  W3 EX89 no. 106B 1994 / WW 140 I61 1994a]
  RE68.I56   1994
  617.7'1--dc20
  DNLM/DLC
  for Library of Congress   94-35302
                                                            CIP

Printed in the Netherlands

FOREWORD

This volume represents the corpus of scientific reports presented at the 6th International Symposium on the Immunology and Immunopathology of the Eye (IIPE), which took place on the campus of the National Institutes of Health in Bethesda, Maryland, from June 22-24, 1994. The IIPE is the oldest international congress devoted to the study of the immunology of the eye. During this meeting, we had the great pleasure to honour Dr. Arthur Silverstein, one of the pioneers in our area of study. Dr. Silverstein was present at the first IIPE, held in Strasbourg in 1974, and has witnessed the extraordinary advances that have occurred in our field during the past 20 years. The international flavor has always been one of the major characteristics of the IIPE Symposia, and we believe the reader will find that this characteristic again holds true for this meeting, with researchers from all continents and from 18 countries present. Scientists have contributed over 110 reports to this text and this volume represents the most up-to-date collection of information concerning the status of ocular immunology the interested reader can find. The mixture of clinical as well as basic research reflects the broad scope of the subject matter. It will also be clear to the reader that ocular immunology's various models for organ specific immune responses are remarkably adept at yielding information that has import to all in immunology, and not just those working in the field of ocular immunology. We sincerely hope that this volume will be an often-used reference for all those interested in ocular immunology and immunopathology, and that it will be a solid foundation for future work in the field.

Robert B. Nussenblatt, M.D.
Scott M. Whitcup, M.D.
Rachel R. Caspi, Ph.D.
Igal Gery, Ph.D.

CONTENTS

1. Ocular Immunology and Inflammation
b. ACAID and related processes

1. Ocular Immunology and Inflammation
c. Therapeutic approaches

2. Ocular Infection: Mechanisms of Disease and Therapeutic Approaches

II. CLINICAL PRACTICE
1. Inflammatory Disease
a. Mechanisms, manifestations and diagnosis

I. BASIC SCIENCE
1. Ocular Immunology and Inflammation
a. Mechanisms of disease: Molecules, cells and processes they induce

© 1994 Elsevier Science B.V. All rights reserved.
Advances in Ocular Immunology
R.B. Nussenblatt, S.M. Whitcup, R.R. Caspi and I. Gery, eds.

Tumor necrosis factor synthesis by resident retinal cells from uveitis-susceptible and resistant rat strains; synthesis and regulation of nitric oxide from Lewis rat retinal Müller cells

Y. de Kozak[a], O. Goureau[b], J. Bellot[a], M. C. Naud[a], J. P. Faure[a] and D. Hicks[c]

[a]INSERM U 86, 15 rue de l'Ecole de Médecine, 75270 Paris 06, France.
[b]INSERM U 118, 29 rue Wilhem, 75016 Paris, France.
[c]INSERM CJF 9202, BP 426, 67091 Strasbourg, France.

ABSTRACT

Tumor necrosis factor (TNF) production was examined in two resident ocular cell types cultured *in vitro*. We show that the retinal Müller glia (RMG) and retinal pigmented epithelium cells isolated from Lewis and Lewis x BN F1 rats (susceptible to develop ocular inflammation) and stimulated *in vitro* by combined treatment with IFN-γ and LPS synthesized large amounts of TNF. In contrast, the amount of TNF produced by cells from BN and Long Evans rats (resistant or poorly susceptible) was much lower or remained undetectable. Nitric oxide (NO) release was detected in supernatants from in vitro stimulated Lewis RMG. Addition to the medium of anti-TNF antibody inhibited TNF activity while specific inhibitors of NO synthesis and TGF-β blocked cytokine-induced NO production. Since TNF and NO are involved in tissue necrosis, their inhibition during ocular inflammatory processes could contribute to the modulation of ocular pathologies.

INTRODUCTION

Experimental autoimmune uveitis (EAU) and endotoxin-induced uveitis (EIU) are models for several ocular inflammatory diseases collectively termed uveitis. EAU induced in rodents following immunization with purified retinal proteins [1] is characterized by ocular inflammation and photoreceptor cell destruction. It can be transferred by Th1-like cell lines [2] producing interferon-γ (IFN-γ) and interleukin (IL)-2 but not IL-4 and can be protected by Th2-like cells expressing IL-4 mRNA [3]. EIU is induced in rodents by a systemic injection of endotoxin (lipopolysaccharide (LPS) from gram-negative bacterial outer membranes) [4]. It is characterized by a massive invasion of activated PMN and macrophages, mainly into the anterior segment of the eye but also into the posterior segment [5]. The local release of mediators and cytokines in the aqueous humor and the vitreous, mainly IL-6 and TNF [6-9] is responsible for the breakdown of the blood ocular barriers, the attraction of inflammatory cells into the retina resulting in ocular inflammation and destruction of the photoreceptor cell layer in EAU. Different strains of rodents differ in the degree of disease susceptibility or resistance to EAU [10] and EIU [4,6]. TNF is present in high amounts in aqueous humor and vitreous of diseased Lewis (Lew) rats (highly susceptible to develop immune reactions) while absent in serum. In contrast, low levels of TNF are detected in aqueous humor and vitreous from Brown-Norway (BN) and Long Evans (LE) rats (resistant or poorly susceptible strains) [7]. We have previously shown that ocular resident cells: retinal Müller glial (RMG) and pigment epithelial (RPE) cells prepared from retinas of Lew rats and stimulated *in vitro* with LPS and IFN-γ synthesize tumor necrosis factor (TNF) [8] indicating that TNF present in aqueous humor and vitreous from EAU and EIU-presenting Lew rats originates at least partly by local synthesis. Interestingly, LPS, IFN-γ and TNF have been shown to stimulate nitric oxide (NO) synthesis in different cell types [11]. NO is a reactive gas, synthesized from L-arginine by NO synthase (NOS). We have shown that bovine RPE [12] and rat RMG [13] can express nitric oxide synthase (NOS) and synthesize NO after *in vitro* treatment with various stimulants.

We show in this study that RMG and RPE cells from rat strains susceptible to develop ocular inflammation secrete large amounts of TNF while cells from resistant rats secrete low or undetectable quantities. Moreover, the *in vitro* stimulation of RMG cells from the highly susceptible Lew rat strain leads to the release of NO which could play role in local inflammatory processes.

MATERIALS AND METHODS

Cell culture

RMG and RPE (2-3 passages) were established from young rats [14, 15]. Cells prepared from different rat strains were incubated for 72 h (average density: 2×10^5 cells/well) with stimulatory agents in DMEM containing 2% FCS: recombinant mouse IFN-γ (100 U/ml) followed after 6 h with *Salmonella typhimurium* LPS (100 ng/ml) in 6 well plates. Supernatants were collected after stimulation, centrifuged to remove cells and stored at -70 until TNF and nitrite titration. The purity of cells was controlled by immunocytochemical studies on cells grown on coverslips in parallel with the assay plates [14]. RMG and RPE were estimated as 95% pure and no cells with fibroblastic morphology was detected in both types of cell culture. Three independent cultures of RMG and RPE for each strain were established for TNF determination.

TNF bioassay

Levels of TNF were determined in the RMG and RPE supernatants in a bioassay using L-929 mouse fibroblasts in which the concentration of TNF is proportional to fibroblast cytolysis [16]. This assay does not distinguish between TNF-α and TNF-β, with a TNF detection of 20 to 50 pg/ml.

Nitrite determination

As nitrite and nitrate are a stable end product of NO metabolism, NO synthesis was determined as nitrite release in supernatants from cells treated with LPS and cytokines using the spectrophotometric method based on the Griess reaction [12].

RESULTS AND DISCUSSION

TNF production by cultured RMG and RPE

TNF was not detected in supernatants from non-stimulated RMG and RPE cells or cells stimulated by LPS or IFN-γ alone [8]. TNF synthesis was strongly induced in Lew and Lew x BN F1 hybrids RMG and RPE by combined treatment with IFN-γ (100 ng/ml) and LPS (100 U/ml). Though variability between experiments was observed due probably to the use of cells at 2nd and 3rd passage and in different stages of the cell cycle, the amount of TNF released from BN rats was always low compared to

Lew cells. Cells from LE rats did not release detectable amounts of TNF (Figure 1 A). Inhibition of TNF activity was observed when increasing amounts of a hamster mAb anti-murine TNF (previously shown to neutralize TNF activity) were added to supernatants from stimulated RMG Lew and RPE BN cells (Figure 1 B).

Though different mechanisms have been suggested to explain the variations in susceptibility to develop EAU and EIU [17, 10, 18-20], susceptibility to develop ocular immune responses could also be related to the differential intraocular production of TNF.

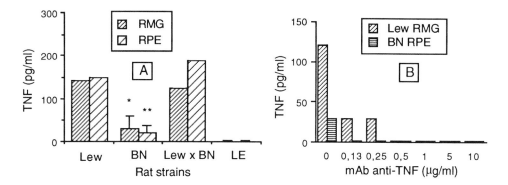

Figure 1.A. Concentration of TNF in supernatants from cultured RMG and RPE from the different strains. Cells were stimulated for 72 h by combined treatment with IFN-γ (100 U/ml) and LPS (100 ng/ml). Values are mean for three different experiments. * p=0.07; ** p=0.04 (Mann -Whitney U test).

Figure 1.B. Inhibiting effect of increasing amounts of hamster mAb anti recombinant mouse TNF on TNF produced by Lew RMG and BN RPE cells.

Nitrite production from Lew RMG cells stimulated by LPS and cytokines

RMG cells stimulated with LPS, IFN-γ or TNF alone did not release nitrite. (Figure 2 A). The highest levels of nitrite were obtained after co-stimulation with LPS, IFN-γ and TNF. Specific NOS inhibitors, N^G-monomethyl-L-Arginine (L-NMMA) and Nω-nitro-L arginine (L-NitroA) or transforming growth factor-β (TGF-β) or cycloheximide co-incubated with NOS inducers (LPS/IFN-γ/TNF-α) blocked cytokine-induced nitrite formation (Figure 2B).

Immunologic and inflammatory stimuli induce NO production via the expression of the inducible form of NOS (11). It has been recently reported that repeated intraperitoneal injection of N^G-nitro-L-arginine methyl ester (L-NAME), a NOS inhibitor, reduced the inflammatory manifestations of EIU [21]. We have shown the expression of an inducible form of NOS in Lew RMG cells stimulated in vitro [13] and the inhibition of EIU and local NO production by L-NAME injection (J. Bellot et al., this meeting).

Since RMG and RPE have been shown to play roles in local ocular immune responses [22-25], therapeutics aimed at inhibiting TNF and NO release by retinal resident cells could represent potential means of modulating inflammatory and autoimmune ocular manifestations.

6

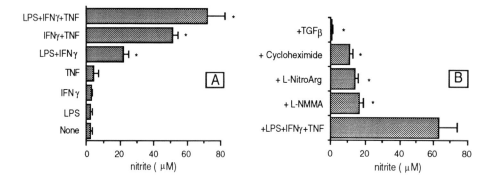

Figure 2.A. Nitrite level (Griess reaction) in supernatants from Lew RMG stimulated for 72 h with IFN-γ (100 U/ml), LPS (1 μg/ml) or TNF-α (100 U/ml) alone or in combination. Values are mean ±SD for five independent cultures.
* p< 0.001 (Student's *t* test).

Figure 2.B. Inhibition of cytokine-induced nitrite formation due to cellular stimulation with 100 U/ml IFN-γ, 1 μg/ml LPS and 100 U/ml TNF-α, by L-arginine analogues, cycloheximide or TGF-β.

REFERENCES

1   Faure JP, In: Bona CA , et al. eds. The Molecular   Pathology of Autoimmune Diseases. Harwood Academic Pub., Langhorne, PA, 1993; 651-672.
2   Caspi RR., Roberge FG, Mc Allister CC, El Saied M, et al. J Immunol 1986;136: 928-933.
3   Saoudi A, Kuhn J, Huygen K, de Kozak Y, et al. Eur J Immunol 1993; 23:3096-3103.
4   Rosenbaum JT, McDevitt HO, Guss RB, Egbert PR. Nature1980; 286: 611-613.
5   Ruiz-Moreno JM, Thillaye B, de Kozak Y. Ophthalmic Res 1992; 24:162-168.
6   Hoekzema R, Verhagen C, van Haren M, Kijlstra A. Invest Ophthalmol Vis Sci1992;33: 532-539.
7   De Vos A F, van Haren MAC, Verhagen C, Hoekzema R, et al. Invest Ophthalmol Vis Sci 1994; 35: 1100-1106.
8   de Kozak Y, Hicks D, Chatenoud L, Bellot J, et al. Reg Immunol 1994 (in press).
9   Planck SR, Huang XN, Robertson JE, Rosenbaum JT. Invest Ophthalmol Vis Sci 1994; 35: 924-930.
10   Caspi RR. Reg Immunol1992; 4: 321-330.
11   Nathan CF. FASEB J 1992; 6: 3051-3064.
12   Goureau O, Lepoivre M, Becquet F, Courtois. Y Proc Natl Acad Sci USA 1993; 90: 4276-4280.
13   Goureau O, Hicks D, Courtois Y, de Kozak Y. J Neurochem, 1994 (in press).
14   Hicks D, Courtois Y. Exp Eye Res1990; 51: 119-129.
15   Malecaze F, Mascarelli F, Bugra K, Fuhrmann G, et al. J Cell Physiol1993; 154: 631-642.
16   Ferran C, Sheenan K, Dy M, Schreiber R, et al. Eur J Immunol 1990; 20: 509-515.
17   Mochizuki, M, Kuwabara, T, Chan CC, Nussenblatt RR, et al. J Immunol1984; 133: 699-1701.
18   Li Q, Whitcup SM, Fujino Y, Nussenblatt RB, et al. Invest Ophthalmol Vis Sci1993; 34: 256-259.
19   Mirshahi M, de Kozak Y, Gregerson DS, Stiemer R, et al. In: M. Usui, S. Ohno, K Aoki, eds. Ocular Immunopathology Today, Excerpta Medica, Amsterdam,1990;195-198.
20   Calogero A E, Sternberg E M, Bagdy G, Smith C, et al. Neuroendocrinology 1992;55: 600-608.
21   Parks DJ, Cheung MK, Chan CC, Roberge FG. Arch Ophthalmol 1994; 112: 544-546.
22   Caspi RR, Roberge FG, Nussenblatt RB. Science 1987; 237: 1029-1032.
23   Roberge FG, Caspi RR, Nussenblatt RB. J Immunol 1988;140: 2193-2196.
24   Percopo CM, Hooks JJ, Shinohara T, Caspi RR, et al. J Immunol1990;145: 4101-4107.
25   Liversidge J, McKay D, Mullen G, Forrester JV. Cell Immunol 1993; 149: 315-330.

Advances in Ocular Immunology
R.B. Nussenblatt, S.M. Whitcup, R.R. Caspi and I. Gery, eds.

EVALUATION OF CYTOKINE-MEDIATED CHEMOTAXIS OF Ia+ LANGERHANS CELLS (LC) INTO THE CENTRAL CORNEA OF MICE: Effect of Cyclosporine A (CsA), Transforming Growth Factor (TGF)-β and Interferons (IFNs)-α,β and γ.

S.P. Epstein,MD[a], M.S. Jan, L.S. Skittone, T. Small,MSIV and P.A. Asbell,MD[a].

[a]Department of Ophthalmology, Mount Sinai Medical Center, New York, NY, USA

INTRODUCTION:

Under normal conditions, the central cornea is devoid of Ia+ Langerhans cells (LC; 1,2). Recent research has indicated that the presence of LC therein disturbs the normal immunosuppressive microenvironment of the eye and can lead to decreased visual acuity via corneal opacification/scarring.

A variety of stimuli have been shown to induce the migration of peripheral LC into the cornea, which is known to elaborate a variety of cytokines. It was logical to assume that a single chemical mediator, most likely a cytokine, is released by the corneal epithelium and induces the centripetal migration of LC from the conjunctiva.

To determine whether each of the cytokines studied acts directly on LC or via induction of a secondary mediator, we first investigated whether Cyclosporine A (CsA) could inhibit the induction of Ia on LC. We reasoned that signals acting through the production of other cytokines might be rendered inoperative by the presence of CsA, enabling it to differentiate between direct- and indirect-acting chemotactic cytokines. Indeed, previous reports have shown that: 1)CsA is particularly effective in inhibiting cytokine production (3,4), and 2)CsA has been successful in distinguishing direct-acting cytokines from those which evoke a response through the induction of intermediaries (indirect-acting cytokines, 5).

Transforming growth factors (TGF)-β are known to be produced in corneal cells (6), effecting various immunologic functions (7) by promoting the development of suppressor T cells (8). Because CsA shares many of these activities with TGF-β [reviewed in (8)], and given this author's prior findings concerning the effect of both CsA (5) and TGF-β (9) on cytokine-induced expression of Ia antigen (Ag) on LC in skin, we were curious about what effect TGF-β might have on LC chemotaxis.

Interferons (IFNs) have been also documented as possessing inhibitory activities (10), so it was considered possible that IFN-γ might be inhibitory for direct- and/or indirect-acting cytokines. Those cytokines found to be chemotactic for LC were therefore also injected simultaneously with IFN-γ.

MATERIALS AND METHODS:

Animals: Female 2-3 month old BALB/c, C57BL/6 and C3H/HeJ mice (Charles River Breeding Laboratories Inc., Kingston, NY).

Cytokines: Recombinant (r) human (hu) IFN-α, r murine (mu) interleukins (IL)-1α, 1β, 2 and 6, natural (n) mu granulocyte macrophage-colony stimulating factor (GM-CSF) and n hu tumor necrosis factor (TNF)-α were obtained from Collaborative Biomedical Products (Becton Dickinson, Bedford, MA). The dosage of each of the cytokines used in these experiments was determined from dose-response curves in mouse skin; the lowest dosage that reliably gave maximal enhancement was used.

Increased LC chemotaxis into the cornea at higher dose levels was never observed.

Intracorneal injection of cytokines: 0.004U IL-1α or β, 250U IL-2, 1000U IL-6 or IFN-α, 15U GM-CSF or 10U TNF-α was intracorneally injected using a 10μl Hamilton Syringe, 30 gauge needle and dissecting microscope. Injections utilizing glass pipets drawn out to micron diameters failed to evoke any different response.

Each cytokine was diluted in 0.9% normal saline (NS). All intracorneal injections were performed with and without the simultaneous intraocular application of CsA (5 μg/eye, courtesy of Dr. Paul Nadler & Ms. Kathleen Roskaz, Sandoz, Inc., East Hanover, NJ), 41.5ng n TGF-β or 500IU r hu IFN-γ (Collaborative Biomedical Products, Becton Dickinson, Bedford, MA) administered as ophthalmic drops:

CsA: dissolved in minimum volume of ethanol. Tears Naturale II (Alcon Laboratories, Fort Worth, TX) slowly added to a final concentration of 10mg/ml which was filtered and the alcohol allowed to evaporate.

TGF-β & IFN-γ: dissolved in Tears Naturale II. Final pH adjusted to ≈6.0.

Preparation of corneal samples and positive controls: After 16 hours, the animals were euthanized and the corneas, as well as a small depilated skin sample, were harvested. Corneal epithelium and epidermal sheets were prepared by incubation in 0.5M NH_4SCN (in 1M Phosphate Buffer, pH 6.5, 25 min, 37°C).

Enumeration of Ia$^+$ LC: Both the experimental samples (corneas), as well as the positive controls (epidermal sheets), were fixed in ethanol (20 mins, 4°C) and the specimens stained with monoclonal anti-mouse Ia clone M5/114 (Boehringer Mannheim, Indianapolis, IN, 11) via an indirect immunoperoxidase technique (12).

The number of LC/cornea was determined microscopically in a blinded fashion. Prior research has shown that LC, but neither corneal epithelial cells nor corneal keratocytes, acquire Ia Ag (unpublished observations).

Statistics: Statistical differences were determined using a Student's t test.

RESULTS:

Negative Controls: In our hands, the normal unstimulated mouse cornea, as well as those of the negative controls, were each found to contain from 0 to 3 Ia$^+$ LC in the peripheral cornea (see Table I) with none in the central or paracentral.

Effect of cytokines on Ia$^+$ LC chemotaxis: The intracorneal injection of neither IL-1α nor GM-CSF successfully induced the migration of greater than 3 Ia$^+$ LC (see Table I); while IL-1β, IL-6, and TNF-α, consistently induced the migration of between 6 and 15 Ia$^+$ LC (see Table I). Surprisingly, IL-6 yielded the migration of the smallest number of Ia$^+$ LC into the murine corneas, while IL-1β and TNF-α were each approximately equally potent. In BALB/c, C57BL/6 and C3H/HeJ mice, IL-2 induced the chemotaxis of a statistically larger number of Ia$^+$ LC as compared to that of the other cytokines studied (see Table I, p<0.01). Neither longer incubations nor higher doses elicited any higher chemotactic levels.

Effect of CsA on cytokine-mediated Ia$^+$ LC chemotaxis: The intracorneal injection of IFN-α, IL-1β nor IL-6, was chemotactic for LC when intracorneally injected with 5μg CsA (see Table I), while both IL-2 and TNF-α maintained their chemotactic effect upon LC in the presence of CsA (see Table I). The addition of CsA upregulated the level of IL-2-induced Ia$^+$ LC chemotaxis in C57BL/6, but not C3H/HeJ, mice to that of BALB/c mice (see Table I).

TABLE I:

STRAIN-RELATED DIFFERENCES IN CYTOKINE-MEDIATED CHEMOTAXIS OF Ia⁺ LANGERHANS CELLS INTO THE CORNEA

* Ia⁺ LC/CORNEA ± STANDARD DEVIATION (n)

CYTOKINE	MODUL-ATOR	BALB/c	C57BL/6	C3H/HeJ
None	None	0.17 ± 0.41 (12)	0.33 ± 0.49 (12)	0.82 ± 0.75 (11)
None	5 µg CsA	0.17 ± 0.41 (12)	0.63 ± 0.74 (12)	1.08 ± 0.95 (13)
None	42ngTGF	0.25 ± 0.45 (12)	0.17 ± 0.39 (12)	0.70 ± 0.67 (10)
None	500U IFN	0.67 ± 0.82 (15)	0.56 ± 0.73 (16)	0.92 ± 0.67 (12)
IL-1β	None	8.67 ± 2.53 (12)	13.81 ± 1.91 (12)	9.55 ± 1.21 (11)
IL-1β	5 µg CsA	0.67 ± 0.78 (12)	0.58 ± 0.79 (12)	1.25 ± 1.22 (12)
IL-1β	42ngTGF	0.25 ± 0.62 (12)	0.33 ± 0.65 (12)	0.80 ± 0.79 (11)
IL-1β	500U IFN	29.28 ± 2.08 (18)	29.08 ± 1.38 (13)	28.67 ± 1.44 (12)
IL-2	None	30.00 ± 2.30 (12)	11.56 ± 1.36 (12)	17.00 ± 1.41 (11)
IL-2	5 µg CsA	24.17 ± 4.63 (12)	27.58 ± 4.03 (12)	17.23 ± 1.54 (13)
IL-2	42ngTGF	29.67 ± 1.23 (12)	28.00 ± 1.60 (12)	17.09 ± 1.13 (11)
IL-2	500U IFN	29.00 ± 1.51 (23)	29.42 ± 1.24 (12)	28.50 ± 1.31 (12)
IL-6	None	6.83 ± 1.64 (12)	8.19 ± 1.33 (12)	10.08 ± 1.89 (13)
IL-6	5 µg CsA	0.75 ± 1.06 (12)	0.25 ± 0.62 (12)	1.19 ± 0.83 (16)
IL-6	42ngTGF	28.58 ± 1.73 (12)	0.58 ± 0.67 (12)	0.90 ± 0.74 (10)
IL-6	500U IFN	28.67 ± 2.23 (15)	28.89 ± 1.62 (9)	28.75 ± 1.06 (12)
TNF-α	None	9.67 ± 0.89 (12)	13.13 ± 1.78 (12)	10.40 ± 1.51 (10)
TNF-α	5 µg CsA	8.92 ± 1.73 (12)	12.83 ± 1.99 (12)	10.25 ± 1.54 (12)
TNF-α	42ngTGF	28.33 ± 1.44 (12)	15.50 ± 0.24 (12)	0.00 ± 0.00 (00)
TNF-α	500U IFN	28.50 ± 2.38 (14)	28.82 ± 0.98 (11)	28.55 ± 1.51 (11)
IFN-α	None	11.78 ± 3.07 (9)	8.00 ± 1.26 (6)	9.00 ± 1.60 (12)
IFN-α	5µg CsA	1.00 ± 1.00 (6)	1.00 ± 0.89 (6)	0.75 ± 0.75 (12)
IFN-α	42ngTGF	0.20 ± 0.42 (10)	0.30 ± 0.48 (10)	0.70 ± 0.67 (10)
IFN-α	500U IFN	28.70 ± 1.16 (10)	29.10 ± 2.02 (10)	29.33 ± 1.03 (6)

The results show that: 1)IFN-α, IL-1β and IL-6 failed to have any effect in the presence of 5µg CsA, 2)IL-2 and TNF-α were at least as active in the presence of CsA than in the absence of CsA and 3)in C57BL/6 mice, IL-2 had a significantly greater effect in the presence, than in the absence, of CsA (p = 0.01).

Effect of TGF-β on cytokine-mediated Ia⁺ LC chemotaxis: As seen in Table I, IFN-α and IL-1β, in the presence of TGF-β, failed to be chemotactic, while IL-2, TNF-α and IL-6 in BALB/c mice all not only remained chemotactic for LC, but were elevated to levels of chemotaxis previously only attainable by IL-2 (p≥0.26). TGF-β with IL-6 in C57BL/6 and C3H/HeJ mice abrogated the chemotactic effect of IL-6 alone (see Table I; p<0.01).

Effect of IFN-γ on cytokine-mediated Ia⁺ LC chemotaxis: When injected with IFN-γ, each of the cytokines studied induced the migration of ≈28.9±1 Ia⁺ LC (n=162), substancially upregulating the chemotaxis afforded by the individual cytokines alone to a point previously only attainable by IL-2 in BALB/c mice (p>0.22).

CONCLUSIONS:

The normal peripheral cornea contains from 0 to 3 Ia⁺ LC (none paracentrally or centrally). Neither IL-1α, GM-CSF, CsA, TGF-β nor IFN-γ are chemotactic for of Ia⁺ LC in mouse corneas, while IFN-α, IL-1β, IL-6 and TNF-α are all equally chemotactic: IL-2 inducing the equal number as IFN-α, IL-1β, IL-6 and TNF-α in only C57BL/6 mice. IL-2 induces the chemotaxis of more LC into the corneas of C3H/HeJ, than in C57BL/6, mice, but less than in BALB/c. CsA abrogates IFN-α-,

C3H/HeJ, than in C57BL/6, mice, but less than in BALB/c. CsA abrogates IFN-α-, IL-1β- and IL-6-mediated chemotaxis in all 3 species, but has no effect on IL-2 and TNF-α.

TGF-β abrogates the chemotactic effect of IL-1β upon Ia$^+$ LC in BALB/c, C57BL/6 and C3H/HeJ mice, but has no apparent effect upon the IL-2-induced chemotaxis of Ia$^+$ LC in BALB/C mice, and actually upregulates the effects of both IL-6 and TNF-α to levels previously only attainable by IL-2. In C57BL/6 and C3H/HeJ mice, the presence of TGF-β elevates the chemotactic effect of IL-2 upon Ia$^+$ LC to levels attained in BALB/c mice. In all species, the effect of IL-6 is abrogated by TGF-β, while it has no effect upon TNF-α-induced chemotaxis. IFN-γ, on the other hand, synergizes with all cytokines studied and potentiates their chemotactic effects up to a level only attainable with IL-2. It has no effect upon IL-2-mediated chemotaxis.

Although the identical cytokines were chemotactic for Ia$^+$ LC in the three strains of mice studied, each cytokine appeared to induce a statistically different number of Ia$^+$ LC to migrate into the corneas of each of the three strains.

SPECULATIONS:

IL-2 and TNF-α are directly chemotactic for LC, while IFN-α, IL-1β and IL-6 act through induction of IL-2, TNF-α or both. In BALB/c, TGF-β appears to upregulate LC chemotaxis via the inhibition of biofeedback mechanism(s); which either do not exist, or are not functioning, in C57BL/6 and C3H/HeJ mice. TGF-β seems to differentiate between directly and indirectly acting cytokines by rendering inoperative those signals presented via cytokine receptors. IFN-γ, on the other hand, inhibits some sort of a self-regulatory "biofeedback-type" of mechanism, upregulating the maximum level of chemotaxis attainable by other cytokines to that normally attainable only by IL-2. There appear to be a variety of strain-related differences in the induction pathway of cytokine-mediated Ia$^+$ Langerhans cell chemotaxis.

REFERENCES:

1. Klareskog L, Forsum U, Tjernlund UM, Rask L, et al. Invest Ophthalmol Vis Sci 1979; 18: 310.
2. Bergstresser PR, Fletcher CR, Streilein JW. J Invest Dermatol 1980; 74: 77.
3. Abbud-Filho M, Kupiec-Weglinski JW, Araujo JL, et al. J Immunol 1984; 133: 2582.
4. Espevik T, Figari IS, Shalaby MR, GA, et al. J Exp Med 1987; 166: 571-.
5. Belsito DV, Epstein SP, Schultz JM, et al. J Immunol 1989; 143: 1530-1536.
6. Wilson SE, Lloyd SA, He YG. Invest Ophthalmol Vis Sci 1992; 33: 1987.
7. Roberts AB, Sporn MB. Adv Cancer Res 1988; 51: 107.
8. Quere P, Thorbecke GJ. Cell Immunol 1990; 129: 468.
9. Epstein SP, Baer RL, Thorbecke JG, Belsito DV. J Immunol 1991; 96: 832.
10. Pene J. Int Arch Allergy Appl Immunol 1989; 90 Suppl 1: 32.
11. Bhattacharya A, Dorf ME, Springer TA. J Immunol 1981; 127: 2488.
12. Xue B, Dersarkissian RM, Baer RL, et al. J Immunol 1986; 136: 4128.

© 1994 Elsevier Science B.V. All rights reserved.
Advances in Ocular Immunology
R.B. Nussenblatt, S.M. Whitcup, R.R. Caspi and I. Gery, eds.

Corneal endothelial cells block IL-2 production, but not IL-2 receptor upregulation of T cells[1]

HIDETOSHI KAWASHIMA and DALE S. GREGERSON

Department of Ophthalmology, University of Minnesota
Minneapolis, Minnesota, 55455, U.S.A.

ABSTRACT

We previously reported that monolayers of LEW rat corneal endothelial (CE) cells did not induce proliferation of MHC compatible T cell lines or IL-2 production by hybridomas, and inhibited T cell proliferation when added to conventional assays with APC. Here we report that T cells activated in the presence of CE cells were responsive to exogenous IL-2, and upregulate IL-2R. However, IL-2 production by these T cells was inhibited by CE cells, which is consistent with the lack of proliferation. Hybridoma growth inhibition was not prevented by the CE cells, indicating that the APC provide TCR occupancy, despite the lack of subsequent IL-2 production.

INTRODUCTION

We have been interested in the role that CE cells might play in the regulation of immune responses in the eye, including the phenomena of anterior chamber immune privilege and the high success rate of corneal allografts. We previously reported that CE cells suppress in vitro lymphocyte proliferative responses to antigen and Con A, but the mechanisms of the inhibitory activity were unclear [1, 2]. Here we report evidence showing that CE cells inhibit T cell proliferation following activation by dissociating IL-2 secretion and IL-2R expression. T cells activated in the presence of CE cells were found to upregulate IL-2R expression and IL-2 responsiveness, but their IL-2 secretion was substantially inhibited.

RESULTS

CE cells do not inhibit the T cell response to exogenous IL-2

Although CE cells inhibit conventional in vitro T cell proliferation assays, the inhibition is reversed by the addition of exogenous IL-2 (Table 1). Since we have shown that CE cells do not inhibit the growth of T cells preactivated in the absence of CE cells, and then transferred onto CE cells, these results show that functional IL-2R are expressed by T cells activated in the presence of CE cells, and that these IL-2R can successfully signal for cell growth. Delivery of that signal leads to T cell growth that is not susceptible to inhibition by the CE cells.

CE cells do not inhibit upregulation of IL-2R

The R1170 T cell line and several other rat T cell lines make IL-2 in response to conventional stimulation and are also responsive to IL-2 [2]. We have observed that lymphocytes in proliferation assays done in the presence of CE cells become blast-like and enlarged, but do not divide [2]. These

Table 1
CE cells do not block responsiveness to exogenous hrIL-2 after activation on APC and Ag.

Culture conditions				cpm x 10⁻³	
APC	S-Ag	CE cells	hrIL-2	Exp. I	Exp. II
+	−	−	−	4 ± 1	8 ± 1
+	+	−	−	71 ± 7	63 ± 7
+	+	+	−	28 ± 2	26 ± 7
+	+	+	+	87 ± 4	80 ± 4
−	−	+	+	24 ± 2	8 ± 1
−	+	+	+	19 ± 1	7 ± 1

All wells contain 20 x 10³ retinal S-Ag-specific R1507/1513 T cells/well [1, 2]. Indicated wells also contained 0.5 x 10⁶ splenic APC's irradiated with 2000 R, 0.5 µM S-Ag, CE cells, or 20 U/ml of hrIL-2. After 48 hr, 1 µCi/well [³H]-thymidine was added, followed by harvesting after another 18 hr. The CE cells were isolated from LEW rat corneas as described, and grown to confluent monolayers prior to the addition of other components.

observations suggested that the T cell-antigen-APC interaction occurred, but that a subsequent event was blocked. CE cells were tested to determine their effect on IL-2R expression in response to Ag stimulation. Either with or without CE cells, Ag-specific stimulation of line cells led to upregulation of IL-2R (Fig. 1, panels II & III). CE cells alone, however, did not lead to IL-2R upregulation (panel IV).

CE cells allow IL-2R downregulation

CE cells, with or without Ag, do not induce upregulation of IL-2R (Fig. 1) nor induce IL-2 responsiveness [2]. Conversely, they allow unstimulated line cells to survive and downregulate IL-2R (Fig. 1, panel IV), and to lose responsiveness to exogenous IL-2 by day 2, unless restimulated with Ag and APC [2]. It should be noted that downregulation of the IL-2 responsiveness of T cells on a CE monolayer is not due to toxic effects of CE cells, since T cells recovered after 6 days from a monolayer of CE cells did not lose Ag-specific proliferative capacity [1]. Instead, enhanced T cell viability is observed in the presence of CE cells [1].

Effect of CE cells on growth inhibition and IL-2 secretion by a T cell hybridoma

Occupancy of T cell receptors on T cell hybridomas has differing outcomes including the secretion of IL-2, and also the induction of apoptosis [3]. IL-2 production by the hybridoma 1C3.4 was found to be suppressed when stimulated with Ag and splenic APC in the presence of CE cells. Cells from the same wells were also pulsed and harvested for evidence of growth inhibition.

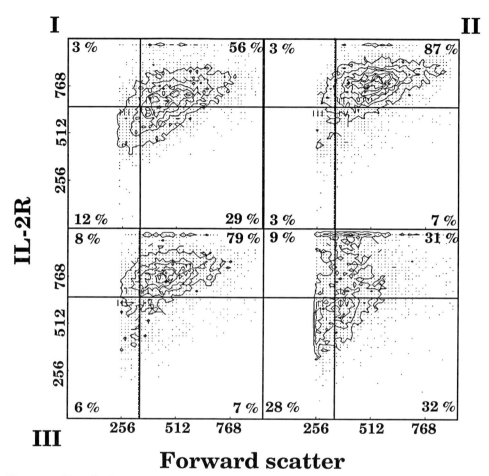

I ... **II**

3 % ... 56 %   3 % ... 87 %

768

512

256

12 % ... 29 %   3 % ... 7 %

8 % ... 79 %   9 % ... 31 %

768

512

256

6 % ... 7 %   28 % ... 32 %

256   512   768   256   512   768

III

IL-2R

Forward scatter

Figure 1. CE cells do not prevent IL-2R expression by Ag-stimulated rat T cells. The R1507/1513 line cells were prepared on day 2 after culture setup according to the legend of Table 1. Panel I, T cells incubated without a monolayer of CE cells; Panel II, line cells activated with Ag and APC without a monolayer; Panel III, line cells activated together with a CE cell monolayer; Panel IV, T cells kept on a CE cell monolayer. Viable T line cells (1 x 10⁶) were incubated with PE-conjugated mouse α-rat CD25 for 30 min on ice in 200 μl of PBS containing 2% FCS and 0.02% sodium azide. After incubation, cells were washed, and analyzed on a FACStar PLUS (Becton-Dickinson, Sunnyvale, CA).

As shown in Table 2, hybridoma growth was inhibited both in the absence and presence of CE cells, but IL-2 production was inhibited in the presence of CE cells. These data show that the hybridomas received activation signal(s) from Ag-specific TCR occupancy, and that CE cells did not interfere with this step. In the absence of APC's, CE cells did not induce growth inhibition or IL-2 production despite preinduction of class II expression [1].

Table 2
CE cells do not prevent T cell hybridoma growth inhibition, but do inhibit IL-2 production by hybridomas and splenic lymphocytes.

Conditions of stimulation			Hybridoma 1C3.4			Splenic T cells
			Growth inhibition		IL-2 production	IL-2 production
APC	Ag	CE	cpm x 10^{-3}	(%)	cpm x 10^{-3}	cpm x 10^{-3}
+	−	−	55 ± 8	0	31 ± 1	8 ± 1
+	+	−	7 ± 2	100 ± 5	134 ± 14	83 ± 21
+	+	+	9 ± 1	96 ± 3	17 ± 1	26 ± 1
−	+	+	72 ± 8	− 35 ± 16	14 ± 4	not done

Forty thousand 1C3.4 hybridoma cells were seeded into wells with or without splenic APC's (0.4 x 10^6), in the absence or presence of a CE monolayer and Ag (0.5 µM bovine S-antigen peptide 273-289) in a 1:1 mixture of RPMI 1640 and modified Click's medium with 10% FCS. After 18 hr, 30 µl of supernatant was collected from each well for IL-2 bioassay on CTLL cells as described below. The plate was then pulsed with 1 µCi/well [^{3}H]-thymidine, incubated for 18 hr, and harvested for the growth inhibition assay. Supernatants to be assayed for IL-2 were collected 24 hr after initiation of the assay and diluted in 96 well plates. IL-2-dependent CTLL indicator cells were added (20 x 10^3/well) to a final volume of 150 µl in RPMI 1640 with 10% FCS. CTLL cells were cultured for 18 hr, pulsed with 1 µCi/well [^{3}H]-thymidine, and harvested after another 18 hr. The T cell hybridoma clone 1C3.4 responds to residues 273-289 of bovine retinal S-antigen [4].

DISCUSSION

In this paper, we provide further evidence that CE cells inhibit lymphocyte proliferation by blocking a discrete step in the activation sequence following TCR occupancy. The results presented here, together with previous results [1, 2], allow analysis of the inhibitory effect of CE cells on the physical/temporal sequence of events leading to T cell growth following receptor occupancy.

Our results show that events leading up to and including TCR occupancy are not inhibited by CE cells. Also, TCR-dependent activation signals up to and including hybridoma growth inhibition and IL-2R upregulation (see below) are not inhibited. T cells activated on a monolayer of CE cells by Ag and APC were found to be quite responsive to exogenous IL-2 [2]. Together, the results show that CE cells do not inhibit upregulation of IL-2R following activation, nor do they inhibit responsiveness to IL-2.

IL-2 production by lymphocytes is dependent on signals resulting from both TCR occupancy and costimulation [5]. Since CE cells inhibit IL-2 secretion by the 1C3.4 and E3 hybridomas, which do not require costimulation, the block is at a distal event in TCR signalling. Although this block was effective, the inhibition was reversible, by simply recovering and washing the lymphocytes.

Since the growth of preactivated T cells is not inhibited, whether assessed by [^{3}H]-thymidine incorporation or direct count of viable cells, when transferred onto a CE monolayer after normal activation [1], it argues that once the T cell has received the necessary signals for division, it is no longer susceptible to the CE cell inhibitory activity.

Although it has not yet been possible to characterize or identify the inhibitory activity at the molecular level, the results presented here reveal another mechanism by which an IL-2-linked T cell unresponsiveness can be induced, further underscoring the importance of peripheral regulatory mechanisms and the variety of mechanisms used for local immunoregulation.

REFERENCES

1 Obritsch WF, Kawashima H, Evangelista A, Ketcham JM, Holland EJ, Gregerson DS. Cell Immunol 1992; 144:80-94.
2 Kawashima H, Gregerson DS. Corneal endothelial cells block T cell proliferation, but not T cell activation or responsiveness to exogenous IL-2. (submitted)
3 Nabavi N, Freeman GJ, Gault A, Godfrey D, Nadler LM, Glimcher LH. Nature 1992; 360:266-268.
4 Fling SP, Gold DP, Gregerson DS. Cell Immunol 1992; 142:275-286.
5 Jenkins MK, Pardoll DM, Mizuguchi J, Chused TM, Schwartz RH. Proc Natl Acad Sci USA 1987; 84:5409-5413.

Advances in Ocular Immunology
R.B. Nussenblatt, S.M. Whitcup, R.R. Caspi and I. Gery, eds.

Human retinal pigment epithelial cells secrete cytokines in response to inflammatory mediators

Chandrasekharam N. Nagineni, Barbara Detrick* and John J. Hooks

Immunology & Virology Section, Laboratory of Immunology, National Eye Institute, NIH, Bethesda, MD 20892

*Department of Pathology, The George Washington University Medical Center, Washington, D.C.

INTRODUCTION

Clinical and experimental studies have demonstrated that cytokines play a vital role in a variety of inflammatory eye diseases. In inflammatory and autoimmune diseases of the eye, breakdown of the blood-tissue barrier system and infiltration of lymphocytes and macrophages into the anterior and posterior segments of the eye are the initial events.

Activated leukocytes secrete IFN-γ, TNF-α, IL-2, IL-1 and other cytokines that would initiate and perpetuate immune reactions (1-4). In laboratory animals, direct inoculation of endotoxin, TNF-α, IL-1 or IL-6 into the anterior or posterior compartments of the eye was reported to induce uveitis (5-7). In human studies, significant levels of IL-6, IL-1, TNF-α and IFN-γ were found in the vitreous aspirates of patients with PVR, uveitis and other inflammatory eye diseases (8-10). In addition, increased expression of the intercellular adhesion molecule-1(ICAM-1), a cell surface adhesion molecule upregulated during inflammation, was found in retinal pigment epithelium (RPE), vascular cells and in epiretinal membranes in uveitis and PVR patients (11,12). Soluble ICAM-1was also detected in serum and vitreous of these patients (13,14).

RPE plays an important role in degenerative and inflammatory diseases of the eye by expressing MHC class I and class II molecules and by processing and presenting antigen to T cells (15,16). The potential role of RPE in the secretion of IL-6 and ICAM-1 is examined by exposing human RPE cultures to inflammatory mediators.

MATERIALS & METHODS

Cell cultures

Primary cell lines of human RPE (HRPE) were established from RPE-choroid explants derived from donor eyes (17). Growth medium consists of MEM supplemented with 10% FCS, non-essential amino acids and antibiotic- antimycotic mixture (GIBCO, Grand island, NY). Cytokeratin mab (Sigma, St. Louis, MO) was used for immunostaining of the cells for the detection of cytokeratins. RPE cultures at passages 6 to 10 were used in this study.

IL-6 & ICAM-1 assays by ELISA

The effects of inflammatory mediators on HRPE cells were studied in serum-free medium (SFM). SFM was used to prevent the interaction and interference of serum derived factors with cytokine action and with ELISA assays. Cultures were grown to confluence in 8 well glass chamber slides (Nunc, Naperville, IL) in MEM containing 10% FCS. Cultures were subsequently washed with SFM twice and incubated in SFM (control) or SFM containing LPS (S.typhosa), rIFN-γ, rTNF-α, rIL-1α or rIL-1β for 24 hr. Media were collected, centrifuged and used for IL-6 and ICAM-1 determinations. IL-6 and ICAM-1 were measured by commercially available ELISA kits (AMAC, Westbrook, ME & Endogen, Cambridge, MA).

RESULTS

Phase contrast photomicrographs of live cultures of HRPE are shown in figure 1. HRPE lost pigmentation gradually and upon second passage no visible pigment was noticed. Cells form monolayers with a typical epithelial shape and intercellular boundaries when the cells

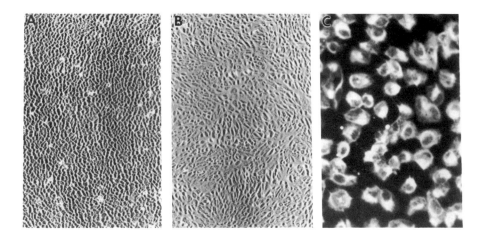

Figure 1. Photomicrographs of human retinal pigment epithelial cultures at passage 6. (A) after 4 days in culture, (B) after 2 weeks in culture. Fluorescent images of cells stained with mab to cytokeratin (C).

reach confluence (Fig. 1A). During 2 to 6 weeks of culture, cells divide and form compact sheets with less clear intercellular junctions (Fig. 1B). All of the cells examined between passages 2 to 12 stained positively for cytokeratins (Fig 1C), an epithelial-specific cytoskeletal proteins, suggesting homogeneous population of RPE cells without contamination of choroid derived fibroblasts and endothelial cells.

IL-1α, IL-1β, TNF-α, LPS and IFN-γ are all capable of stimulating IL-6 secretion by HRPE cells. IL-1α and IL-1β are the most potent inducers of IL-6 production (Fig.2A).

Stimulation of RPE cells with IFN-γ resulted in the lowest levels of IL-6 secretion. However, IFN-γ exhibited synergistic effects in the secretion of IL-6 by RPE cells stimulated with IL-1 or TNF-α. In fact, combinations of TNF-α and IFN-γ were the most potent inducers of IL-6 production (data not shown).

IL-1α, IL-1β, TNF-α and IFN-γ were all capable of stimulating ICAM-1 secretion by HRPE cells (Fig. 2B). All of these cytokines induced similar amounts of ICAM-1 (9 -14 ng/million cells). In contrast, LPS, an inducer of IL-6 secretion, did not induce ICAM-1 secretion.

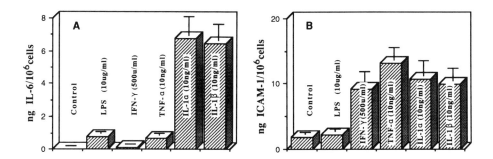

Figure 2. Effect of inflammatory mediators on IL-6 and ICAM-1 secretion by HRPE cells.

DISCUSSION

IL-6, a multipotent cytokine, regulates immune responses by inducing lymphocyte proliferation, differentiation and production of antibodies. ICAM-1 is an adhesive glycoprotein with five immunoglobulin like extracellular domains, a single transmembrane region and a short cytoplasmic tail. ICAM-1 mediated cell adhesion is essential for several immunological functions such as T cell mediated B cell activation and cytotoxic T cell function. Circulating levels of IL-6 and ICAM-1 were found to be elevated in a variety of inflammatory and infectious diseases. Increased levels of IL-6 and ICAM-1 in the vitreous aspirates of patients with uveitis, PVR and other inflammatory eye disorders are reported (8-10,13,14). Production of IL-6 and ICAM-1 by ocular resident cells could be responsible for local elevation of these molecules in the eye.

Cytokines play an essential role in maintaining normal physiological states and in modulating responses to aberrant conditions. The presence of cytokines within the eye during pathologic states and the induction of ocular pathology following administration of cytokines suggest a critical role for these molecules in ocular diseases. These studies provide evidence that cytokines and inflammatory mediators can act alone or synergistically with IFN-γ to activate RPE cells and dramatically increase the expression and secretion of IL-6 and ICAM-1. Future studies that define the specific mechanisms by which cytokines regulate IL-6 and ICAM-1 secretion by RPE cells in normal and disease states may provide important insights into biologic mechanisms to modify inflammatory processes in retinal inflammation, degenerations and retinal-RPE transplantation.

REFERENCES

1 Deschenes J, Char HD, Kaleta S. Br J Ophthalmol 1988; 72: 83-87.
2 De Vos AF, Hoekzema R, Duff GW. Curr Eye Res 1992; 11: 581-597.
3 Hooks JJ, Chan CC, Detrick B. Invest Ophthalmol Vis Sci 1988; 29:1444-1451.
4 Wakefield D, Lloyd A. Cytokine 1992; 4: 1-5.
5 Rosenbaum JT, Howes EL, Rubin RM, Samples JR. Am J Pathol 1988; 133: 47-53.
6 Hoekzema R, Verhagen C, Horen MV, Kijilstra A. Invest Ophthalmol Vis Sci 1992; 33: 532-539.
7 Fleisher LN, Ferrell JB, McGahan MC. Invest Ophthalmol Vis Sci 1992; 33: 2120-2127.
8 De Boer JH, Van Hren MAC, de Vries-Knoppert WAEJ, Baarsma GS, et al. Curr Eye Res 1992; 11: 181-186.
9 Franks WA, Limb GA, Stanford MR, Ogilive J, et al. Curr Eye Res 1992; 11: 187-191.
10 Limb GA, Little BC, Meager A, Ogilive JA, et al. Eye 1991; 5: 686-693.
11 Whitcup SM, Chan CC, Li Q, Nussenblat RB. Arch Ophthalmol 1992; 110: 662-666.
12 Heidenkummer HP, Kampik A. Arch Clin Exp Ophthalmol 1992; 230: 483-487.
13 Arocker-Mettinger E, Steurer-Georgiew L, Steurer M, Huber-Spitzy V, et al. Curr Eye Res 1992; 11 (suppl): 161-166.
14 Esser P, Bresgen M, Heimann K, Wiedmann P. Invest Ophthalmol Vis Sci 1994; 35: 2039 (abstract).
15 Detrick B, Newsome D, Percopo C, Hooks JJ. Clin Immunol Pathol 1985; 36: 201-211.
16 Percopo C, Hooks JJ, Shinohara T, Caspi R, Detrick B. J Immunol 1990; 145: 4101-4107.
17 Nagineni CN, Detrick B, Hooks JJ. Clin Diag Lab Immunol 1994; in press.

© 1994 Elsevier Science B.V. All rights reserved.
Advances in Ocular Immunology
R.B. Nussenblatt, S.M. Whitcup, R.R. Caspi and I. Gery, eds.

The role of tumor necrosis factor-alpha in the induction of experimental autoimmune uveoretinitis in mice

S. Nakamura[a], T. Yamakawa[b], M. Sugita[a], M. Kijima[a], M. Ishioka[a], S-i. Tanaka[b], and S. Ohno[a]

[a]Department of Ophthalmology and [b]Third Department of Internal Medicine, Yokohama City University School of Medicine, Yokohama, Japan.

INTRODUCTION

Experimental autoimmune uveoretinitis (EAU) has been actively investigated in recent years as an animal model of human endogenous uveitis. Although the immunopathogenic mechanisms of EAU are still controversial, it is reported that not only the major histocompatibility complex (MHC) but also non-MHC genes control the disease susceptibility.[1] In recent years, evidence has been assembled that tumor necrosis factor-alpha (TNF) may be involved in inflammatory processes. We previously reported that TNF plays an important role in the pathogenesis of uveoretinitis in Behçet's disease.[2] In this report, we investigated the relationship between susceptibility to EAU and the ability to produce TNF in congenic mice.

MATERIALS

B10.A and B10.D2 male mice were used when they were 8-10 weeks old. All experiments were adhered to the ARVO Statement for the Use of Animals in Ophthalmic and Vision Research.

Interphotoreceptor retinoid-binding protein (IRBP) was prepared from bovine retinas according to the method of Redmond et al.[3] Complete Freund's adjuvant (CFA), *Mycobacterium tuberculosis* H37R (MT), and lipopolysaccharide (LPS) from E. Coli 055 : B5 were purchased from Difco Laboratories, Detroit, MI. Purified *Bordetella pertussis* toxin (PT) was purchased from SIGMA, St. Louis, MO. Recombinant human TNF (rhTNF) was kindly provided by Asahi Chemicals Co., Tokyo, Japan.

METHODS

Measurement of TNF production

We measured the LPS-stimulated TNF production in B10.A and B10.D2 mice *in vivo*. Six mice of both strains were injected with $50\mu g$ of lipopolysaccharide (LPS) intravenously. Blood was collected 90 minutes after the injection, when maximum TNF production was observed.[4] After preservation for 24 hours at 4°C, sera were obtained by centrifugation for 10 minutes. The levels of TNF in sera were assayed by using LM cells, L929, as target cells. Statistical analysis was done by Student's t-test.

Immunization for EAU

Both B10.A and B10.D2 mice were divided to four groups by different immunization protocols. Each group of both strains was consisted of 5 mice.

Group 1. To compare the incidence and severity of EAU, we immunized mice with the method according to the single-dose induction protocol.[1] Mice were immunized with a dose of 100 μg of IRBP in 0.2 ml emulsified CFA supplemented with additional MT at a final concentration of 2.5 mg/ml. They were additionally given 1 μg of PT in 0.2 ml intraperitoneally as an adjuvant.

Group 2. To evaluate the role of MT in the immunization, we tried to produce EAU without additional MT in CFA.

Group 3. To study the influence of TNF in EAU, we injected two times of 3,000 U of rhTNF in 0.2 ml of saline subcutaneously at day 0 and day 2. In this group, we did not add any MT in CFA.

Group 4. To estimate the potential of TNF to induce inflammatory changes in eyes of mice, mice were immunized with CFA without IRBP and injected with rhTNF.

Evaluation of disease

Mice were killed two weeks after the immunization. Enucleated eyes were immediately fixed for 24 hours in cacodylic acid formaldehyde and embedded in paraffin. Sections were cut at 4 μm through the pupillary-optic nerve plane and stained with standard hematoxylin and eosin. Severity of EAU was graded from 0 to 3.

RESULTS

TNF production of mice

LPS-stimulated TNF production was significantly higher ($p<0.01$) in B10.A mice than in B10.D2 mice (Table 1.).

Table 1
LPS-stimulated TNF production in B10.A and B10.D2 mice[*]

mice	n	TNF[†]
B10.A	6	24.9 ± 7.0[§]
B10.D2	6	4.1 ± 0.5[§]

[*] Mice were injected with 50μg of lipopolysaccharide (LPS) intravenously. Blood was collected 90 minutes after the injection. Sera were obtained by centrifugation for 10 minutes. The levels of tumor necrosis factor-alpha (TNF) in sera were assayed by using LM cells.
[†] average ± SD (U/ml)
[§] $p<0.01$: statistical analysis was done by Student's t-test.

Severity and incidence of EAU

The severity and incidence of EAU experiment were shown in Fig. 1. Three of 5 B10.A mice in the group 1 developed mild to moderate EAU. There were only traces of iritis and cyclitis. The remainders, however, did not develop any EAU-related changes. One of 5 B10.D2 mice in the group 1 developed mild EAU, but the other 4 did not. None of 5 mice of either strain immunized without MT (group 2) developed EAU. All B10.A mice injected with rhTNF (group 3) developed severe EAU. Most of them showed not only extensive retinal inflammation but also choroiditis, vitritis, iritis, and cyclitis. Three of 5 B10.D2 mice developed mild EAU when injected with 6,000 U of rhTNF (group 3). In contrast, none of 5 mice of either strain injected with 6,000 U of rhTNF and CFA without IRBP (group 4) developed EAU.

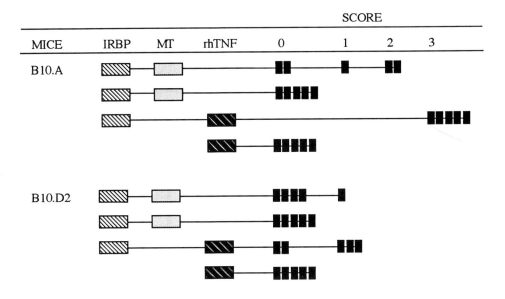

Figure 1. Severity and incidence of EAU
■ = one mouse.
IRBP : interphotoreceptor retinoid-binding protein, CFA : complete Freund's adjuvant, MT : *Mycobacterium tuberculosis*, rhTNF : recombinant human tumor necrosis factor-alpha
All mice were injected with purified *Bordetella pertussis* toxin intraperitoneally at the time of immunization.

DISCUSSION

The immunopathogenic mechanisms of EAU have been actively investigated in recent years, whereas the role of other cytokines such as TNF is still obscure. TNF is a monocyte-macrophage derived protein whose major biologic function was presumed to be the mediation of cytotoxicity to tumor cells. Yokota et al[5] reported the activation of T cells by TNF, facilitating their capacity to proliferate in response to mitogens and antigens. Induction of surface antigen such as VCAM-1,[6] ICAM-1 and HLA-DR[7] in vascular endothelial cells and, as a result, enhancement of polymorphonuclear neutrophils adhesion and suppression of migration[8] were also reported as functions of TNF. In a previous study, we measured the *in vitro* production of TNF of peripheral blood monocytes from patients with Behçet's disease and suggested the possible participation of this inflammatory cytokine in the pathogenesis of Behçet's disease.[2]

In this study we aimed to elucidate the pathogenic role of TNF in the development of EAU in mice.

It has been recommended to add MT to CFA (or add excessive MT to incomplete Freund's adjuvant) to develop EAU in mice.[1,9,10] MT was reported to induce the production of TNF from human T cells.[11] Therefore we hypothesized that the enhancement of TNF production with MT is necessary to raise the disease susceptibility to EAU in mice.

Moreover, it is likely that disease susceptibility based on the genetic background may be, in some part, the reflection of ability to produce TNF in response to immunization.

To confirm this hypothesis, we measured LPS-stimulated TNF production in different strains of B10 congenic mice *in vivo*.

Serum TNF levels after the stimulation with LPS were significantly higher in B10.A mice than in B10.D2 mice. There was also marked difference in susceptibility to EAU between these two strains. Freund et al reported that certain strain of mice susceptible to toxoplasmic encephalitis (TE) expressed elevated levels of TNF mRNA in brain tissue after infection of TE while resistant strain did not.[12] This data implicates that the ability to produce TNF may strongly correlate to the susceptibility to inflammatory diseases.

In this study, some mice immunized with IRBP and CFA supplemented with MT developed mild to moderate EAU whereas none of 10 mice immunized with IRBP and CFA, without additional MT, developed EAU. We consider that the insufficient production of TNF caused by the lack of additional MT in the induction phase might be responsible for this phenomenon. From this standpoint of view, we prepared mice which were immunized with CFA containing IRBP, but not MT, and received injection of 6,000 U of rhTNF (group 3). These mice showed marked increase of incidence and severity of EAU in both strains examined. These results indicate that rhTNF strongly increased the immune response to IRBP, whereas MT increased it moderately. In addition, rhTNF itself does not have any potential to induce EAU. rhTNF therefore seems to enhance the immune responses to IRBP in EAU in mice.

It is conceivable that the genetic control of the disease susceptibility may have relevance to sensitivity to TNF or production of TNF by macrophages in response to antigens.

REFERENCES

1 Caspi RR, Grubbs BG, Chan CC, Chader GJ, and Wiggert B.J Immunol. 1992;148:2384-2389.
2 Nakamura S, Sugita M, Tanaka S-i, and Ohno S. Acta Soc Ophthalmol Jpn. 1992;96:1282-1285.
3 Redmond TM, Wiggert B, Robey FA, et al. Biochem. 1985; 24:787-793.
4 Tanaka S-i, Seino H, Satoh J, et al. Clin Immunol Immunopathol. 1992;62:258-263.
5 Yokota S, Geppert TD, and Lipsky PE. J Immunol. 1988;140:531-536.
6 Carlos TM, Schwartz BR, Kovach NL, et al. Blood. 1990;76:965-970.
7 Detmar M, Tenorio S, Hettmannsperger U, Ruszczak Z, and Orfanos CE. J Invest Dermatol. 1992;98:147-153.
8 Salyer JL, Bohnsack JF, Knape WA, Shigeoka AO, Ashwood ER, and Hill HR. Am J Pathol. 1990;136:831-841.
9 Caspi RR, Roberge FG, Chan CC, et al. J Immunol. 1988;140:1490-1495.
10 Caspi RR, Chan CC, Wiggert B, and Chader GJ. Curr Eye Res. 1981; 9(suppl):169-174.
11 Barnes PF, Abrams JS, LU S, et al. Infect Immunol. 1993;61:197-203.
12 Freund YR, Sgarlato G, Jacob CO, et al. J Exp Med. 1992;175.683-688.

Advances in Ocular Immunology
R.B. Nussenblatt, S.M. Whitcup, R.R. Caspi and I. Gery, eds.

Interleukins enhanced neural regeneration of axotomized retinal ganglion cells in adult mammals

M. Takano[1], H. Horie[2], T. Takenaka[2] and S. Ohno[1]

Departments of [1]Ophthalmology and [2]Physiology, Yokohama City University School of Medicine, 3-9 Fukuura, Kanazawa-ku, Yokohama 236, Japan

INTRODUCTION

Recent studies clarified that the expression of interleukins in brain increased after axonal injury [1]. The interleukins might play a role of regulating functions in the central nervous system (CNS), but their precise mechanism on axonal regeneration has been still unclear. We introduced *in vitro* model of adult retina to clarify the effect of interleukins on neural regeneration in the CNS.

MATERIALS AND METHODS

Thirteen male Wistar rats aged 9 weeks, weighing 200-220 g, were used for this study. The rats were anesthetized with an intraperitoneal of pentobarbital (40 mg/kg body weight), and left optic nerve (ON) was intraorbitally transected at a distance of 5 mm from eye ball without affecting the retinal blood supply. At 7 days after ON transection, the rats were killed by ether and their retinas were dissected from the enucleated left eyes under sterile conditions. Then the retina located 250-750 μm apart from the optic disc was used and cut into sixteen pieces (approximately 500 μm squares) by using a sharp blade. The retinal pieces were carefully embedded into collagen gel as every 4 pieces per dish that was precoated with 10 μg/ml poly-L-lysine (Sigma). The embedding procedure followed that in our previous study [2]. The explants were cultured in serum-free media that based minimum essential medium (MEM, Sigma) containing 4.5 mg ml^{-1} glucose, 5 μg ml^{-1} insulin, 8 μg ml^{-1} putrescine, 792 μg ml^{-1} bovine serum albumin (BSA, Sigma), 4.3 ng ml^{-1} Na$_2$SeO$_3$, 3.7 mg ml^{-1} NaHCO$_3$, and 3.6 mg ml^{-1} Hepes. Several concentrations of recombinant human interleukin-1β (IL-1β, GZM) (1-100 U/ml) and interleukin-6 (IL-6, GZM) (0.1-10 U/ml) were applied to the cultures. To maintain the cultures, the media were replaced with fresh media every 3 days in 37°C an incubator that was kept 5% CO$_2$ and 95% air atmosphere. The number of outgrowing neurites was counted under phase contrast optics using inverted microscope.

RESULTS

Neurites with spreading growth cones first appeared from retinal explants within 24 hr after culture. Immunohistochemical studies verified that the origins of these neurites were the regenerating axons from the retinal ganglion cells (RGCs) [2-3]. The neurites survived and elongated for distances of over 3.0 mm by 7 days after explantation. The numbers of outgrowing neurites per explant were 51.0 with IL-1β (10 U/ml), 55.8 with IL-6 (1 U/ml), and 36.8 without interleukins at 5 days in culture, respectively. The relative numbers of outgrowing neurites were shown in table 1. Numbers of regenerating neurites were increased approximately 40% by application of either IL-1β or IL-6 *in vitro*. These enhancements on neurite outgrowth continued to 7 days in culture.

Table 1
Effects of interleukins on relative numbers of regenerating neurites

	Days in culture		
	3	5	7
IL-1β (10 U/ml)	1.54 ± 0.28	1.38 ± 0.13	1.41 ± 0.18
IL-6 (1 U/ml)	1.28 ± 0.25	1.48 ± 0.25	1.42 ± 0.22

* control = 1

DISCUSSION

After brain injury, the level of IL-1β and IL-6 secreted from microglia and astrocyte rapidly increased *in vivo* [1]. The IL-1β then activates astrocyte to secrete nerve growth factor (NGF) and the other neurotrophins [4] which might promote neural regeneration. The IL-6 similarly stimulates astrocytes [5] and promotes the survival of cultured neurons *in vitro* [6]. The activated astrocytes might also promote the axonal sprouting after injuries [7]. Thus the interleukins were associated with the reactive changes after injuries. Though the interleukins were thought to enhance neural regeneration in the CNS, which had not been defined *in vivo* and even *in vitro*. However, our findings using the *in vitro* model showed that both IL-1β and IL-6 clearly enhanced neurite regeneration from the RGCs. Since the retinal explants in the collagen gel preserved their structures and cell to cell interactions, the mechanism of the activation of neural regeneration induced by interleukins might be due to the reactive changes.

CONCLUSION

The application of both IL-1β and IL-6 increased the numbers of regenerating neurites from adult rat retinal explants, suggesting these interleukins have a biological activity to enhance neural regeneration of axotomized RGCs *in vitro*. These results indicate that the interleukins might play a critical role in regeneration of injured CNS neurons *in vivo*.

REFERENCES

1 Woodroofe MN, Sarna GS, Wadhwa M, et al. J Neuroimmunol 1991; 33: 227-236.
2 Horie H, Ito S, Takano M. Brain Res Bull 1994 (in press).
3 Takano M, Horie H. Neurosci Lett 1994 (in press).
4 Spranger M, Lindholm D, Bandtlow C, et al. Eur J Neurosci 1990; 2: 69-76.
5 Frei K, Malipiero UV, Leist TP, et al. Eur J Immunol 1989; 19: 689-694.
6 Kushima Y, Hama T, Hatanaka H. Neurosci Res 1992; 13: 267-280.
7 Gage F, Olejniczak P, Armstrong DM. Exp Neurol 1988; 102: 2-13.

© 1994 Elsevier Science B.V. All rights reserved.
Advances in Ocular Immunology
R.B. Nussenblatt, S.M. Whitcup, R.R. Caspi and I. Gery, eds.

Significance of the secretion of plasminogen activators in normal and chronic granulomatous uveitis eyes.

Yafei Wang, David M. Smalley, J.W.-P. Wang, Robert E. Cone and James O'Rourke

Vision Immunology Center, Department of Pathology, University of Connecticut Health Center, Farmington, CT 06030-3105.

Abstract

Uninhibited plasminogen activator activity in ocular fluids may play a major role in metalloenzyme activation, matrix proteolysis, clots lysis and aqueous outflow. Two patterns of intraocular PA secretion have been identified: a continuous basal release of tissue plasminogen activator [t-PA] mainly from uveovascular endothelium, and a sharply increased secretion of presumed urokinase [u-PA] activity by activated macrophages, monocytes and fibroblasts in the late stages of granuloma formation. The onset of cell mediated uveitis induced by mycobacterial antigen is attended by an initial depression of the basal t-PA activity, followed by a sharp rise in presumed u-PA activity as macrophage and monocyte populations increase.

Text

Plasminogen activators [PA] are serine proteases that cleave plasminogen to form plasmin. Plasmin is an aggressive, versatile, trypsin-like protease able to activate enzymes such as collagenases and TGF-b, as well as regulate matrix proteolysis, fibrinolysis and aqueous outflow [1,2].

The two major types of PA are tissue plasminogen activator [t-PA] and urokinase [u-PA], both of which are closely regulated in all tissues by an excess of inhibitors, principally PAI-1. Hence, the free uninhibited fraction of PA activity available to effect the above functions approximates 10 percent of the total released antigen.

Tissue plasminogen activator [t-PA[is a 68 kD protein whose major source is microvascular endothelium, principally precapillary arterioles and post capillary venules. t-PA activity is greatly amplified when bound to fibrin, but is minimally active in plasma and other fluids where, in the absence of fibrin binding, it is almost entirely bound to excess PA1-1 [3].

Urokinase is expressed by several cell types including activated macrophages, monocytes and fibroblasts at sites of wound healing, and by proliferating endothelium during angiogenesis. Like t-PA its activity is also closely regulated by excess PAI-1 [4].

Until recently it has been difficult to identify and assay the free PA activity in ocular fluids, meaning aqueous and vitreous humors, and to follow these during immunological disorders of the eye, such as uveitis. Normal aqueous humor contains higher levels of PA activity and much lower inhibitor levels than plasma, which balance may allow activity to persist longer in aqueous [5,6]. Plasma half-life for t-PA is between 2 and 5 minutes [3]. The PA activity present in aqueous is predominantly t-PA, the major sources of which are uveovascular, corneal and trabecular endothelia, based on immunohistochemical localizations [2].

t-PA activity has been quantified in aqueous humor by a modified two stage amidolytic assay, using the synthetic plasmin substrate, S2251, in the presence of excess plasminogen and soluble fibrin. Normal values are 0.07 - 0.47 I.U/ml. Total antigenic levels are assayed by ELISA; normal range is 2.1-5.8 ng/ml [2]. Relative changes in unspecified PA activity during the evolution of granuloma formation in chronic mycobacterial-induced uveitis [CMIU} have been assessed using I-125 plasminogen substrate cleavage and gel electrophoresis [6]. These show an initial depression of basal PA activity during initial stages of the uveitis, followed by a sharp increase in presumed u-PA activity as vitreous granuloma formation is consolidated [7].

Recent advances in plasminogen activator research suggest two patterns of PA activity secretion that may occur in the eye: under physiological conditions a continuous basal secretion of t-PA and PAI-1 inhibitor from endothelial source cells provides free PA activity in excess of that found in plasma, which balance may facilitate several proteolytic functions; e.g. metalloenzyme activation, clot lysis, aqueous outflow, matrix remodeling. The vascular endothelium believed most active in this t-PA secretion is that of the precapillary arterioles, and venules, but not that of large vessels and capillaries [8]. The capacity of isolated choroidal eyecup organ cultures to continually secrete significant amounts of free t-PA albuminally into the vitreous cavity is an important example of this source, and suggests that uveovascular endothelium is the major intraocular supplier of t-PA activity [unpublished data]. A second pattern of PA secretion is shown by the initial depression of basal activity, followed by a sharp PA secretion during the late stages of vitreous granuloma formation [5,6] [Fig. 1]. The correspondence of this increase to the proliferation of activated macrophages, monocytes, and fibroblasts in the granuloma suggests a probable late surge of free u-PA secretion [Fig. 2] that is sufficient to overcome the normal excess of inhibitor, since these cells when activated secrete u-PA but not t-PA [4]. Mechanisms of each type of secretion, as well as identification of PA release pathways within cells remain unelucidated.

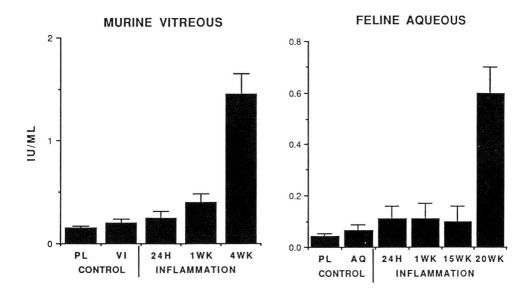

Figure 1. Changes in free uninhibited PA activity in murine vitreous and feline aqueous during maturation of vitreous granulomas induced by intravitreal injection of killed BCG organisms [4, 7]. Plasma levels (PL) unchanged during chronic uveitis.

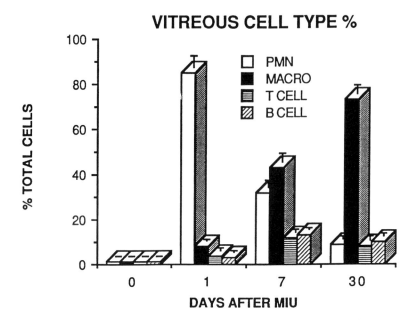

Figure 2. Changes in murine vitreous cell composition during mycobacterial induced uveitis (MIU) and granuloma formation induced by intravitreal injection of killed BCG organisms [7].

References

1.   Matrisian LM, Hogan BL. Curr Topics in Developmental Biology 1990; 24:219-259.
2.   Wang Y, Taylor DM, Smalley D.M., Cone RE, O'Rourke J. Increased basal levels of free plasminogen activator activity found in human aqueous humor. Invest Ophthalmol Vis Sci (in press).
3.   van Hinsbergh VWM. In: Kluft C, ed. Tissue plasminogen activator (t-PA): physiological and clinical aspects. Vol II. Boca Raton FL (USA): CRC Press, 1988; 3-20.
4.   Schafer BM, Maier K., Eikhoff U, Todd RF, Kramer MD. Am J. Pathol 1994; 144: 1269-1280.
5.   O'Rourke J, Moore M, Kreutzer DL. Curr Eye Res 1985; 4: 569-578.
6.   O'Rourke J, Wang WP, Donnellly L, Wang E, Kreutzer DL. Am J. Pathol 1987; 126: 334-342.
7.   Wang JW-P. Regulation of local plasminogen activator (PA) and PA inhibitor (PAI) activities during murine uveitis. (Unpublished thesis), University of Connecticut.
8.   Levin EG, del Zoppo GJ. Am. J. Pathol 1994; 144:855-861.
9.   O'Rourke J, Wang JW-P, Wang E, Kreutzer DL. Curr Eye Res 1989; 7:1207-1219.

© 1994 Elsevier Science B.V. All rights reserved.
Advances in Ocular Immunology
R.B. Nussenblatt, S.M. Whitcup, R.R. Caspi and I. Gery, eds.

Transforming growth factor-beta (TGF-ß), TGF-ß-binding proteins and ocular immunoseclusion

Asad Abrahamian, Mu Shi Xi, John J. Donnelly, William V. Williams and John H. Rockey
Departments of Ophthalmology and Rheumatology, University of Pennsylvania, 51 N. 39th Street, Philadelphia, PA 19104

ABSTRACT

Mixed leukocyte response-human corneal fibroblast (MLR-HCF) coculture assay, RT-PCR, radioreceptor assay (RRA), receptor binding inhibition assay (RIA), bioassay (BIA) and mink cell-HCF (MC-HCF) co-culture assay showed that HCF produced TGF-ß in culture, and interferon-γ up-regulated their higher-affinity TGF-ß receptors ($K_D = 0.2$ pM) and TGF-ß output. HCF may use TGF-ß-dependent mechanisms to inhibit T-cell activation (e.g. by alloantigens) and maintain corneal immunoseclusion. Media-borne TGF-ß-binding proteins were considered responsible for the discrepancy between the TGF-ß values measured by RIA and BIA. Exclusion of binding proteins from aqueous humor may be crucial to TGF-ß-dependent intra-ocular immune privilege.

INTRODUCTION:

The T-cell alloresponse is inhibited by human corneal fibro-blasts in MLR-HCF co-culture assays[1]. The inhibition is contact-independent, indomethacin-insensitive and augmentable by pre-treatment of HCF with interferon-gamma (IFN-γ)[1]. IFN-γ also induces MHC Class-II (HLA-DR, -DP, -DQ) antigens and very high-affinity TGF-ß receptors on HCF[1,2]. In this paper, we show that IFN-γ increases TGF-ß output of HCF. HCF may use TGF-ß-dependent mechanisms to maintain corneal immunoseclusion. The in vitro and in vivo biologic signifi-cance of a TGF-ß-binding protein is defined.

MATERIALS AND METHODS:

Cells: HCF cell lines were maintained in culture medium (DMEM + 10% FBS), and used in experiments between the 4th and 12th passages[1,2]. Mink lung epithelial (Mv-1 Lu) cells from sub-confluent cultures were used in bioassay (BIA) or co-culture experiments.

Mixed Leukocyte Response-Human Corneal Fibroblast (MLR-HCF) Coculture Assays: The PGE$_2$-independent inhibition of T-cell allo-response by HCF was demonstrated by MLR-HCF co-culture assay[1]. IFN-γ-treated (0.0 or 500 U/ml, 4 days) HCF were overlaid with responder and stimulator human peripheral blood lymphocytes (PBL) and incubated (7 days) in the presence of 0 - 10 ug/ml indomethacin. T-cell alloresponse was determined by [^{3}H]-thymidine uptake during the final 18 hours of incubation[1].

Reverse Transcriptase-Polymerase Chain Reaction (RT-PCR): The capacity of HCF to express TGF-ß mRNA was assessed by combined RT-PCR. Total RNA (5 μg), from IFN-γ-treated and untreated HCF, was converted to cDNA in 40 μl PCR buffer, and 2 μl of cDNA library was amplified (25 cycles) by PCR, using _Thermus aquaticus_ DNA-polymerase, molar excesses of specific sense and anti-sense primers for TGF-ß1 and TGFß2, and proper controls. Primers were designed so that a splice junction was included in the amplified DNA sequence.

Amplified DNA bands were visualized by ethidium bromide staining in agarose gel. For PCR semi-quantitative (comparative) assay, PCR-amplified samples were diluted five times to the equivalent of 24, 23, 22, 21, and 20 cycles, and compared for the intensity of DNA bands on agarose-gel. A 612 base-pair actin DNA band was used as an internal control.

Measurement of TGF-ß Output of HCF by Bioassay (BIA) and Radioreceptor Assay (RIA): Culture supernatants from IFN-γ-treated (0.0 or 500 U/ml) HCF monolayers in 100 mm dishes were obtained by incubating the cells with fresh culture medium (8 ml) for 4 days[1]. Samples were stored at -70°C. To convert latent media-borne TGF-ß to bioactive forms, sample pH was lowered to 2.5 with 2 N HCl for 20 minutes at room temperature, and restored to 7.4 with 2 N NaOH. The highly sensitive standard mink cell assay system was utilized to examine whether HCF can produce TGF-ß and if IFN-γ affected their TGF-ß output. Mv-1 Lu cells (0.5×10^5) were incubated for 24 hours with increasing concentrations of TGF-ß1 (0.0 - 300 pg/ml) or test samples (0.05 - 50%, V:V) in 200 μl final volume. Cell growth was assessed by [^{3}H]-thymidine uptake during the final 6 hours of incubation and counts per minute (cpm ± SD) was plotted as a function of TGF-ß1 (standard) or test sample concentration. The high-affinity receptors (K_D = 17 pM) of HCF were utilized for measurement of TGF-ß by RIA[2]. HCF monolayers were incubated (4°C, 3 hours) with 0.2 ng/ml [^{125}I]-TGF-ß1, and increasing concentrations of unlabeled TGF-ß1 (0 - 120 ng/ml), or test samples (0.1 - 80%, V:V)[2].

Mink Cell-Human Corneal Fibroblast (MC-HCF) Co-culture Assay: The ability of HCF to produce bioactive TGF-ß was assessed by MC-HCF co-culture assay. IFN-γ-treated (500 U/ml) monolayers of HCF, pre-treated with mitomycin-C (25 μg/ml), were co-cultured with Mv-1 Lu cells (0.5×10^5/well) for 36 hours, and cell growth was assessed by [^{3}H]-thymidine incorporation (final 6 hours). In these assays, the Mv-1 Lu cells were physically separated from HCF by a porous membrane.

RESULTS AND DISCUSSION:

The results of MLR-HCF co-culture assays showed that, regardless of indomethacin concentration, HCF inhibited T-cell alloresponse. The inhibition was significantly enhanced by pretreatment of HCF with IFN-γ. The results of RT-PCR revealed that HCF express TGF-ß1 and TGF-ß2 mRNA. The level of TGF-ß1 message was approximately 8 times that of TGF-ß2 by comparative assays. Scatchard analysis of the [^{125}I]-TGF-ß1 binding data revealed that HCF constitutively express 8000 high-affinity (K_D = 17 pM) receptors/cell. After IFN-γ treatment, in addition to the high-affinity receptors, HCF also expressed a new population (300/cell) of very high-affinity (K_D = 200 fM) receptors. The results of BIA, extrapolated from 50% growth inhibition points, showed that the TGF-ß content of acidified culture medium and 4-day culture supernatants from HCF, before and after treatment with IFN-γ, were 0.2, 1.7 and 3.1 ng/ml, respectively. These results indicated that the net TGF-ß output of HCF increased from 1.5 to 2.9 ng/ml (100%) after IFN-γ treatment. TGF-ß production by HCF was confirmed by RIA. The total TGF-ß contents of culture medium, before and after acidification, and acidified 4-day culture supernatants from IFN-γ-treated HCF, extrapolated from 50% binding inhibition points, were 0.8, 6, and 15 ng/ml, respectively. The results of MC-HCF co-culture assays revealed that IFN-treated HCF were capable of reducing mink cell growth. Maximum growth inhibition obtained was 70%. These results suggest that TGF-ß production by HCF, and its upregulation by IFN-γ, may be part of a homeostatic cytokine-dependent mechanism that maintains corneal immunoseclusion and preserves corneal optical competency.

The net TGF-ß content of IFN-γ-treated HCF culture supernatants by RIA (9 ng/ml) was three times the level of TGF-ß measured by BIA in the same sample. The observed discrepancy between the results of BIA and RIA may be explained by the presence of a TGF-ß-binding protein in the test samples. Evidence in support of a binding protein was primarily drawn from the results of RIA. While the standard RIA curve reached its maximum binding inhibition at 15 ng/ml TGF-ß1, and higher concentrations of TGF-ß1 (30 - 120 ng/ml) resulted in a binding inhibition plateau (212 ± 35 cpm), the binding inhibition curves of the acidified culture medium (4.8 ng/ml TGF-ß at 80% V:V), and 4-day culture supernatants from IFN-γ-treated HCF (12.8 ng/ml at 80% V:V), did not plateau. The maximum binding inhibition points of the samples (40 ± 35 cpm) at 80% V:V were significantly lower than the plateau of the standard curve (p < 0.02). While in the standard assay, 120 ng/ml TGF-ß1 was unable to eliminate the plateau, the test samples with TGF-ß values less than 15 ng/ml resulted in complete binding inhibition of [^{125}I]-TGF-ß1. The phenomenon can be explained by the presence of a TGF-ß-binding protein in the test samples. Such binding proteins would bind and progressively remove [^{125}I]-TGF-ß1 from the free compartment of the assay system.

The effect of binding proteins on the measurement of TGF-ß by RIA would be one of overestimation, because the protein-bound radio-labeled TGF-ß1 would be erroneously measured as if it was displaced by media-borne TGF-ß. In contrast, in the BIA the binding proteins progressively remove a greater fraction of the free bioactive TGF-ß available for interaction with the receptors of Mv-1 Lu cells, resulting in a reduction in growth inhibition. Thus, the BIA would underestimate the concentration of TGF-ß in biologic materials. The presence of TGF-ß-binding proteins in the MLR-HCF co-culture assay may also explain the incomplete neutralization obtained with anti-TGF-ß antibodies. A TGF-ß-binding protein may absorb significant fractions of bioactive TGF-ß, only to dissociate and release it into the co-culture system, "buffering" the effect of added antibody (Figure 1). In addition to their interference with TGF-ß assessment by BIA and RIA and with antibody neutralization, TGF-ß-binding proteins may have important pathobiologic implications in vivo. The exclusion of binding proteins from the intraocular fluids, made possible by blood-eye barrier, may be important in maintenance of TGF-ß-dependent ocular immunoseclusion. Anterior chamber-associated

34

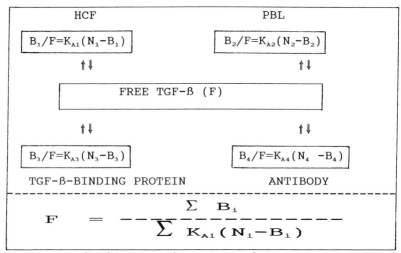

Figure 1: Effect of binding protein, and antibody on concentration of free TGF-ß in a system with multiple binding components. Binding equation is expressed in terms of bound TGF-ß (B_i), binding sites (N_i), and association constant (K_{Ai}) for each component.

immune deviation (ACAID), reportedly can be induced if antigen is injected intracamerally (not intravenously), or by adoptive transfer of syngeneic eusplenic mice with macrophages pulsed with antigen in presence of aqueous humor or TGF-ß[3]. The crucial difference between the intraocular and intravenous routes of antigen delivery may be the absence of TGF-ß-binding proteins from the eye. Disruption of blood-eye barrier, such as occurs in ocular injury/hemorrhage, may result in elevation of intraocular TGF-ß-binding protein levels and abrogation of TGF-ß-dependent immune privilege.

ACKNOWLEDGEMENT:
Supported by USPHS/NIH Grant EY06616, by a grant from Tissue Banks International, and by the Mackall fund. We thank Doctor Stephen Orlin for human corneal tissues.

REFERENCES:
1. Donnelly JJ, Xi MS, and Rockey JH; A Soluble Product of Human Corneal Fibroblasts Inhibits Lymphocyte Activation. Enhancement by IFN-γ: Exp. Eye Res. (1993); 56, 157-165.
2. Abrahamian A, Xi MS, and Rockey JH; Interferon-gamma Induces High-Affinity Transforming Growth Factor-beta Receptor Expression on Corneal Fibroblasts: Curr. Eye Res. (1994) (13), 213-17.
3. Wilbank GA, Mammolenti M and Streilein JW: Studies on the induction of anterior chamber-associated immune deviation (ACAID): III: Induction of ACAID depends upon intraocular transforming growth factor-ß: Eur. J. Immunology, (1992), 22, 165-173.

Advances in Ocular Immunology
R.B. Nussenblatt, S.M. Whitcup, R.R. Caspi and I. Gery, eds.

Effect of Interferon α and γ on HLA expression of uveal melanoma cells.

I. de Waard-Siebinga, J. Kool, M.J. Jager

Dept. of Ophthalmology, Leiden University, PO Box 9600, 2300 RC Leiden,
The Netherlands

Introduction

Interferons are known to have a direct anti-proliferative effect on tumour cells as well as an immunomodulatory effect (1,2). These characteristics make interferons interesting drugs for the systemic treatment of skin melanoma metastases. Interferon α has recently been accepted as the cytokine of choice in combination with cytotoxic drugs for a European study to treat metastases of ocular melanoma. Interferon α is known to increase the expression of HLA Class I antigens on skin melanoma cells, but not of Class II, while interferon γ induces both, even on Class II negative melanoma cell lines (3,4). Incubation of skin melanoma cells with interferon γ increases the susceptibility of the tumour cells to lysis by tumour infiltrating lymphocytes (5).

The induction of HLA antigens may not only stimulate immune responses against tumour cells in vitro but may also contribute to a better anti-tumour immune response in vivo. This may also be the case with regard to ocular melanoma cells. Melanomas originating from the choroid or ciliary body are the most common intraocular malignancy in adult Caucasians, and up to 50% of the patients will die of metastases (6). An effective treatment for either the prevention or the treatment of metastases is therefore essential and interferon α may be applicable. However, although much is known about the effect of interferon α on skin melanoma cells, we do not yet know which effect the interferons have on ocular melanoma cells. We already know that uveal melanomas vary greatly in their expression of the HLA class I and II antigens (7). We recently showed that ocular melanomas show a great variability in the level of expression of the allele-specific HLA class I molecules as well: expression of HLA-B antigens was much lower than of HLA-A antigens (8). In addition, we performed short-term in vitro cultures of uveal melanoma cells, and observed the same low expression of HLA-B antigens on uveal melanoma cells in vitro. Since the HLA molecules bind tumour-specific proteins that can be targets of cytotoxic T cells, lack of expression of the HLA Class I molecules is likely to inhibit a CTL attack (9). We set out to test the hypothesis that, similar to the situation with skin melanoma cells, interferons might induce HLA antigen expression on cultured uveal melanoma cells.

Materials and methods

The human uveal melanoma celline 92.1 was established in our own laboratory. The HLA type of this cell line is HLA-A2, A3, B51, B12, Bw4.

Cells were maintained in culture in petri dishes in RPMI 1640 medium (Gibco, UK) supplemented with penicillin-streptomycin, L-glutamine, and fetal bovine serum. Cells were seeded in 6-well plates at a density of 1-3 x 10^5 cells per well in a total volume of 1.5 ml. Cells were incubated with recombinant interferon γ (specific activity 2 x 10^7 IU/mg protein) or recombinant human interferon α-2b (specific activity 1.66 x 10^8 IU/mg protein) at concentrations of 50, 200 and 500 IU/ml. After 2 and 5 days cells were harvested by trypsinisation (0.01 % trypsin) and cytospin preparations were made. The cytospin preparations were stained by immunohistology with specific monoclonal antibodies.

Results

The allele-specific HLA-A2 antigen was present on 69 % of the cultured uveal melanoma cells before addition of cytokines. Addition of all three different concentrations of interferon α and γ increased the expression to 95-100% of the uveal melanoma cells after 2 days in culture (Figure 1). A similar increase was observed after 5 days of culture with the cytokines.

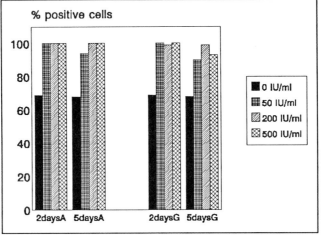

Figure 1. Influence of interferon α and γ on expression of HLA-A2 after 2 and 5 days.

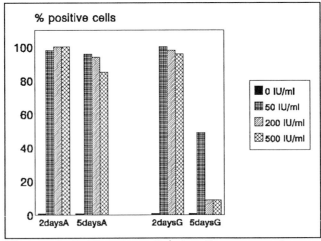

Figure 2. Influence of interferon α and γ on expression of HLA-Bw4 after 2 and 5 days.

The HLA-B-allele Bw4 is normally absent on cultured 92.1 cells. Addition of interferon α induced expression of HLA-Bw4 on almost all cells after two days (Figure 2). The highest concentration showed a decrease in expression after five days. This phenomenon was also observed with interferon γ: interferon γ induced expression of Bw4 after two days, but showed an impressively lower level after five days.

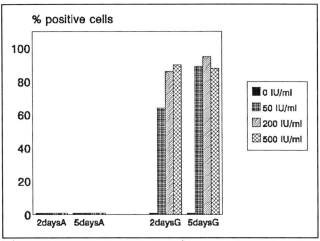

Figure 3. Influence of interferon α and γ on expression of HLA-DR after 2 and 5 days.

Finally, we tested the effect on HLA-Class II antigens, since tests on skin melanoma had previously shown that only interferon γ and not interferon α influences expression of Class II on skin melanoma cells. The 92.1 cells did not constitutively express Class II antigens, and while interferon α did not have any effect, interferon γ did induce expression. The effect was dose-dependent on day 2, but not on day five (Figure 3).

Discussion

Our data show that interferon α increases HLA Class I but not Class II expression on uveal melanoma cells in vitro, while interferon γ induces both. This is similar to the findings on skin melanoma cells. An unusual observation was made with regard to the higher concentrations of interferon γ and the inducible HLA-Bw4 expression: although after two days expression was over 90% at all concentrations of interferon γ, the level of expression had decreased again after 5 days. This test has been repeated several times with similar results (unpublished). Since interferon does not only have an immunomodulatory effect but also a direct cytotoxic effect, the lack of expression may be due to a sublethal effect on these cells. Since only live (adherent) cells were obtained for preparing the cytospins, cell death was not responsible for decrease in expression. However, sublethal damage may result in a decreased functioning of the Golgi-apparatus and intracellular protein transport molecules and thereby decrease the level of expression of the HLA antigens. Expression of HLA Class II antigens was not decreased after five days, indicating that HLA Class I and II proteins have different pathways of induction in uveal melanoma cells. It had already been shown for skin melanoma that interferon γ needs de novo protein synthesis, while this is not the case for interferon α (4).

Our results show that interferon α and γ do indeed influence the level of expression of the antigen-presentation molecules and that their application may stimulate local immunological anti-melanoma responses.

References

1. Krasagakis K, Garbe C, Orfanos CE. Cytokines in human melanoma cells: synthesis, autocrine stimulation and regulatory functions- an overview. Melanoma Research 1993, 3, 425.

2. Garbe C, Krasagakis K. Effects of interferons and cytokines on melanoma cells. J Invest Dermatol 1993, 100, 239S.

3. Carrel S, Schmidt Kessen A, Giuffre L. Recombinant interferon-gamma can induce the expression of HLA-DR and -DC on DR-negative melanoma cells and enhance the expression of HLA-ABC and tumor-associated antigens. Eur J Immunol 1985, 15, 118.

4. Giacomini P, Aguzzi A, Pestka S, Fisher PB, Ferrone S. Modulation by recombinant DNA leukocyte (alpha) and fibroblast (beta) interferons of the expression and shedding of HLA- and tumor-associated antigens by human melanoma cells. J Immunol 1984, 133, 1649.

5. Wiebke EA, Custer MC, Rosenberg SA, Lotze MT. Cytokines and target cell susceptibility to lysis: evaluation of non-major histocompatibility complex-restricted effectors reveals differential effects on natural and lymphokine-activated killing. J Biol Response Mod 1990, 9, 113.

6. Jensen OA. Malignant melanoma of the human uvea. 25 year follow-up of cases in Denmark, 1943-1952. Acta Ophthalmol. 1982, 60: 161.

7. Jager MJ, Pol JP van der, Wolff-Rouendaal D de, Jong PTVM de, Ruiter DJ. Decreased expression of HLA Class II antigens on human uveal melanoma cells after in vivo X-ray irradiation. Am J Ophthalmol 1988, 105, 78.

8. Jager MJ, Waard-Siebinga I de, Kool J. Allele-specific HLA expression on uveal melanoma. Inv Ophthalmol Vis Sci (suppl) 1993, 34, 890.

9. Melief CJM, Kast WM. Lessons from T cell responses to virus induced tumours for cancer eradication in general. Cancer Surveys 1992, 13, 81.

© 1994 Elsevier Science B.V. All rights reserved.
Advances in Ocular Immunology
R.B. Nussenblatt, S.M. Whitcup, R.R. Caspi and I. Gery, eds.

ANTIBODIES AGAINST CELL ADHESION MOLECULES INHIBIT PROLIFERATION OF UVEITOGENIC LYMPHOCYTES IN VITRO

S. Ishimoto, N.P. Chanaud III, A.T. Kozhich, A. Fukushima, I. Gery, and S.M. Whitcup

National Eye Institute, NIH, Bethesda, MD.

Abstract

To study the role of cell adhesion molecules (CAMs) in the pathogenic process of experimental autoimmune uveoretinitis (EAU), we examined the effect of monoclonal antibodies (mAbs) against lymphocyte function-associated molecule-1 (LFA-1;CD11a/CD18) and very late antigen-4 (VLA-4;CD49d) on lymphocyte proliferation. MAbs against CD11a/CD18 effectively inhibited the proliferative response of lymphocytes to retinal antigens. In contrast, mAb against CD49d had minimal inhibitory effect. These data suggest that LFA-1, which binds to intercellular adhesion molecule-1 (ICAM-1;CD54) on antigen presenting cells, is important for optimum lymphocyte proliferation in vitro, and that VLA-4, which binds to vascular cell adhesion molecule-1 (VCAM-1; CD106) on vascular endothelium, is not integral to the process.

Introduction

Cell adhesion molecules (CAMs) are involved not only in recruitment of leukocytes to areas of inflammation, but also in the interaction of lymphocytes and antigen presenting cells during lymphocyte activation. The integrins are a family of heterodimeric leukocyte proteins consisting of an α- and ß-chain. LFA-1 (CD11a/CD18) is a β_2 integrin that binds to ICAM-1 and is involved in a variety of adhesion-dependent lymphocyte functions including the interaction of antigen presenting cells (APCs) and lymphocytes, cytotoxic T cell-mediated killing of target cells, and lymphocyte adhesion to the vascular endothelium [1,2]. VLA-4 (CD49d/CD29) is a β_1 integrin that interacts with VCAM-1 which is induced on vascular endothelium at sites of inflammation [3]. Monoclonal antibodies (mAbs) against CAMs were previously shown to inhibit experimental autoimmune uveoretinitis (EAU) in animals [4,5], suggesting that CAMs play a pivotal role in the pathogenesis of human uveitis. This study examined the effect of the mAbs against the α-chain (CD11a) and ß-chain (CD18) of LFA-1 and against VLA-4 on lymphocyte proliferation, a process that involves interaction between lymphocytes and APCs.

Materials and Methods

Immunization of animals and derivation of cells
Female Lewis rats (Charles River, Wilmington, MA), 8-11 weeks old, were immunized with 50 µg of bovine retinal soluble antigen (S-Ag) emulsified (1:1)

mg/ml *Mycobacterium tuberculosis* H37Ra. A volume of 0.1 ml was injected into the hind footpad. Cells were harvested from draining lymph nodes (popliteal and inguinal) 21 days after immunization. The use of animals conformed to the ARVO statement.

MAbs

MAbs against rat CD11a (TA-3; mouse IgG2a) [6], rat CD18 (TA-4; mouse IgG2a) and rat CD49d (TA-2; mouse IgG1) [7] mAbs were kindly provided by Seikagaku Co. (Rockville, MD). Purified mouse IgG (Pierce, Rockford, IL) was used as a control antibody.

Inhibition assay of lymphocyte proliferation by mAbs

Lymph node cells (3×10^5) in 0.2 ml of RPMI 1640 medium (Mediatech, Herndon, VA) supplemented with 100 U/ml penicillin, 100 µg/ml streptomycin, 5×10^{-5}M 2-mercaptoethanol and 1% syngeneic rat serum were seeded in triplicate cultures in 96-well, flat-bottomed microculture trays with 5 µg/ml of S-Ag and the tested of antibodies at 10, 2, 0.4 and 0 µg/ml. The cultures were incubated at 37°C in 5% CO_2 for 4 days and pulsed with 0.5 µCi ^{3}H-thymidine/well (New England Nuclear, Boston, MA) during the last 14 h. Incorporated radioactivity was measured by liquid scintillation counting. The results were presented as the percent of the stimulation index in control cultures in which no antibody or globulin was added.

Results

Figure 1 is showing the effect of the antibodies on lymphocyte proliferation in vitro. Anti-CD11a mAb inhibited the lymphocyte proliferative response by 65.2%, 40.5% and 22.6% at concentrations of 10, 2 and 0.4 µg/ml, respectively, when compared to the control cultures. Anti-CD18 mAb also effectively inhibited lymphocyte proliferation by 52.7%, 40.7% and 34.9%, respectively.

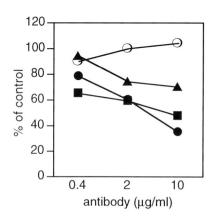

Figure 1. Inhibition of lymphocyte proliferation by mAbs against CD11a, CD18 and CD49d. Triplicate aliquots of limph node cells (3x105) were cultured in supplemented RPMI 1640 medium with the indicated antibodies [CD11a (●), CD18 (■), CD49d (▲) and mouse IgG (○)] for 4 days, and cell proliferation were measured using a 3H-thymidine incorporation assay. Shown are the percent control of stimulation index by the indicated antibodies.

Anti-CD49d mAb was less inhibitory, reducing the response by 30.2%, 26.1% and 5.9%, respectively. In contrast, the control antibody (mouse IgG) had practically the same proliferative response as the cultures without antibody.

Dicussion

MAbs against CD11a and CD18 effectively inhibited the proliferative response of lymphocytes in a dose dependent manner. The inhibitory effect in this study is possibly due to inhibition of costimulatory signals between lymphocytes and APCs. T cell activation requires antigen contact with the T cell receptor (TCR) in the presence of costimulatory signals provided by APCs. Thus, TCR signaling alone in the absence of costimulatory signals not only appears to be insufficient to induce lymphocyte proliferation and cytokine production, but also may render specific T cell clones anergic [8]. Indeed, the interference with CAMs during Ag contact using mAbs against CD2, LFA-3, LFA-1 and ICAM-1 can cause inactivation of Ag specific T cells [1]. Furthermore, Vistica et al. [9] showed that anti-LFA-1 and anti-ICAM-1 mAbs inhibited the proliferation of a uveitogenic T cell line in the presence of Ag and APCs. Our data indicate that blocking of the LFA-1/ICAM-1 interaction by mAbs against CD11a and CD18 down-regulates the proliferative responses of the T cells to S-Ag.

Recently, mAbs against LFA-1 and ICAM-1 were reported to prevent the development of EAU [3,4]. EAU is predominantly a cell mediated immune response and can be induced by uveitogenic T lymphocytes. In addition, these T cells may be activated and have increased expression of CAMs on their surface. Therefore, mAbs against CAMs can inhibit the development of EAU by several mechanisms. Anti-CAM mAbs can interfere with Ag-APC induced uveitogenic T cell stimulation and suppress the homing of the uveitogenic T cells to the activated endothelium of ocular vessels [1,2]. Our findings suggest that the inhibitory effect of mAbs against CD11a and CD18 on the development of EAU is partially explained by their effects on lymphocyte activation.

Our study also showed that anti-CD49d (VLA-4) mAb had minimal effect on lymphocyte proliferation. The ligand for VLA-4 is VCAM-1, expressed on endothelial cells [2], and fibronectin, the extracellular matrix [10]. Although VLA-4 might augment the binding of lymphocytes to activated endothelium at inflammatory sites, it would not be expected to play a role in lymphocyte proliferation.

References

1. Bohming GA, Kovarik J, Holter W, Pohanka E, Zlabinger G. J Immunol 1994; 152: 3720-3728
2. Nakajima H, Sano H, Nishimura T, Yoshida S, Iwamoto I. J Exp Med 1994; 179: 1145-1154
3. Whitcup SM, DeBarge LR, Caspi RR, Harning R, Nussenblatt RB, Chan CC. Clin Immunol Pathol 1993; 67: 143-150
4. Uchio E, Kijima M, Tanaka S, Ohno S. Invest Ophthalmol Vis Sci 1994; 35: 2626-2631
5. Issekutz TB, Wykretowicz A. J Immunol 1991; 147: 109-116

6. Issekutz TB. Transplantation 1993; 55: 1196-1199

7. Vyth-Dreese FA, Dellemijin TAM, Frijhoff A, Kooyk Y, Figdor CG. Eur J Immunol 1993; 23: 3292-3299

8. Schwartz RH. Science 1990; 248: 1349-1356

9. Vistica V, Gery I, Chan CC, Nussenblatt RB, Whitcup SM. Invest Ophthalmol Vis Sci 1993; 34 (Suppl): 1144

10. Shimizu Y, Seventer GV, Horgan KJ, Saw S. J Immunol 1990; 145: 59-67

Advances in Ocular Immunology
R.B. Nussenblatt, S.M. Whitcup, R.R. Caspi and I. Gery, eds.

ADHESIVE MECHANISMS OF HUMAN RETINAL PIGMENT EPITHELIAL CELLS

D. Lahiri-Munir[a], T. Li[b], C.A. Garcia[b] and R.M. Franklin[b]

[a]Department of Ophthalmology, University of Texas Health Science Center,
[b]Bob Hope Eye Research Center, St. Joseph Hospital, Houston, TX.

INTRODUCTION

Retinal pigment epithelium (RPE) forms a blood-retina barrier analogous to the blood-brain barrier, thus regulating the access of circulating blood components into the neural retina. Due to its key position, the RPE may be critical in initiation and propagation of ocular inflammation(1) in proliferative vitreoretinopathy (2), uveoretinitis (3) and others.

Neuropeptides released from sensory neurons following certain stimuli can directly or indirectly modulate neurogenic inflammation. Neuropeptides can produce rapid and marked effects within the eye including vasodilation, miosis, prostaglandin release and breakdown of the blood aqueous barrier. Examples of peptides are substance P, neurokinin A (NKA), calcitonin gene-related peptide (CGRP), vasoactive intestinal peptide (VIP), neuropeptide Y(NPY) and others (4).

ICAM I (intercellular adhesion molecule)is a cell surface receptor for the leukocyte function antigen-1 (LFA-1) and is believed to regulate the binding of leukocytes to other cells and thereby can regulate leukocyte "trafficking" in tissues. Previous studies have shown that interactions between intercellular adhesion molecules (ICAMs) I and II LFA-1 and 3 are necessary for leukocyte migration and antigen presentation (5, 6). In addition, synergistic expression of major histocompatibility complex (MHC) antigens I and II and ICAM-I is necessary for antigen presentation. In this study, we have examined adhesive interactions between the RPE and T lymphocytes and the involvement of cell adhesion molecules such as ICAMs under the influence of interferon γ (IFN), the pro-inflammatory cytokine, VIP and the lectin concanavalin A (Con A).

METHODS

RPE culture: Human fetal eyes ranging from 10-16 wk gestational age were obtained following therapeutic abortion. RPE was dissected and transferred to 35mm tissue culture dishes in medium 199 supplemented with 15 % fetal calf serum, 1% antimycotic-antibiotic agent and other additives (7, 8).

Lymphocyte Isolation: Blood from volunteers was collected in sodium heparin vacutainers and diluted 1:15 in Hank's balanced salt solution (HBSS). 50 ml tubes were filled with 20 ml Lympholyte M and 30 ml diluted blood without disturbing the interface and centrifuged for 30 min at 2000 rpm. The interface with lymphocytes was harvested and washed 3 time with HBSS.

Adherence Assay: For adherence assays RPE cultures from passage 2 were used. Con A (5 µg/ml), VIP (5×10^{-7} µg/ml), IFN γ (10^3 U/ml) were added to the experimental wells and cultured for 4 days. Unstimulated wells were used as control. Stimulated cultures were washed 3 times with HBSS. Freshly isolated human lymphocytes (1x10⁵) were added to each RPE well and co-cultured for 24 hrs. The plates were then gently rotated (60 rpm) on a circular shaker bath for 30 mins at 25°C, then gently washed 4 times by aspirating and filling each well with 1 % glutaraldehyde in HBSS. The number of adherent lymphocyte on RPE cells was counted at a constant magnification of 400x in separate fields.

Immunocytochemistry: Control and stimulated cultures were subjected to immunocytochemical analysis for adhesion molecules ICAM I, ICAM II, LFA1-α, LFA1-β and MAC-1, using a standard ABC technique with AEC as the chromogen.

RESULTS

Adherence assays: Cultured RPE cells showed distinct binding of lymphocytes that increased significantly over the control after stimulation with IFN γ, Con A and VIP. The increase in adherence of T lymphocytes on fetal RPE cells was highest when cells were stimulated with IFN γ. Percent control binding values after stimulation with IFN γ, con A and VIP were 53-72%, 41-49% and 35-49% (Figs 1a, 1b) respectively in contrast to 10% in the untreated cultures, thus activation with IFN γ increased adhesion by 40 to 60 % whereas pretreatment with VIP led to 25-40% increase in adhesion. Cultures activated with con A characteristically contained large homoptypic aggregates of lymphocytes in selected areas on the plate. The T-lymphocytes retained a 75-80% viability throughout the period of the assay.

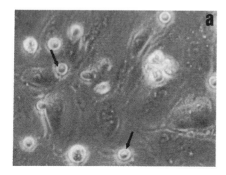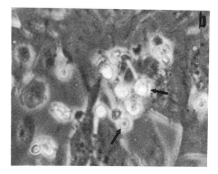

Figure 1a and 1b demonstrate binding of T-lymphocytes (arrows) to human fetal RPE cells after stimulation with IFN-γ and VIP respectively.

Immunocytochemistry: RPE cells stimulated with IFN γ demonstrated robust staining with a delicate granular reaction product with anti-ICAM I (40%)(Figs 2a, 4). Concentrated pockets of expression rather than an uniform distribution of cells positive for ICAM I were present. In comparison to ICAM I, positive staining for ICAM II was at a reduced level. RPE cells when stimulated with VIP showed selective and restricted expression of ICAM I(Figs 2b, 4). VIP did not induce expression of ICAM II. Untreated cultures failed to show any staining with either antibody and thus were used as negative controls for comparison. RPE cells were negative for mABs to MAC-1, LFA-1α, LFA-1β.

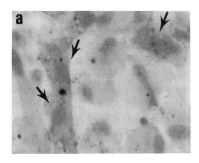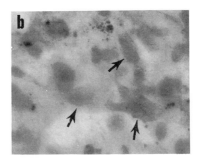

Figure 2a and 2b demonstrate RPE cells stained with anti-ICAM-I (arrows) after treatment with IFN-γ and VIP respectively.

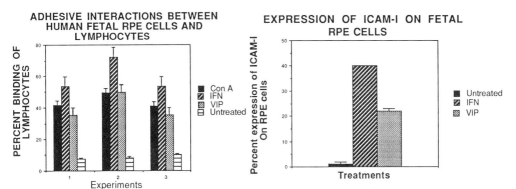

Figure 3 demonstrates percent binding of lymphocytes to RPE cells after stimulation.
Figure 4 demonstrates percentage of cells stained with ICAM-I following stimulation.

DISCUSSION

Our studies are the first to demonstrate ICAM-1 expression by human fetal RPE cells *in vitro*. We have also shown that these cells can be activated by cytokines like IFN γ and induced to express ICAM I and II. Moreover, pretreatment with vasoactive intestinal peptide (VIP) a 28-residue polypeptide hormone, also activates RPE cells to express ICAM I but not ICAM II. Our adherence assays represent ICAM I dependent binding of lymphocytes by RPE as shown by Liversidge et al., 1990 (9), following activation by con A, IFN γ and VIP.

ICAM I is the major ligand for LFA-1(5). Therefore, the presence of ICAM I on RPE suggests its active role in T-cell recruitment and infiltration into the retina and choroid by binding LFA-1 receptors on leukocytes (10). It is apparent from our control studies that ICAM I is not constitutively expressed on fetal RPE cells, however it is inducible following activation by IFN γ as well as VIP. Such potential of the fetal cells suggests the possible availability of pathways dependent on such adhesion molecules at an early developmental stage. Further, the availability of ICAM dependent pathways at an early gestational age may imply that these molecules may also be subject to activation in order to participate in cell to cell interactions during other developmental events.

VIP is synthesized by neurons in the central and peripheral nervous systems (11) and has multiple functional attributes, some of which include stimulation of acinar cell secretion in pancreas and parotid, stimulation of glycogenolysis in neuronal and hepatic tissue and others. This peptide has been found to also have a role in immune modulation in the intestine (12). VIP is found to be ubiquitous in all ocular tissues but is present in highest concentrations in the choroid/sclera of all species indicating an important and conserved regulatory role in the eye. The evidence from our present study elucidates the induction of ICAM I on RPE following pretreatment with VIP thus indicating a regulatory effect of this peptide on the expression of these molecules on RPE.

Furthermore, it has been shown previously that ICAM I is strongly expressed on ocular tissue including the RPE, vascular endothelium and retinal glial cells in human eyes with posterior uveitis and other forms of ocular inflammation (10, 13, 14). It is also known that experimental autoimmune uveitis can be inhibited by monoclonal antibodies to ICAM-1. Thus the inductive influence of a neuropeptide such as VIP on ICAMs suggests a possible correlation of RPE with ocular inflammation regulated by VIP. VIP containing nerves that arise from the ocular parasympathetic nerve supply of the facial origin, have been demonstrated in the ciliary body, posterior uvea and choroid (15, 16). Therefore, at present it is feasible to speculate that some forms of ocular inflammation may regulated by VIP via a pathway involving ICAMs and the retinal pigment epithelium.

ACKNOWLEDGEMENT This work was supported by grants from Knights Templar Eye Foundation, Research to prevent blindness, William Stamps Farish Fund and NEI RO1-EYO3028.

LITERATURE CITED
1. Chan CC, Detrick B, Nussenblatt R, et al. Arch Ophthalmol 1986; 104:725.
2. Baudoin C, Fredj-Reygrobellet D, Lapalus P et al. Am J Ophthalmol 1988; 105:383.
3. Chan CC, Nussenblatt R, Detrick B. Curr Eye Res 1986; 5:325.
4. Nilsson SFE, Anders B. Acta Physiol Scand 1984; 121:385.
5. Springer TA, Dustin ML, Kishimoto TK et al. Ann Rev Immunol; 5: 223.
6. Dougherty GJ, Murdoch S and Hogg N. Eur J Immunol 1988; 18:35.
7. Nicolaissen BJ, Allen C, Nicolaissen A, et al. Acta Ophthalmol 1988; 64:1.
8. Aronson, JF. In vitro 1983; 19:642.
9. Liversidge J, Sewell HF and Forrester JV. Immunol 1990; 71: 390.
10. Elner SG, Elner VM, Pavilack MA, et al. Lab Invest 1992; 66:200.
11. Larsson LI, Fahrenkrug H, Schaffalitzky de Muckadell O, et al. Proc Natl Acad Sci USA 1976; 73:3197.
12. Stanisz AM, Befus D and Bienenstock J. J Immunol 1986; 136:152.
13. Whitcup SM, DeBarge LR, Caspi RR, et al. Clin Immunol Pathol 1993; 67:143.
14. Forrester JV, Liversidge J and Dua HS. Curr Eye Res 1990; 9:183.
15. Miller AS, Coster DJ, Costa M, et al. Aust J Ophthalmol 1983; 11:185.
16. Stone RA, Tervo T, Tervo K, et al. Acta Ophthalmol 1986; 64:12.

© 1994 Elsevier Science B.V. All rights reserved.
Advances in Ocular Immunology
R.B. Nussenblatt, S.M. Whitcup, R.R. Caspi and I. Gery, eds.   47

EXPRESSION OF CELL ADHESION MOLECULES IN THE TRABECULAR MESHWORK AND AQUEOUS OUTFLOW PATHWAYS

Joel S. Schuman, MD, Nan Wang, MD, Dan L. Eisenberg, MD

New England Eye Center, Tufts University School of Medicine, Boston, MA.
Address correspondence to Joel S. Schuman, MD, New England Eye Center, 750 Washington
Street, Box 450, Boston, MA, 02111. Telephone 617-956-7950, Facsimilie 617-956-4866.

INTRODUCTION

Glaucoma, a leading cause of blindness in the United States, is characterized by what many believe to be a causal relationship between impaired aqueous humor outflow through the TM leading to elevated intraocular pressure, which apparently damages the axons that comprise the optic nerve. TM cells may play a major functional role in the maintenance of the outflow pathway, either through cell-cell interactions involved in paracellular fluid transport from the anterior chamber to Schlemm's canal, transcellular transport, or cellular production of extracellular matrix, which may have a place in aqueous outflow resistance.[1,2] Aberrations in the integrity or function of TM cells may result in increased resistance to aqueous outflow. CAMs are surface proteins which have an important role in cell adhesion and migration and so might be expected to affect the regulation of aqueous outflow in normal and diseased states.

CAMs in the category of the immunoglobulin gene superfamily perform essential functions in a wide range of immune responses in the eye. Expression of intercellular adhesion molecule-1 (ICAM-1), which binds leukocyte function antigen-1 (LFA-1) on endothelial and epithelial cells, fibroblasts and leukocytes, have been found in human cornea [3-5], iris, choroidal blood vessels and retinal pigment from patients with uveitis [6,7], as well as TM [8]. Other cell surface proteins, such as HLA class-I and II antigens have also been reported to be present on TM cells; CAM expression can be induced on these cells with cytokines [9]. Finally, CAMs could mediate cell binding and promote the migration of leukocytes to areas of ocular inflammation. Whitcup et. al. demonstrated that ICAM-1 is expressed in the eye before clinical or histologic signs of inflammation, and monoclonal antibodies against ICAM-1, LFA-1 and Mac-1 are effective in inhibiting experimental autoimmune uveitis in mice [10,11].

METHODOLOGY

Isolation of tissues and cultivation of cells.

Normal human eyes are obtained from the NDRI (National Disease Research Interchange) and New England Eye Bank. The eyes are enucleated within 2-4 hour of death, stored in moist chamber at 4 °C, and used in the laboratory 20-36 hours after death. Fresh calf eyes are obtained from a local slaughterhouse. Trabecular meshwork tissue from glaucomatous eyes is obtained from cadaver and trabeculectomy specimens. Specimen dissection and processing is carried out under aseptic conditions in a laminar air flow hood. The TM is dissected free from neighboring tissues as described previously [12-15]. The anterior segment is removed and divided into 4 segments after the lens is removed. For cell culture, incisions are made at the anterior and posterior edges of the TM and the TM is gently lifted away from Schlemm's canal, and soaked in 10% antibiotic-antimycotic solution (penicillin, streptomycin and amphotericin B). The tissue is then washed in several changes of culture medium with 1% antibiotic-antimycotic. The underlying Schlemm's canal endothelium is then dissected free and cultured in a manner similar to the TM. The dissected tissues are examined under light and phase-contrast microscope to ascertain the absence of other neighboring tissues. In addition, a portion of the neighboring corneal endothelium, sclera, iris and ciliary muscle are cut from same segment. For tissue section, intact corneoscleral tissue containing TM is dissected and embedded in optimum cutting temperature compound (OCT) and immediately snap frozen in dry ice and 95% alcohol, then stored at -80°C.

The explants are placed in T-25 culture flasks filled with complete culture medium [For human tissue: Dulbecco's modified Eagle's medium (DMEM) supplemented with 15% fetal bovine serum (GIBCO BRL); 1% 200 mM glutamine; 1% antibiotic-antimycotic. For bovine tissue: Eagle's minimum essential medium (MEM) supplemented with 5% fetal bovine serum, 2.5% calf serum; 1% essential aminoacids, 0.5% non-essential aminoacids (GIBCO BRL); 1% 200 mM glutamine, 1% antibiotic-antimycotic].The explants are incubated at 37°C in 5% CO_2 humidified atmosphere. Media are changed every there days. After 2-3 weeks in culture the explants are removed with sterile forceps and the culture flasks are returned to the incubator. When confluency is reached, cells are trypsinized and subcultured.

Staining with biotin-labeled antibody

Immunohistochemical staining is performed by means of an avidin-biotin-peroxidase complex "A B C" technique. Monoclonal antibody is used to determine the distribution of CAMs and other cell surface molecules. Fourth passage human and bovine TM cells, scleral fibroblasts and iris pigment epithelial cells, as well as human Schlemm's canal endothelial cells, are cultured on sterile coverslips until confluence. 4µm thick frozen sections are placed on poly-l-Lysine treated glass slides and are air dried. Both cells in culture and frozen sections are fixed in 100% acetone for 10 minutes, and washed in Tris-saline buffer for 3 minutes 3 times each. After rinsing with Tris-saline, non-specific background staining is blocked by immersion of the coverslips and slides in 10% normal horse serum in PBS for 20 minutes. The primary antibodies include monoclonal antibodies against LFA- 1a (CD 11a), LFA-1ß (CD 18), ICAM-1 (CD 54), VCAM-1 (INACAM-110), N-CAM-16 (CD 56) N-cadherin (A-CAM), ELAM-1 (E-selectin), GMP-140 (CD 62, P-selectin), Integrin a2 (CD 49b), integrin a3 (CD 49c), integrin a4 (CD 49d), HPCA-2 (CD 34) (BECTON DICKINSON, San Jose, CA), PECAM-1 (CD 31), HLA-class1 (HLA-ABC) and HLA-class 2 (HLA-DR) (DAKO, Carpinteria, CA). The slides are covered with the primary antibody for one hour. Mouse IgG (VECTOR, Burlingame, CA) is the control primary antibody; it is incubated for one hour with biotinylated horse-anti-mouse IgG (VECTOR, Burlingame, CA). Cells and sections are washed in Tris-saline for 3 minutes 3 times each. 0.1% Tween-20 is added in buffer after incubation with the primary and secondary antibodies. 0.3% hydrogen peroxide is used for 15 minutes to block endogenous peroxidase activity. Following a wash in Tris-saline buffer 3 times for 5 minutes each time, the cells and the sections are covered with ABC reagent (DAKO, Carpinteria, CA) and incubated for 45 minutes. After rinsing with Tris-saline, cells and sections are developed in DAB (3'3 diaminobenzine) reagent (KPL, Gaithersburg, MD) and washed in distilled water for 5 minutes. Following alcohol dehydration (70%-80%-95%-100%), counterstaining is done with 1% methyl green for 2-4 minutes. Coverslips and slides are mounted with aquamount.

RESULTS

We reviewed 6 human cadaver eyes (age range 50-81) and 3 human cadaver glaucoma eyes, 3 human glaucomatous trabeculectomy specimens (age range 49 - 86) and 3 bovine eyes. We examined 8-24 sections per eye per stain. With regard to TM cells in culture, we reviewed 3 human and 2 bovine cell lines, examining 4 coverslips per stain. The results are summarized in TABLE 1.

One fascinating finding was that some CAMs, such as HLA-1 and VCAM-1, show staining that extends from the TM toward the corneal endothelium, *staining Schwalbe's line*, but not staining the corneal endothelium. This indicates that the Schwalbe's line cells are expressing different CAMs than corneal endothelium, and perhaps may represent a pluripotential cell line, as suggested by other investigators.

TABLE 1: EXPRESSION OF CAMs IN HUMAN AND BOVINE TM SECTIONS.

Antibody	Tissue	TM	Schlemm's Canal	Sclera		Cornea	
				Fibro	Vessel	Epi	Endo
LFA-1a	H	-	-	-	-	-	-
	B	-		-	-	-	-
LFA-1b	H	-	-	-	-	-	-
	B	-		-	-	-	-
ICAM-1	H	+	+	-	+	++	+/-
	B	+		-	-	+	+/-
VCAM-1	H	+	+	-	-	+	-
	B	+		-	-	+	-
N-CAM-16	H	+++	+++	-	-	++	+
	B	+++		-	-	++	+/-
N-Cadherin	H	-	-	-	-	-	-
	B	-		-	-	-	-
ELAM-1	H	-	-	-	-	-	-
	B	-		-	-	-	-
GMP-140	H	-	-	-	-	-	-
	B	-		-	-	-	-
Integrin-a2	H	-	-	-	-	++	+/-
	B	-		-	-	+	+/-
Integrin-a3	H	++	++	-	+	++	+/-
	B	+		-	-	+	+/-
Integrin-a4	H	-	-	-	-	+	-
	B	-		-	-	+	-
HPCA-2	H	-	+	++	+	+	-
	B	-		-	-	+	-
PECAM-1	H	-	+	-	+	-	-
	B	-		-	-	-	-
HLA-1	H	++	+++	+	+	+++	-
	B	+		+	+	++	-
HLA-2	H	-	+	-	+	-	-
	B	-		-	+/-	-	-

H: human   (+++) intense (++) moderate (+) light (+/-) trace (-) negative
B: bovine

DISCUSSION

We found that CAMs were expressed differently by the various cell types in the outflow pathway and hypothesize that they may play a role in determining outflow facility. Previous work in this laboratory suggests that CAMs may be involved in the increase in resistance to outflow in leukemic glaucoma.[16] It seems likely from the work of Whitcup and others that CAMs play a role in the development of uveitis[7,10,11] and from our laboratory that they may be involved in white cell related glaucomas, such as inflammatory and leukemic glaucomas. Even if CAMs have no role in outflow facility under normal circumstances, modification of CAM expression or function may provide a means by which outflow facility could be modulated, perhaps providing a new avenue for glaucoma treatment.

We showed similar staining in tissue and cell culture comparing human and bovine samples; bovine specimens may be useful in future investigations of outflow pathway CAM expression and its modulation.

Finally, our work with CAM staining revealed differences between cell types in the outflow system not revealed with other staining techniques. Future investigators may utilize this differential CAM staining in order to distinguish between cell types in tissue section and in cell culture.

REFERENCES

1. Bill A, The drainage of aqueous humor. Invest. Ophthalmol. Vis. Sci. 1975 14: 1-3.
2. Polansky JR,Wood I, Maglio MT, Alvarado JA. Trabecular meshwork cell culture in glaucoma research: Evaluation of biological activity and structural properties of human trabecular cells in vitro. Ophthalmol. 1984 91: 580-595.
3. Elner VM, Elner SG, Pavilack MA, et. al. Intercellular adhesion molecule-1 in human corneal endothelium modulation and function. Amer. J. Pathol. 1991 138: 525-535.
4. Pavilack MA, Elner VM, Elner SG, et. al. Differential expression of human corneal and perilimbal ICAM-1 by inflammatory cytokines. Invest. Ophthalmol. Vis. Sci. 1992 33: 564-573.
5. Kaminska GM, Niederkorn JY, and McCulley JP. Intercellular adhesion molecule-1(ICAM) expression in normal and inflamed human cornea: Induction by recombinant interferon gamma and interleukin-1. Invest. Ophthalmol. Vis. Sci. 1991 suppl. 32: 51-23.
6. Wakefield D, McCluskey and Palladinetti P. Distribution of lymphocytes and cell adhesion molecules in iris biopsy specimens from patients with uveitis. Arch. Ophthalmol 1992 110: 121-125.
7. Whitcup SM, Chan CC, LI Q, Nussenblatt RB. Expression of cell adhesion molecules in posterior uveitis. Arch. Ophthalmol 1992 110: 662-666.
8. Klett ZG, Elner SG, Pavilack MA, et. al. Expression of intercellular adhesion molecule-1 (ICAM) by human trabecular meshwork cells. Invest. Ophthalmol. Vis. Sci. 1992 suppl. 33: 2377-52.
9. Lynch MG, Peeler JS, Brown RH and Niederkorn JY. Expression of HLA class I and II antigens on cells of the human trabecular meshwork. 1987 94: 851-857.
10. Whitcup SM, DeBarge R, Rosen H, et. al. Monoclonal antibody against CD11b/CD18 Inhibits endotoxin-induced uveitis. Invest. Ophthalmol. Vis. Sci. 1993 34 673-681.
11. Whitcup SM, DeBarge R, Caspi RR, et. al. Monoclonal antibody against ICAM-1 (CD54) and LFA-1 (CD11a/CD18)Inhibits experimental autoimmune uveitis. Clin. Immun. & Immunopath. 1993 67: 143-150.
12. Alvarado JA, Wood I, and Polansky JR. Human trabecular cells II. Growth pattern and ultrastructural characteristics. Invest. Ophthalmol. Vis. Sci. 1982 23: 464-478.
13. Tripathi RC, Tripathi BJ. Human trabecular Endothelium, corneal endothelium, keratocytes, and scleral fibroblasts in primary cell culture. A comparative study of growth characteristics, morphology, and phagocytic activity by light and scanning electron microscopy. Exp. Eye Res. 1982 35: 611-624.
14. Southern AL, Gordon GG, Munnangi PR, et al Altered cortisol metabolism in cells cultured from trabecular meshwork specimens obtained from patients with primary open-angle glaucoma.Invest. ophthalmol. Vis. Sci. 1983 24: 1413-1417.
15. Yue BYJT, Kurosawa A, Elvart JL, et. al. Monkey trabecular meshwork cell in culture: growth, morphologic, and biochemical characteristics. Graefe's Arch. Clin. Exp. Opthalmol. 1988 226: 262-268.
16. Wang N, Schuman JS, Woods WJ, Yang H, Eisenberg DL: Observations on the Effects of Outflow Facility of Leukemic Cells. *Investigative Ophthalmology and Visual Science* 1993 (ARVO suppl); 34:3369.

Advances in Ocular Immunology
R.B. Nussenblatt, S.M. Whitcup, R.R. Caspi and I. Gery, eds.

Immunohistochemical Localization of Platelet-Endothelial Cell Adhesion Molecule-1 in Rat Eyes

J. Zhang[a], V.K. Kalra[b,] G.S. Wu[a], and N.A. Rao[a]

[a]Doheny Eye Institute and Departments of Ophthalmology and

[b]Biochemistry, University of Southern California School of Medicine, Los Angeles, California 90033, USAA

INTRODUCTION

Platelet endothelial cell adhesion molecule-1 (PECAM-1), also known as CD31 or endoCAM, is a 130 kDa transmembrane glycoprotein [1-3]. It is expressed on the surface of endothelial cells at intercellular junctions, and to a lesser extent on the surface of platelets and leukocytes [1-3]. Known functions of PECAM-1 include initiation of endothelial cell contact, and transmigration of neutrophils and monocytes across vascular endothelium during acute inflammation [4,5]. Constitutive or inducible expression of PECAM-1 in vascular endothelium of the eye, and its role in induction/amplification of uveitis have not been elucidated.

Retinal pigment epithelium (RPE), in addition to its phagocytic capability, is known to mediate some functions that are proinflammatory. For example, cultured RPE cells express MHC class II molecules [6] and present antigen to sensitized T-cells following stimulation [7]. RPE cells also express adhesion molecules (CD54 and ICAM-1) and release cytokines, including IL-1, IL-6 and IL-8 [8,9]. The present study was designed to study the expression of PECAM-1 in the eye, more specifically in the RPE, in association with experimental uveitis.

MATERIALS AND METHODS

Uveitis was induced in Lewis rats by foot-pad injection of 60 μg of S-antigen in complete Freund's adjuvant. On day 17 postimmunization, these animals and a group of normal control rats were killed, and eyes enucleated and snap frozen. Frozen sections (7 μ thickness) of the globes were used for immunohistochemistry. The primary antibody (1:10 dilution) used was mouse monoclonal antibody directed to bovine PECAM-1 [1-2]. A biotinylated goat anti-mouse IgG was used as the secondary antibody; this was preabsorbed with normal rat serum to eliminate cross-reaction with rat IgG. The avidin-biotin-complex method was used to detect a positive reaction. Similar immunohistochemical studies were carried out using cultured mouse RPE cells. Mouse RPE culture was obtained according to the published procedure [10]. For controls, sections were processed similarly except that phosphate buffered saline was used in place of the primary antibody.

RESULTS

In normal rat eyes, positive staining was noted in the vasculature of the retina, choroid and uvea, primarily along the abluminal surface of the endothelium. There was intense staining of the RPE from inflamed (S-antigen-induced uveitis) and non-inflamed (control) eyes of the Lewis rats and in cultured mouse RPE cells. There was no obvious difference in the staining intensity or pattern between inflamed and non-inflamed eyes. In the inflamed eyes, however, some of the inflammatory cells, including lymphocytes and neutrophils, were also positively stained.

DISCUSSION

Our results show that relatively high levels of constitutive PECAM-1 are expressed on the RPE and endothelium of normal eyes. This positive staining appears to be selective, as it is limited to only these two cell types. In the inflamed eyes with experimental uveitis, positive staining was noted also on the inflammatory cells, but there was no up-regulation of PECAM-1 on the RPE or endothelium. These results are consistent with those of other investigators who reported recently that PECAM-1 is expressed constitutively on endothelium [3], and that the expression of PECAM-1 on leukocytes is not altered significantly following activation [11].

The role of PECAM-1 in transendothelial migration of leukocytes has been well established [4,]. The PECAM-1 mediated interactions of these two types of cells include 1) expression of PECAM-1 on the surface of both leukocytes and endothelial cells, and alignment of the two types of cells to effect adhesion; and 2) the concentration of PECAM-1 expressed at the junction increases from luminal to abluminal surface in preparation for transendothelial migration [4]. The functional expression of PECAM-1 in RPE, however, is more difficult to delineate. RPE cells are thought to play pivotal role in inflammation, and cultured RPE cells do express adhesion molecule CD54 and intercellular adhesion molecule-1, which are important in leukocyte trafficking [8]. PECAM-1 could also belong to this category of molecule, the sole function being mediation of adhesion and migration of inflammatory cells across RPE monolayers. The absence of up-regulation of PECAM-1 in uveitis, as seen in the present study, could be due partly to a complex interplay between various soluble factors and cytokines generated by the RPE [8,9].

CONCLUSIONS

1) PECAM-1 is expressed constitutively in the RPE on the abluminal surface of retinal and choroidal vasculature.

2) PECAM-1 in RPE may function as an adhesion molecule and may be required for transmigration of leukocytes, as is the case in endothelium.

3) The surface expression of PECAM-1 in the RPE and endothelium is not up-regulated in experimental uveitis; this could be due to a complex interplay between various RPE cytokines and soluble factors.

REFERENCES

1   Jaffe S, Oliver PD, Farooqui SM, Novak PL et al. Biochim Biophys Acta 1987; 898:37-52.
2   Kalra VK, Banerjee R, Sorgente N. Biotech Appl Biochem 1990;12:579-585.
3   Delisser HM, Newman PJ, Albelda SM. Curr Top Microbiol Immunol 1993;184:37-45.
4   Muller WA, Weigl SA, Deng X, Phillips DM. J Exp Med 1993;178:449-460.
5   Vaporciyan AA, Delissr HM, Yan HC, Mendiguren II et al. Science 1993;262:1580-1582.
6   Detrick B, Newsome DA, Percopo CM, Hooks JJ. Clin Immunol Immunopathol 1985;36:201-211.
7   Percopo CM, Hooks JJ, Shinohara T, Caspi R, et al. J Immunol 1990;145:4101-4107.
8   Elner SG, Elner VM, Pavilack MA, Todd RF, et al. Lab Invest 1992;66:200-211.
9   Planck SR, Dang TT, Graves D, Tara D, Ansel JC, Rosenbaum JT. Invest Ophthalmol Vis Sci 1992;33:78-82.
10 Mayerson PL, Hall MO, Clark V, Abrams T. Invest Ophthalmol Vis Sci 1985;26:1599-1609.
11 Torimoto Y, Rothstein DM, Dang NH , Schlossman SF et al. J Immunol 1992;148:388-396.

Advances in Ocular Immunology
R.B. Nussenblatt, S.M. Whitcup, R.R. Caspi and I. Gery, eds.

TH1 AND TH2 LYMPHOCYTES IN EXPERIMENTAL AUTOIMMUNE UVEORETINITIS.

RACHEL R. CASPI.
National Eye Institute, NIH, Bethesda, MD 20892, USA.

Introduction

Experimental autoimmune uveoretinitis (EAU) is mediated by CD4+ T cells. Distinct subsets of CD4+ T cells can be distinguished on the basis of the lymphokines they secrete. It is thought that uncommitted T cells (Th0) secreting a mixed lymphokine profile can differentiate along one of two pathways: Th1 cells that secrete IL-2, IFNg and lymphotoxin, and mediate delayed hypersensitivity, or Th2 cells that secrete IL-4, IL-10, IL-5 and IL-6, and are involved in immediate hypersensitivity. Responses of these two T cell subsets are antagonistic, and it is believed that they regulate each other in vivo to maintain a balanced immune response (1-3). Both subsets have been implicated in different forms of autoimmunity. Our group has been studying cellular mechanisms involved in ocular autoimmune disease using the model of experimental autoimmune uveoretinitis (EAU) induced with retinal antigens, or with retinal antigen-specific T cell lines, in mice and in rats. The uveitogenic proteins used in this study are interphotoreceptor retinoid binding protein (IRBP), the retinal soluble antigen (S-Ag), and their pathogenic peptides. This report will briefly review our current notions concerning the possible role of Th1 and Th2 cells in EAU.

Lymphokine profile of uveitogenic T cells in vitro and in vivo

Uveitogenic long-term T cell lines isolated from Lewis rats primed with retinal antigens appear to be primarily of the Th1 phenotype, in that they characteristically secrete high amounts of IL-2 and IFNγ (4, 5 and Savion et al, submitted). IL-4 production could not be detected using the mouse IL-4-responsive CT.4S line. In contrast, uveitogenic T cell lines of mice secrete a mixed lymphokine profile. The lymphokines secreted by a uveitogenic T cell line specific to bovine IRBP derived from B10.A mice, and by a uveitogenic line specific to peptide 161-180 of human IRBP derived from B10.RIII mice, included IL-2, IL-4, IL-5, IL-10, IFNγ and TNFα (6 and Rizzo et al, in preparation). Thus, these lines appear to be of the Th0 phenotype, or possibly a mixture of Th1 and Th2. A clone that was isolated from the anti-IRBP B10.A line exhibited the same unrestricted lymphokine profile, suggesting that at least some Th0 cells were present in the parent line.

Despite the fact that murine uveitogenic T cell lines exhibit a mixed lymphokine profile in vitro, only Th1-specific lymphokine mRNA's could be identified in retinas of mice in which EAU was induced by an adoptive transfer of these cells (7). The mice were extensively perfused through the carotid artery with a physiological solution to flush out lymphocytes present in retinal vasculature. Reverse transcriptase-polymerase chain reaction (RT-PCR) analysis of RNA isolated from the retinas 11 days after cell transfer (soon after onset of disease) revealed the presence of IL-2 and IFNγ mRNA, but not IL-4 or IL-10 mRNA. Assuming that the mRNA's detected originated from the transferred cells, it is unclear whether this might reflect a differentiation event from a non-Th1 to a Th1 type cell, or a selective entry of Th1 cells into the eye. The observation that such a lymphokine profile restriction also occurred following transfer of the uveitogenic clone described above would tend to support the former possibility.

Kinetics of expression of lymphokine mRNA in the uveitic mouse retina: early expression of Th1-type and late expression of Th2-type lymphokines

Rizzo et al. performed a time-course study of lymphokine mRNA's expressed during the development and resolution of EAU in mice that were actively immunized with IRBP (7). The results showed that retinas harvested 14 and 21 days after immunization expressed abundant amounts of IL-2 and IFNγ mRNA. In contrast, retinas collected 28 and 35 days after immunization expressed high amounts of mRNA for IL-4 and IL-10. Thus, acute-stage disease was correlated with presence of elevated Th1-type lymphokine mRNA's, whereas the resolution stage was associated with Th2-type mRNA's.

We asked the question whether the emergence of a Th2-type response during the resolution phase of EAU merely reflected a temporal association, or whether it could be indicative of a role for these cells in the downregulation of the disease. We addressed this question by treating IRBP-immunized mice with IL-10 or with a combination of IL-10 + IL-4 during the first 5 days after immunization, with the purpose of skewing the developing immune response towards the Th2 pathway (2, 3). EAU was suppressed in animals receiving the IL-10 treatment, and the combination of IL-10 and IL-4 was even more potent than IL-10 alone in preventing disease development (Stiff et al., in preparation). It is unlikely that the injected Th2-type lymphokines directly suppressed the expression stage of EAU, because their short half-life in the circulation would largely exclude the possibility of significant levels remaining until the onset of disease, over a week later. Rather, it is likely that the treatment enhanced differentiation of Th2-type cells, which subsequently suppressed the development of disease. In either case, the results are compatible with an interpretation that a Th2 response would be conducive to a state of resistance against EAU.

Peyer's Patch cells of mice protected from EAU by oral tolerance to IRBP produce Th2-type lymphokines

Additional support for the hypothesis that a Th2-type response contributes to disease suppression was obtained in studies of protection from EAU by induction of oral tolerance. Feeding of the eliciting autoantigen before and/or after immunization has been used to suppress a variety of experimental autoimmune diseases. Evidence from numerous studies, that cannot be discussed here due to space considerations, has led to the conclusion that protection from autoimmune disease can be achieved through anergy of the autopathogenic lymphocytes, or through active suppression mediated by regulatory cells that are elicited by the tolerogenic regimen (8, 9). We have recently shown that three feedings of 0.2 mg IRBP each are not sufficient to induce protection from EAU, however, an appropriately timed treatment with as little as 1000 U of IL-2, converted the nonprotective feeding regimen to a protective one. Peyer's Patch cells of protected mice produced IL-4, IL-10 and TGFβ, whereas Peyer's Patch cells of unprotected mice produced low or undetectable quantities of these cytokines (10 and Rizzo et al., these Proceedings). Thus, protection from EAU induced by this regimen of oral tolerance was associated with production of Th2-type cytokines. These results suggest that a Th2-type regulatory cell may be involved in suppression of EAU.

Genetic susceptibility to EAU in the Lewis rat is correlated with an elevated interferon-gamma response

Finally, we asked the question whether a genetic predisposition to mount a Th1-dominated immune response might underlie susceptibility to EAU, and conversely, whether a predisposition to mount a Th2-dominated response might underlie genetic resistance to EAU. This question was addressed by comparing the responses of the Lewis and Fischer 344 (F344) rat strains. These two strains are MHC class II-identical, and consequently recognize the same epitopes in a uveitogenic molecule. However, the Lewis strain is susceptible to EAU induced by S-Ag, IRBP, or their peptides, whereas the F344 is relatively resistant (11). Interestingly, lymph node cells of Lewis and F344 rats that had been immunized with the R16 peptide of IRBP proliferated similarly in vitro to the peptide, indicating that equivalent numbers of primed lymphocytes were being generated by both strains. However, the lymph node cells of Lewis efficiently transferred EAU to naive syngeneic recipients, whereas those of the F344 did not. Analysis of lymphokines produced by these cells in response to antigenic stimulation revealed that the Lewis cells produced at least three times more IFNγ than did F344 cells (as evaluated by ELISA and by RT-PCR), whereas the IL-10 response (by PCR) was of similar magnitude in both (Caspi et al, in preparation). This result supports the hypothesis that a genetic propensity to develop a Th1-dominated response is correlated with susceptibility to uveitis. Experiments in known EAU-susceptible and EAU-resistant strains of mice (12) are currently being carried out to further test the validity of this hypothesis.

Conclusions

Taken together, the data summarized above point to the conclusion that the pathogenic cells in EAU are of the Th1 phenotype, whereas Th2-type lymphocytes might serve as regulatory cells capable of conferring protection from disease. Thus, a directed enhancement of the Th2 arm of the immune response may represent a viable strategy for immunotherapy of ocular autoimmune disease.

References

1. Romagnani S. *Int J Clin Lab Res* 1991; 21:152-8.

2. Hsieh CS, Heimberger AB, Gold JS, O'Garra A, Murphy KM. *Proc Natl Acad Sci U S A* 1992; 89:6065-9.

3. Powrie F, Menon S, Coffman RL. *Eur J Immunol* 1993; 23:3043-9.

4. Caspi RR, Roberge FG. *J Autoimmun* 1989; 2:709-722.

5. Savion S, Grover S, Kawano Y, Caspi RR. *Invest Ophthalmol Vis Sci* 1992; 33(Suppl.):932 (Abstract).

6. Rizzo LV, Silver PB, Hakim F, Chan CC, Wiggert B, Caspi RR. *Invest Ophthalmol Vis Sci* 1993; 34(suppl.):1143.

7. Rizzo LV, Silver PB, Gazzinelli RT, Chan CC, Wiggert B, Caspi RR. *Invest Ophthalmol Vis Sci* 1994; 35(suppl.):1862.

8. Friedman A, Weiner HL. *Proc Natl Acad Sci* 1994; (in press).

9. Gregerson DS, Obritsch WF, Donoso LA. *J Immunol* 1993; 151:5751-61.

10. Rizzo LV, Miller-Rivero NE, Chan CC, Wiggert B, Nussenblatt RB, Caspi RR. *J Clin Invest* 1994; (in press).

11. Caspi RR, Chan C-C, Fujino Y, Oddo S, Najafian F, S. Bahmanyar, Heremans H, Wilder RL, B.Wiggert. *Curr Eye Res* 1992; 11(Suppl.):81-86.

12. Caspi RR, Roberge FG, Chan CC, Wiggert B, Chader GJ, Rozenszajn LA, Lando Z, Nussenblatt RB. *J Immunol* 1988; 140:1490-1495.

© 1994 Elsevier Science B.V. All rights reserved.
Advances in Ocular Immunology
R.B. Nussenblatt, S.M. Whitcup, R.R. Caspi and I. Gery, eds.

T cell traffic and the pathogenesis of experimental autoimmune uveoretinitis

R. A. Prendergast[a], N. M. Coskuncan[a], D. S. McLeod[a], G. A. Lutty[a], and R. R. Caspi[b]

[a]The Wilmer Institute, Johns Hopkins University, 600 N. Wolfe Street, Baltimore, MD 21287

[b]The National Eye Institute, National Institutes of Health, Bethesda, MD 20892

INTRODUCTION

Experimental autoimmune uveoretinitis (EAU) is a well characterized T cell-mediated autoimmune disease induced by clonally expanded T-helper cells specific for retinal S-antigen. This response induces the rapid development of retinal and uveal inflammation in many species including primates (1,2; reviewed in ref. 3). Recent experiments using cultured antigen- and lectin-expanded S-antigen-specific T cells obtained from Lewis rats with EAU have shown that intravenous syngeneic transfer of fewer than 5×10^5 of these cells will induce destructive inflammation (4). The precise mechanism of T cell-mediated disease is not fully understood. Further, the complete temporal sequence of ocular inflammation, including the ultimate chemotaxis and activation of mononuclear cells, is also unclear. The use of S-antigen-specific T cells marked with a very strong fluorescent cell dye enables us to examine this sequence more directly.

MATERIAL AND METHODS

Lewis male rats, 200-250 g, were treated in accord with the NIH Guidelines for the Use of Experimental Animals.

The SP35 T cell line, specific to peptide 341-360 of human S-antigen (4), was stored in the frozen state at -70°C. The cells were rapidly thawed and incubated in complete medium for 4 hr at 37°, Ficoll separated, washed, and labeled at 25×10^6 cells/tube with the cell-linker dye PKH-26 (Sigma, St. Louis) strictly according to the manufacturer's instructions. 10×10^6 labeled T cells in 0.4 ml HBSS were injected into the dorsal vein of the penis and the animals bled and sacrificed at the times shown in Fig. 1.

The retinas were removed from eyes minutes after death and fixed for 3 days in 4% paraformaldehyde in PBS with 6% sucrose at pH 7.2. After washing, the fixed retinas were digested by the method described by Laver et al (5). The total number of free retinal cells isolated by this technique averaged $12 \times 10^6 \pm 7.5\%$ per retina by Coulter counter analysis. Labeled cells were counted using a standard hemocytometer and epifluorescent Zeiss microscopy and a 16x planapochromatic objective. Ficoll-separated PBLs were counted in a similar fashion.

In separate experiments, retinas were fixed in glutaraldehyde, plastic embedded, sectioned at 1 μ, and stained for light microscopy.

RESULTS AND DISCUSSION

Brightly fluorescent S-antigen-specific T cells were counted at 12 hr and then daily for 5 days post-cell transfer. In Fig. 1, a distinct bimodal curve is shown with the first peak of 150 cells/retina at 24 hr, falling at 48 and 72 hr after cell transfer to 30 cells/retina. A sharp second peak at 96 hr was associated with gross edema and vascular dilatation of retinas taken at this time. No gross or microscopic evidence of disease was present in any eye prior to 96 hr after cell transfer. Thus it is seen that the first peak of S-antigen-specific cells is not associated with concomitant disease. Detectable inflammation begins between 72 and 96 hr (hatched area), with a sharp increase of the injected S-antigen-specific T cells together with a massive increase in host inflammatory cells as demonstrated below. It should be noted that, while the number of labeled T cells in the peripheral blood fell rapidly during the first hour post-injection, they stabilized at approximately 25,000-30,000 labeled cells/ml through the 5-day course of the experiment. Taken together, these data indicate that activated S-antigen-specific T cells enter the retina briskly, peak at 24 hr, and fall over the next 2 days with no evidence of re-entry of S-antigen-specific T cells or inflammation up to this point. However, at 96 hr, the cell numbers increase very rapidly with concurrent inflammation and retinal destruction.

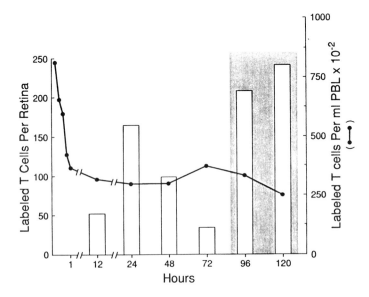

Figure 1

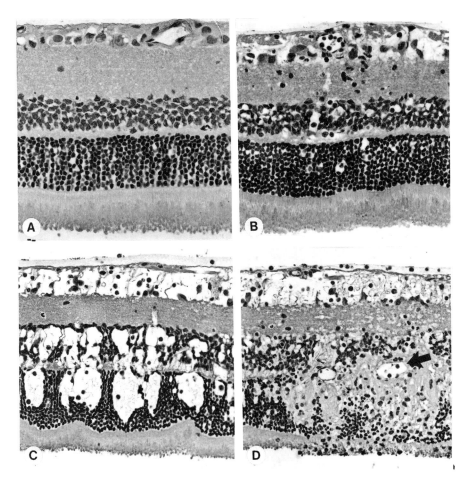

Figure 2 illustrates the temporal sequence of adoptive autoimmune retinal damage in sections from the paracentral retina. The retina is completely normal 48 hr after T cell transfer as shown in Fig. 2A (original magnification 280x). Adhesion and perivascular extravasation of mononuclear cells are seen focally in the edematous nerve fiber layer after 72 hr. Mononuclear cells also penetrate the inner plexiform layer where dilated capillaries penetrate the inner nuclear layer (Fig. 2B; 250x). As inflammation proceeds, both edema and compression of outer nuclear layer elements are prominent (Fig. 2C, 200x). However, it is important to note that the outer photoreceptor layer, the major site of S-antigen concentration, is completely intact at this time. In rats sacrificed after 96 hr, retinal architecture is completely disrupted, most prominently in areas surrounding the outer capillary network (Fig. 2D; 200x). Destruction of both inner and outer nuclear cell layer elements, mononuclear cell infiltrate, and loss of capillary endothelium (arrow) are shown. At this time, the outer photoreceptor layer is involved in the spreading inflammatory process with loss of photoreceptor elements. Large numbers of mononuclear phagocytes are present within the damaged portions of this layer.

The ability to identify and enumerate each injected S-antigen-specific T cell in the entire extravascular disaggregated retinal cell population clarifies certain aspects of this autoimmune model. There is no evidence of any blood-retinal barrier to antigen-activated T cells which rapidly enter retinal tissue. This is seen to be the case using Con A-stimulated syngeneic normal Lewis spleen cells as well (data not shown). Similar results have been demonstrated in models of EAE (6).

Two points are of particular interest in this model of autoimmune ocular disease. The first is the delay in the entry of nonspecific inflammatory cells until 72 hr after S-antigen-specific T cell transfer. Adoptive immunization for both cutaneous DTH responses or for non-ocular autoimmune-induced pathology occurs within 24 hr after cell transfer (7). On the basis of the retinal pathology we describe and evaluation of retinal cell markers, we propose that the delay in mononuclear cell accumulation after T cell transfer is due to the initial lack of class II molecules at the cell surfaces of the presumed antigen-presenting cells (APC). These might include Müller cells, microglia, or vascular endothelial cells. The second area is the delay in inflammation seen at the outer photoreceptor layer, i.e., the sites where S-antigen is in greatest concentration. This occurs only late in the course of retinal pathology. It is likely that APC are not adjacent to the photoreceptor outer segments. Antigen presentation requires a functional and intact class II MHC-peptide complex for effective interaction with T helper cells. Responding T cells then generate and secrete appropriate cytokines which chemotactically attract nonspecific host inflammatory cells and induce adhesion molecules on vascular endothelial cells (8). Future experiments will test this hypothesis.

REFERENCES

1   Wacker WB, Donoso LA, Kalsow CM, et al. J Immunol 1977; 119: 1949-1958.
2   Nussenblatt RB, Kuwabara T, de Monasterio F, Wacker WB. Arch Ophthalmol 1981; 99: 1090-1092.
3   Caspi RR. In: Lightman S, ed. Immunology of Eye Diseases. Dordrecht: Klewer, 1989; 61-86.
4   Beraud E, Kotake S, Caspi RR, et al. Cell Immunol 1992; 140: 112-122.
5   Laver NM, Robison WG, Pfeffer BA. Invest Ophthalmol Vis Sci 1993; 34: 2097-2104.
6   Hickey WF, Hsu BL, Kimura H. J Neurosci Res 1991; 28: 254-260.
7   Werdlin O, McCluskey RT. J Exp Med 1971; 133: 1242-1263.
8   Springer TA. Cell 1994; 76: 301-314.

Advances in Ocular Immunology
R.B. Nussenblatt, S.M. Whitcup, R.R. Caspi and I. Gery, eds.

Diverse lymphocyte responses to determinants of human S-antigen (HS-Ag) in uveitic monkeys and normal humans indicate a lack of shared immunodominant epitopes

A. Fukushima[1], J.C. Lai[1,2], J. Shiloach[3], S.M. Whitcup[1], I. Gery[1] and R.B. Nussenblatt[1].

[1]NEI and [3]NIDDK, NIH, Bethesda, MD, USA and [2]Howard Hughes Medical Institute

INTRODUCTION

Cellular immune responses against whole proteins are targeted at selected (immunodominant) peptide determinants of these molecules (1). Lymphocytes from rats of different MHC backgrounds which were immunized with recombinant HS-Ag (rHS-Ag) responded to selected peptides localized to three areas of the rHS-Ag molecule (2). In contrast, lymphocytic responses of uveitis patients to determinants of human S-antigen have been diverse, with no specific peptides being identified as immunodominant epitopes (3). In this study, we identified the peptides of HS-Ag that are selected as the dominant epitopes by monkeys that developed uveitis following immunization with rHS-Ag. The monkey lymphocyte responses were compared to those of two normal human donors.

MATERIALS AND METHODS

Antigens
Recombinant human S-Ag was prepared as described in reference (4). Forty overlapping 20-mer peptides spanning the entire HSAg sequence (3) were used to identify immunodominant epitopes by their capacity to stimulate lymphocytes.

Monkeys
One male stump tailed macaque (monkey #1) and one female rhesus (monkey #2) were obtained from NIH approved random sources. Both monkeys received a preliminary fundoscopic exam prior to immunization. The nutritional status of the animals was monitored throughout the course of the study. This study was approved by the institutional Animal Care and Use Committee and complies with Public Health Service Policy on Humane Care and Use of Laboratory Animals.

Human Subjects
Blood was collected from two normal male volunteers, ages 23 and 61 years.

Immunization
Both monkeys were immunized by subcutaneous injections at 4-6 sites in the nape of the neck with recombinant H-S-Ag emulsified (1:1) in complete Freund's adjuvant at the dose of 40 ug S-antigen / kg body weight. Both monkeys developed uveitis approximately 40 days after immunization. The monkeys were

64

euthanized by sodium pentobarbital overdose on days 80 and 70 post-immunization, respectively.

Cellular Proliferation Assay
For both monkey and human assays, peripheral blood lymphocytes were isolated on an Isolymph gradient and cultured as described in reference (5). The data recorded here were obtained with peptides at a concentration 100 ug/ml .

RESULTS

The lymphocyte responses of the two monkeys are shown in Figures 1 and 2. Both animals showed strong responses against some of the peptides, with S.I. as high as 20. Interestingly, different peptides produced high responses. Stimulation indices > 10 were found against peptides 25, 36 and 37 in monkey #1 (Fig. 1) and against peptides 3, 4, 9, 10, 12 and 21 in monkey #2 (Fig. 2).

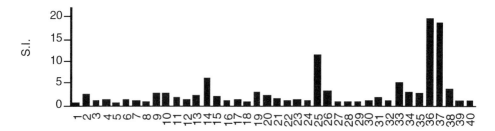

Figure 1

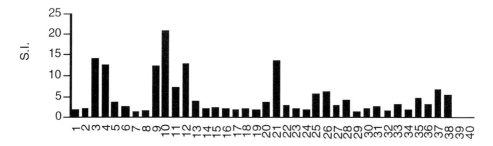

Figure 2

Figs. 1 and 2: Lymphocytic proliferative responses against peptide fragments for monkeys. (SI= mean cpm in cultures with antigen /mean cpm in control cultures without stimulant)

The responses of the two human donors are shown in Figures 3 and 4. These responses were in general lower than those of the immunized and diseased monkeys, with donor #1 showing higher proliferative responses than donor #2. (Please note that different scales were used for the S.I. values in the two figures). Although different patterns of response to the peptides were demonstrated by the two donors, it is noteworthy that both of them responded substantially to peptides 8, 13, and 18.

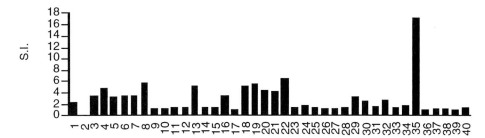

Figure 3

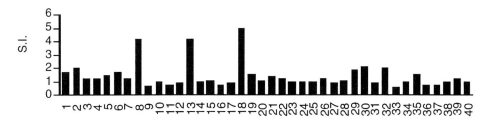

Figure 4

Figs. 3 and 4: Lymphocytic proliferative responses against peptide fragments for humans

DISCUSSION

The present study is the first to report on the immune responses of monkeys immunized with rHS-Ag. It is also of interest that the monkeys developed severe uveitis following immunization with rHS-Ag, an antigen that presumably is highly homologous to the autologous protein.

The analysis of the lymphocyte responses of the two monkeys shows a remarkable level of diversity between the two animals; different peptide determinants were selected by each of the monkeys as the dominant epitopes (Fig. 1 and 2). The differences are attributed to the different MHC backgrounds of the monkeys. Interestingly though, studies have demonstrated the existence of immunodominant epitopes in myelin basic protein that are targets for lymphocyte response in the majority of patients with a different T-cell mediated autoimmune disease, multiple sclerosis (6). The data with the human blood samples showed low but significant lymphocyte responses to selected peptides, suggesting an incomplete thymic deletion of autoreactive T cells. More donors are to be tested in order to examine whether certain peptides of human S-Ag are recognized by a significant group of apparently normal individuals.

CONCLUSIONS

Recombinant H-S-Ag is uveitogenic and immunogenic in primates. However, no common immunodominant peptides were found in uveitic monkeys of different genetic backgrounds. T cell populations capable of recognizing HS-Ag were also present in nonuveitic humans. Susceptibility of humans to uveitis may be determined by the varying reactivities of these T cell populations to uveitogenic antigens.

REFERENCES

1   Sercarz EE, Lehmann PV, Ametani A, Benichour G, et al. Annu Rev Immunol. 1993; 11:729.

2   Chanaud III NP, Shiloach J, Hafler DA, Egwuagu CE, et al. Invest Ophthalmol Vis Sci. 1994; 35 (Suppl):1864.

3   de Smet MD, Wiggert B, Chader GJ, Mochizuki M, et al. Ocular Immunology Today 1990; 285.

4   Oettinger HF, Sabbagh AA, Jingwu Z, LaSalle JM, et al. J Neuroimmunol 44:157.

5   Hirose S, Wiggert B, Redmond TM, Kuwabara T, et al. Exp. Eye Res 1987; 45:695.

6   Ota K, Matsui M, Milford EL,Mackin GA, Weiner HL, Hafler DA. Nature 1990: 346:183.

© 1994 Elsevier Science B.V. All rights reserved.
Advances in Ocular Immunology
R.B. Nussenblatt, S.M. Whitcup, R.R. Caspi and I. Gery, eds.

Nucleotide Sequences Homologous to Retinal S-Antigen in the Rat Thymus Lack a Known EAU Inducing Epitope

Scott W. McPherson and Dale S. Gregerson

Department of Ophthalmology, University of Minnesota, John E. Harris Ophthalmology Research Laboratories, Lion's Research Building, 2001 6th Street S.E., Minneapolis, Minnesota 55455, USA.

Introduction

Rat retinal S-Antigen (S-Ag), a member of the arrestin gene family, is one of several ocular autoantigens that, upon immunization of a susceptible host, can induce the autoimmune disease experimental autoimmune uveoretinitis (EAU) [1]. EAU can also be induced by immunization with S-Ag peptides [2-4] and has been shown to be T cell mediated as evidenced by the fact that naive animals can acquire the disease by transfer of activated CD4+ T cells from immunized animals [5]. Recent studies have described specific S-Ag epitopes responsible for proliferative and/or pathogenic T cell responses [6-8].

In addition to being a model for human uveitis of autoimmune etiology, EAU is also a model for immunological self tolerance. A major mechanism of self tolerance is clonal deletion during thymic maturation of T cells reactive to self antigens. However, the presence of S-Ag reactive T cells in EAU is paradoxical to clonal deletion. In order to resolve this paradox, the thymus of LEW rats was assayed for the expression of S-Ag's and/or arrestins. The nature of the expressed sequences was then analyzed to determine the effect on the T cell repertoire.

Results and Discussion

Expression of arrestins in the thymus

Expression of arrestins in the thymus was assayed by reverse transcriptase-polymerase chain reaction amplification (RT-PCR) of thymus mRNA using mixed (degenerate) oligonucleotide primers (MOP's) corresponding to regions of conserved nucleotide sequence between S-Ag's and other arrestins (Figure 1). Following amplification the products of the reaction were analyzed by Southern [9] blot at high and low stringency using rat S-Ag DNA as the probe. This analysis (Figure 2) revealed that numerous arrestin or arrestin-like sequences were expressed in the thymus. The vast majority of these sequences exhibited only a low or moderate level of relatedness (homology) to S-Ag (65%-80% based on hybridization conditions) and only a few displayed potentially higher levels of relatedness as seen on the high stringency blot.

Rat Retina S-Ag
Position of primers on Rat S-Ag

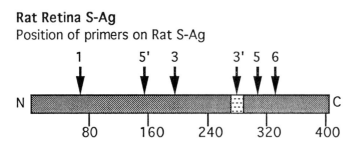

Immunodominant EAU epitope (aa 273-289)

Figure 1. Map of rat retinal S-Ag show the relative position of the MOP's (1,3,5,6) and epitope specific primers (5',3') used in the RT-PCR amplifications. The position of the EAU inducing epitope is indicated.

RT-PCR of Thymus with Arrestin MOP's

Probe: Rat Retina S-Ag DNA

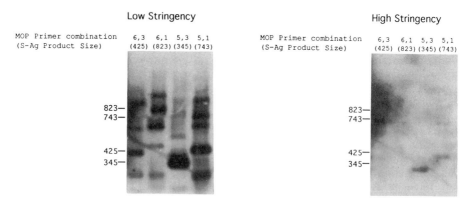

Figure 2. High and low stringency hybridization of rat thymus mRNA RT-PCR amplification products. For reference, the size fragment expected with amplification of retinal mRNA is given.

Sequencing and analysis of arrestins expressed in the thymus
The products of the RT-PCR reaction were randomly cloned into the vector pCRII (Invitrogen, San Diego, CA) and subjected to dideoxy nucleotide [10] sequencing. This analysis indicated the expression in the thymus of the known arrestins rat β arrestin 1 and rat β arrestin 2. This is in agreement with previous studies indicating arrestin expression in peripheral blood leukocytes [11]. Other sequeces related to S-Ag or arrestins were also characterized. These sequences were generally 65% to 75% homologous to one or more members of the arrestin gene family but exhibited the pseudogenic characteristic of occasional termination codons in the reading frame. Cloning and sequence analysis of other arrestin related sequences is continuing.

RT-PCR for S-Ag 273-289 Epitope

Probe: Rat Retina S-Ag DNA, High Stringency

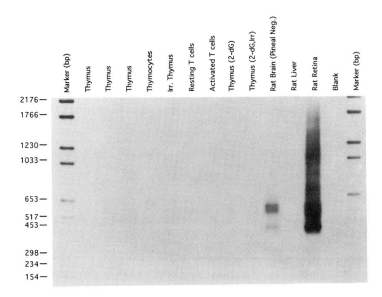

Figure 3. RT-PCR amplification for expression of the S-Ag 273-289 epitope in whole thymus and thymic components. Thymic stroma was prepared by gamma irradiation (Irr) and/or 2-deoxyguanosine (2-dG) treatment of whole thymus.

Analysis for the expression of specific S-Ag epitopes in thymus
A common feature of all the non-photoreceptor arrestin sequences cloned and analyzed was the lack of sequence homology to the primary pathogenic and T cell proliferative epitope of S-Ag (amino acids 273-289).

The presence of T cells of this specificity might be due lack of expression in the thymus of this epitope which, in turn, results in the non-occurrence of clonal deletion. To investigate this possibility the uniqueness of the 273-289 epitope was analyzed and rat thymus was assayed for the expression of this epitope. Computer analysis of GENBANK sequences using TFASTA (Genetics Computer Group, Madison, WI) indicated that the 273-289 epitope sequence was conserved only among S-Ag's. Homology to other arrestins was no greater than to the random sequences that represented the base line level of relatedness as determined by the program's algorithm. Expression of the 273-289 epitope was assayed by RT-PCR using the nucleotide sequence of the epitope as the downstream (3') primer and the nucleotide sequence of S-Ag's amino acids 152-159 as the upstream (5') primer (Figure 1). The sequence of the upstream primer is conserved among S-Ag's but is lacking in other arrestins and is itself a potent T cell proliferative epitope. Whole rat thymus and individual thymic components (lymphocytes or thymic stroma) were assayed. This analysis (Figure 3) revealed no expression of the rat S-Ag epitopes except, as expected, in retina and brain which are the normal sites of S-Ag expression and are immunologically sequestered tissues.

Summary

This study describes the expression of multiple arrestins and arrestin-like sequences in the rat thymus. However, sequence analysis of the expressed arrestins, as well as direct assaying for epitope expression, indicated a lack of expression of a sequence for which there are reactive T cells with that specificity. While multiple arrestin expression in the thymus could drive the clonal deletion of potential arrestin reactive T cells in general, the lack of expression in the thymus of a known epitope (S-Ag 273-289) might account for the presence of pathogenic S-Ag reactive T cells of this specificity.

References

1. Gery, L., et. al. In: Progress in Retinal Research, (Osborne, N. and Chader, J. eds.), Vol. 5. Pergamon Press, New York. 1986. 75-109.
2. Donoso, L.A., et. al. Curr. Eye Res. 1986. 5:995.
3. Gregerson, D.S., et. al. Cell. Immunol. 1990. 128:209.
4. Merryman, C.F., et. al. J. Immunol. 1991. 146:75.
5. Gregerson, D.S., et. al. J. Immunol. 1986. 136:2875.
6. Fling, S.P., et. al. J. Immunol. 1991. 147:483.
7. Fling, S.P., et. al. Cell. Immunol. 1992. 142:275
8. Gregerson, D.S., et. al. Curr. Eye Res. 1992. 11S:67.
9. Southern, E.M. J. Mol. Biol. 1975. 98:503.
10. Sanger, F., et. al. PNAS:USA. 74:5463.
11. Parruti, G. et. al. J. Biol. Chem. 1993. 268:9753

© 1994 Elsevier Science B.V. All rights reserved.
Advances in Ocular Immunology
R.B. Nussenblatt, S.M. Whitcup, R.R. Caspi and I. Gery, eds.

Uveitogenicity and Immunogenicity of IRBP-Derived Peptide in Various Rat Strains

Y. Sasamoto[a], S. Kotake[a], K. Ogasawara[b], K. Onoé[b], B. Wiggert[c], I. Gery[d], and H. Matsuda[a]

[a]Department of Ophthalmology, School of Medicine, and [b]Section of Pathology, Institute of Immunological Science, Hokkaido University, Kita-15, Nishi-7, Kitaku, Sapporo, Hokkaido, 060 Japan

Laboratories of [c]Retinal Cell and Molecular Biology, and [d]Immunology, National Eye Institute, National Institutes of Health, 9000 Rockiville Pike, Bethesda, MD, 20892 USA

INTRODUCTION

Experimental autoimmune uveoretinitis (EAU) is an intraocular inflammation model for certain human endogenous uveitis [1, 2]. EAU can be induced by specific retinal antigen such as interphotoreceptor retinoid-binding protein (IRBP) [2, 3]. IRBP has been sequenced and several determinants of this protein have been identified to be uveitogenic in LEW rats [4, 5]. One of the IRBP-derived determinants, R16 (aa 1177-1191), has strong uveitogenicity in this strain [4]. The present study was aimed at testing the uveitogenicity and immunogenicity of R16 in various strains of rats with different RT1 haplotypes.

MATERIALS AND METHODS

Male rats, 8-10 weeks old, were provided by and maintained at the Institute for Animal Experiments, Hokkaido University School of Medicine. The RT1 haplotypes and allelic specificities of different inbred strains are shown in Table 1 [6]. Rats were immunized with bovine IRBP, or synthetic peptide R16 (aa 1177-1191: ADGSSWEGVGVVPDV) [7, 8]. These antigens were emulsified with equal volume of complete Freund's adjuvant (CFA). *Bordetella pertussis* (10^{10} killed organisms) was injected intravenously concurrently with the immunization. Immunized rats were sacrificed 16-18 days after immunization and the enucleated eyes were examined histologically. The severity of the disease was graded using a scale of 0-4, as described elsewhere [3]. The procedure used for lymphocyte proliferation assay was described in detail elsewhere [9]. Data were recorded as stimulation index (S. I.).

Table 1
RT1 haplotypes and allelic specificities of rat strains used in this study.

Rat	RT1	A	H	B	D
LEW	*l*	*l*	*l*	*l*	*l*
WKAH	*k*	*k*	*k*	*k*	*k*
SDJ	*u*	*u*	*u*	*u*	*u*
BUF	*b*	*b*	*b*	*b*	*b*

RESULTS

The development of EAU in various rat strains immunized with IRBP at 50 µg/rat is summarized in Table 2. Rats of all strains developed EAU. SDJ rats showed mild inflammatory changes, while all other strains (LEW, WKAH, and BUF) developed distinct EAU. Table 3 summarizes the EAU development in rats immunized with R16 peptide at 100 nmol /rat. LEW, WKAH, and BUF rats were also susceptible to EAU induced by the R16. However, quite different susceptibilities were seen among these three strains. Incidence of EAU development was 100 % in LEW, 75 % in WKAH, and 19 % in BUF. Mean histological severities in these susceptible strains were 2.35 in LEW, 1.25 in WKAH, and 0.16 in BUF. SDJ rats showed no EAU development. Lymph node cells from EAU-susceptible rats immunized with R16 showed substantial responses against both R16 peptide and purified protein derivative (PPD) (Table 4). EAU-resistant strain, SDJ, showed no response against R16, while exhibiting significant responses against PPD.

Table 2
IRBP induced EAU in various rat strains.

Rat strain	Total eye	Affected eye	Incidence (%)	Histological severity (mean±S. E.)
LEW	12	12	100	3.83±0.11
WKAH	8	8	100	3.75±0.16
SDJ	8	8	100	1.13±0.13
BUF	8	8	100	3.25±0.25

Table 3
IRBP-derived peptide R16 induced EAU in various rat strains.

Rat strain	Total eye	Affected eye	Incidence (%)	Histological severity (mean±S. E.)
LEW	20	20	100	2.35±0.11
WKAH	16	12	75	1.25±0.16
SDJ	12	0	0	0.00±0.00
BUF	16	3	19	0.16±0.09

Table 4
Lymphocyte proliferation assay in various rat strains immunized with R16

Rat strain	No.	S. I. (mean±S. E.)			
		Concentration of R16 (nmol/ml)			PPD (µg/ml)
		1	10	100	25
LEW	3	4.70±1.08	4.90±1.63	5.17±1.23	15.70±2.57
WKAH	3	2.53±0.29	5.67±1.12	15.30±3.59	16.20±3.78
SDJ	3	1.23±0.23	1.03±0.18	1.27±0.28	8.40±1.17
BUF	3	2.35±0.75	4.10±1.20	5.70±1.70	19.70±4.60

DISCUSSION

The present findings show that all rat strains tested developed remarkable EAU following immunization with IRBP, although these animals carry different RT1 haplotype. This finding supports the postulate that IRBP has several uveitogenic and immunogenic determinants. This broad antigenicity has been thought to be attributable to a number of anchors on IRBP, each of which binds to the specific class II molecule. This hypothesis was supported by other experiments [4, 5, 10]. However, it should be noted that a small synthetic peptide, R16, induced EAU in LEW, WKAH, and BUF. This finding indicates another possibility that R16 can bind to not only class II MHC molecules of LEW, but also those of different RT1 haplotypes. SDJ rats, which showed no EAU development and no lymphocyte proliferation against R16, showed induction of EAU by IRBP, although the EAU was significantly less severe than that seen in other rat strains. Since the response of SDJ against PPD was lowest among the four strains tested, it is considered that SDJ rats are relatively resistant to induction of immunity and diseases.

REFERENCES

1. Wacker WB, Donoso LA, Kalsow CM, Yankeelov JA Jr, et al. J Immunol 1977; 119: 1949-1958.
2. Nussenblatt RB, Palestine AG. Uveitis: Fundamentals and Clinical Practice. Chicago: Year Book Medical Publishers Inc. 1988.
3. Gery I, Wiggert B, Redmond TM, Kuwabara T, et al. Invest Ophthalmol Vis Sci 1986; 27: 1296-1300.
4. Sanui H, Redmond TM, Kotake S, Wiggert B, et al. J Exp Med 1989; 169: 1947-1960.
5. Kotake S, Wiggert B, Redmond TM, Borst DE, et al. Cell Immunol 1990; 126: 331-342.
6. Fujii H, Kakinuma M, Yoshiki T, Natori T. Transplantation 1991; 52: 369-373.
7. Ogasawara K, Wambua PP, Gotohda T, Onoé K. Int Immunol 1990; 2: 219-224.
8. Borst DE, Redmond TM, Elser JE, Gonda MA, et al. J Biol Chem 1989; 264: 1115-1123.
9. Sasamoto Y, Kawano YI, Wiggert B, Chader GJ, et al. Cell Immunol 1993; 152: 286-292.
10. Gery I, Robinson WGJ, Shichi H, El-Saied M, et al. In: O'Connor GR, Chandler JW, eds. Immunology and Immunopathology of the Eye, New York, Masson Publishing, 1985; 242-245.

Advances in Ocular Immunology
R.B. Nussenblatt, S.M. Whitcup, R.R. Caspi and I. Gery, eds.

IDENTIFICATION OF TWO DISTINCT T CELL IMMUNOGENIC DETERMINANT REGIONS IN INTERPHOTORECEPTOR RETINOID-BINDING PROTEIN (IRBP)

M. Takeuchi 1, O. Taguchi 2, J. Sakai 1, T. Kezuka 1, H. Inoue 1, T. Ichikawa 1, T. Takahashi 2, and M. Usui 1.

1 Department of Ophthalmology, Tokyo Medical College Hospital, Tokyo, Japan

2 Aichi Cancer Research Institute, Nagoya, Japan

INTRODUCTION

When the thymus of fetal F344 rats is implanted beneath the renal capsule of BALB/c nude mice (hereafter referred to as TG nude mice), these animals spontaneously develop autoimmune uveoretinitis, with interphotoreceptor retinoid-binding protein (IRBP) as the target antigen (1, 2). IRBP localizes specifically in the retina and the pineal gland (3), and can induce experimental autoimmune uveoretinitis (EAU) in susceptible animals by its immunization (4). Recently, several T cell immunogenic determinants in the IRBP molecule have been identified in Lewis rats (5, 6). We also synthesized several bovine IRBP-derived peptides and found that T cell immunogenic determinants within IRBP in TG nude mice are correspond to the bovine IRBP amino acid residues 1182~1194 (7). This region also shows considerable overlap with the immunogenic determinants for IRBP in the Lewis rat model (which corresponds to the bovine IRBP amino acid sequence 1179~1191) (6). In the present study, we found that the synthetic peptide P518-529, previously identified by us as an immunogenic determinant in Lewis rats (8), clearly stimulated lymphocytes in TG nude mice and also represents a T cell immunogenic determinant in these animals. In addition, we established T cell lines specific to peptides P518-529 and to P1182-1194 in order to study various aspects of these two distinct T cell immunogenic determinants of IRBP. We were able to characterize the Th subsets involved in these peptide-specific T cell lines, and conducted adoptive transfer experiments to compare the relative uveitogenicity of the T cell lines.

MATERIALS and METHODS

1. Animal model
Animals were purchased from Charles River Inc., Hino, Japan. To make TG nude mice, thymus lobes were taken from 15-day-old F344 rat embryos and grafted in pairs under the renal capsules of 4-week-old BALB/c female nu/nu mice (1).

2. IRBP and IRBP-derived synthetic peptides

Table 1 Amino acid sequences of synthetic peptides.

Peptide	Amino acid sequence
P518-529	SHRTATAAEELA
P1182-1194	WEGVGVVPDVAVP

Bovine IRBP was purified as described in detail elsewhere (9). The peptides shown in Table 1 were synthesized with the Applied Biosystems Inc. Model 430A peptide synthesizer, using t-BOC chemistry (10). Their sequences were derived from that of bovine IRBP, as determined and reported by Borst et al (11).

3. Lymphocyte proliferation assay

Spleen cells of TG nude mice were collected 4 to 6 months after thymus grafting. Single-cell suspensions of spleen cells were cultured in triplicate in 96-well flat-bottomed microtiter plates at a density of $5x10^5$ cells/200 ul in RPMI 1640 medium with HEPES, supplemented with 2 mM L-glutamine, 0.1 mM nonessential amino acids, 100 ug/ml streptomycin, 10% fresh fetal calf serum, and $5x10^{-5}$ M 2-mercaptoethanol (conditioned medium). IRBP or individual peptides were added at time zero to the cell cultures. The cultures were then incubated at 37°C in 6% CO_2 for 90 hours, and pulsed with ^{3}H-thymidine (0.5 uCi/10ul/well) 16 hours prior to harvesting.

4. Establishment and maintenance of T cell lines.

T cell lines specific to the synthetic peptides were established from spleen cells of TG nude mice. Single-cell suspensions at a density of $5x10^6$ cells/well were incubated for 7 days (37°C 6% CO_2) with 1 uM of each synthetic peptide in 2 ml of conditioned medium using 24-well culture plates. The cells were then collected, washed three times, and recultured at $1x10^6$ cells/well in 2 ml of conditioned medium with 0.1 uM peptide and syngeneic irradiated spleen cells (1500 rad) at $5x10^6$ cells/well. After incubation for 7 days, 1 ml of supernatant was removed from each well and replaced with 1 ml of conditioned medium enriched with 20 U/ml recombinant IL-2. Following further incubation for 4 days, the cells were collected, washed three times, and recultured at $2x10^5$ cells/ml in 2 ml of conditioned medium with 0.1 uM peptide and $1x10^6$ cells/well of syngeneic irradiated spleen cells. After incubation for 7 days, 1 ml of supernatant was removed from each well and replaced with 1 ml of conditioned medium with 20 U/ml IL-2 and incubated for 4 days. With the cells at $2x10^5$/well and syngeneic irradiated spleen cells at $1x10^6$/well, the cycle of stimulation with peptide (0.1 uM) and expansion with IL-2 was repeated.

5. Cytokine production assay

P518-529 and P1182-1194 specific T cell lines were assayed for IL-2 and IL-4 production. Each cell line was incubated with it specific peptide at a concentration of 1 uM for 48 hours. The supernatants were then removed from each well, and IL-2 and IL-4 dependent cell lines (CTLL-H) were cultured in the supernatants for 24 hours, with a pulse of ^{3}H-thymidine (0.5 uCi/10ul/well) given 6 hours prior to harvesting. Monoclonal antibodies against IL-4 (11B11) were used to assay activity specific for IL-2, while monoclonal antibodies against IL-2 (S4B6) were used to assay activity specific for IL-4.

6. Adoptive transfer of cell lines

Each cell line ($5x10^6$) was injected intraperitoneally into naive recipient BALB/c nude mice after stimulation with Con A for 3 days. Four weeks after injection, the recipients were sacrificed, and the eyes were fixed in Bouin's fixative for histological study.

RESULTS

Figure 1 shows the proliferative response of splenic lymphocytes from TG nude mice when exposed to IRBP or the synthetic peptides shown in Table 1. As expected, the spleen cells of TG nude mice showed a strong proliferative response to IRBP. However in addition, proliferative responses were observed to both P1182-1194 and P518-529, the latter being surprisingly stronger.

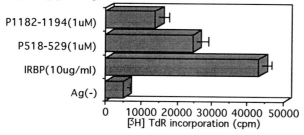

Figure 1. Proliferative responses of splenic lymphocytes to synthetic peptides from TG nude mice with severe uveoretinitis.

We were successful in establishing T cell lines specific for each of the synthetic peptides. As shown in Figure 2, both the P518-529 specific T cell line (Figure 2a) and the P1182-1194 specific T cell line (Figure 2b) elicited proliferative responses to IRBP and each of the synthetic peptides.

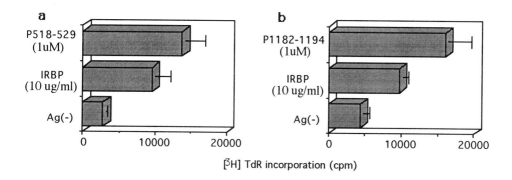

Figure 2. Proliferation responses of P518-529 (a), and P1182-1194 (b) specific T-cell lines against each specific peptides and IRBP.

P518-529 and P1182-1194 specific T cell lines were assayed for IL-2 and IL-4 production. As shown in Table 2, the P518-529 specific T cell line produced only IL-2, while the P1182-1194 specific T cell line produced only IL-4.

5×10^6 cell s from each peptide-specific T cell line were injected intraperitoneally into untreated BALB/c nude mice, and the development of uveoretinitis in these animals was monitored. Uveoretinitis was observed to develop with P518-529 specific T cells but not with P1182-1194 specific T cells.

Table 2 Cytokine production of the peptide-specific T cell lines.

	IL-2 (ng/ml)	IL-4 (ng/ml)
P518-529 specific T cell line	0.86	N.D.
P1182-1194 specific Tcell line	N.D.	0.42

N.D. = These data were not detected.

DISCUSSION

In this paper, we showed that the T cell immunogenic determinant regions of IRBP in TG nude mice lie in the 518~529 amino acid sequence (SHRTATAAEELA) and the 1182~1194 amino acid sequence (WEGVGVVPDVAVP) of bovine IRBP. Although not yet precisely identified, the T cell immunogenic determinant regions of IRBP in TG nude mice appear to be similar to those in Lewis rats. Therefore, it is conceivable that these T cell immunogenic determinant regions of IRBP are not species-dependent, and represent conserved regions of amino acid sequence.

Th1 cells characterized by the secretion of IL-2, IFN-r and TNF-b (12) and Th2 cells characterized by the secretion of IL-4, IL-5, IL-6 and IL-10 (13) are believed to be reciprocally cross-regulated through IFN-r, which inhibits Th2 cells (14), and IL-10, which inhibits Th1 cells (13). It is believed that Th1 cells are responsible for cell-mediated immune reactions (15) while Th2 cells aid in IgE and IgG1 antibody production (16). In our experiments, we found that the P518-529 specific T cell line produced IL-2 and thus consisted of Th1 cells. On the other hand, the P1182-1194-specific T cell line was found to produce IL-4, therefore consisting of Th2 cells. This explains why we were only able to achieve adoptive transfer of uveoretinitis with the P518-529 specific T cell line. We have not excluded the possibility that other immunogenic determinants of IBPB in TG nude mice exist. However, our results suggest that in TG nude mice, T cells reactive to IRBP consist at least of both Th1 cells that are reactive to the amino acid sequence 518-529 and Th2 cells that are reactive to the amino acid sequence 1182-1194.

REFERENCES

1. Taguchi, O., T. Takahashi, M. Seto et al. 1986. J. Exp. Med. 165: 60-71.
2. Ichikawa, T., O. Taguchi, T. Takahashi et al. 1991. Clin. Exp. Immunol. 86: 112.
3. Chader, G. J. 1989. Invest. Ophthalmol. Vis. Sci. 30: 7.
4. Eisenfeld, A. J., A. H. Bunt-Milam, and J. C. Saari. 1987. Exp. Eye Res. 44: 425.
5. Sanui, H., T. M. Redmond, S. Kotake et al. 1989. J. Exp. Med. 169: 1947.
6. Satoshi, K., B. Wiggert, T. M. Redmond et al. 1990. Cell. Immunol. 126: 331
7. Takeuchi, M., O. Taguchi, H. Inoue at el. 1992. Recent Advance in Uveitis: 53
8. Tanaka, T,. H. Inoue, T. Ichikawa et al. 1992. Recent Advance in Uveitis: 57.
9. Redmond, T. M., B. Wiggert, F. A. Robey et al. 1985. Biochemistry 24: 787.
10. Houghtem, R. A. 1985. Proc. Natl. Acad. Sci. USA. 82: 5131.
11. Borst, D. E., T. M. Redmond, J. E. Elser et al. 1989. J, Biol. Chem. 264: 1115
12. Mosmann, T. R. and Coffman, R. L. Adv. Immunol. 1989. 46: 111.
13. Mosmann, T. R. and Moore, K. W. Immunol. Today.1991. 12: A49
14. Gajewski, T.F., and Fitchm, F. W. 1988. 140: 4245
15. Cher, D. J., and Mosmann, T. R. 1987. J. Immunol. 138: 3688
16. Snapper, C. M., Finkelman, F. D. and Paul, W. E. 1988. Immunol. Rev. 1988.

© 1994 Elsevier Science B.V. All rights reserved.
Advances in Ocular Immunology
R.B. Nussenblatt, S.M. Whitcup, R.R. Caspi and I. Gery, eds.

"Uveitogenicity of a polymorphic HLA-class I peptide."
and
"Peripheral T cell response of patients with autoimmune uveitis to a self MHC-peptide."

Gerhild Wildner and Stephan R. Thurau

Section of Immunobiology, University Eye Hospital, Mathildenstr. 8, 80336 München, Germany

Introduction

In endogenous uveitis as with many other autoimmune diseases, correlations with HLA-antigens [1,2] have been found. The immunological mechanism underlying this correlation has not yet been defined.

Cellular responses to peptides in patients

S-Antigen (S-Ag) and S-Ag derived peptides [3] elicit immune responses in uveitis patients [4] and are potent autoantigens in the rat model of experimental autoimmune uveoretinitis (EAU). Sequence homologies between S-Ag- and HLA-peptides are represented by the underlined bold type letters in Table 1. The 14mer peptide B27PD is not only found in HLA-B27, but also in HLA-B51 and various other HLA-B-antigens. In vitro proliferation of PBL from three representative uveitis patients (P1-P3) shows a crossreactivity between the HLA peptide B27PD and the retinal peptide PDSAg (Fig. 1A). Lymphocytes from healthy donors (H1-H2) did not respond to any of these antigens, but did so to the recall antigens PPD and tetanus toxoid (data not shown). The cells of uveitis patients that showed significantly elevated responses to retinal antigens also showed crossreactivity to PDSAg and B27PD. The lymphocytes of patient P1 were obtained immediately before a relapse of disease and, therefore, had the highest reactivity to retinal autoantigens.

In order to test the hypothesis that crossreactivity between HLA- and S-Ag derived peptides is associated with uveitis we performed a series of experiments in the rat model of EAU.

Table 1
Amino acid sequences of retinal S-Ag- and HLA-peptides

Source of peptide	Name	Amino acid sequence	Incidence of uveitis in rat EAU	Comment
S-Ag, 342-355	PDSAg	F **L** G **E** L T **S S** E V **A** T E V	22 / 24 = 92%	acute, severe
HLA-B27, 125-138	B27PD	A **L** N **E** D L **S S** W T **A** A D T	27 / 33 = 82%	mild, relapsing
HLA-B7, 125-138	B7PD	A **L** N **E** D L R **S** W T **A** A D T	0 / 14 = 0%	

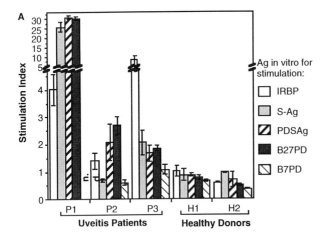

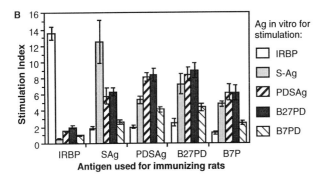

Figure 1. In vitro responses of lymphocytes from uveitis patients (A) and immunized rats (B)
A) Proliferative response of uveitis patients (P1-3) and healthy donors (H1,2) to retinal antigens, peptides and HLA-peptides.
B) Proliferative responses of lymph node cells from groups of 3 to 6 Lewis rats immunized with S-Ag, peptides PDSAg, B27PD and B7PD, and IRBP.

Uveitogenicity and immunogenicity of peptides in EAU

In Lewis rats the S-Ag derived peptide PDSAg was found to be highly uveitogenic (Table 1). Twenty-two out of 24 animals developed an acute, severe form of EAU. A relatively mild, relapsing iritis and chorioretinitis of delayed onset was induced by HLA-peptide B27PD in 27 out of 33 rats. Peptide B7PD, which differs from B27PD by a single amino acid, failed to induce disease in 14 rats. Immunohistochemical staining of $CD4^+$ cells revealed strong signs of uveitis in B27PD-immunized rats (data not shown).

In vitro proliferation assays of lymph node cells from rats immunized with S-Ag, PDSAg, B27PD and B7PD (Fig. 1B) also revealed crossreactivity at the T cell response level of S-Ag, PDSAg and B27PD. B7PD stimulated lower responses when compared to the other peptides.

Induction of oral tolerance

Orally induced tolerance can ameliorate EAU, as shown after feeding of S-Ag [5] or peptide derivative [6]. Prefeeding of rats with peptide B27PD also reduced significantly EAU induced by immunization with whole S-Ag. The tolerizing effect of B27PD was comparable to oral S-Ag and better than oral PDSAg (Fig. 2). Feeding B27PD led to a 25% reduction in IRBP-induced uveitis.In contrast, feeding S-Ag or other peptides failed to suppress, whilst feeding IRBP led to a 75% reduction in disease (data not shown).

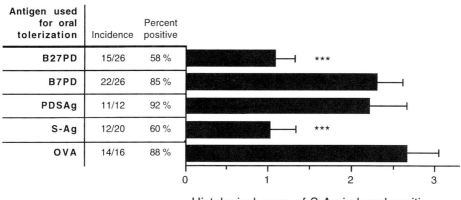

Antigen used for oral tolerization	Incidence	Percent positive
B27PD	15/26	58 %
B7PD	22/26	85 %
PDSAg	11/12	92 %
S-Ag	12/20	60 %
OVA	14/16	88 %

Histological score of S-Ag induced uveitis

Figure 2. Induction of oral tolerance to S-antigen induced EAU by peptide B27PD.
Lewis rats were fed either with S-Ag, Ovalbumin (OVA) or different peptides every other day for a total of three times and immunized with S-Ag 2-3 days after the last feeding.

Discussion

These data suggest there is a functional correlation between HLA-antigens and autoimmune uveitis. All patients that we have investigated to date have HLA-B alleles encoding peptide B27PD. Recent studies have shown that peptides derived from HLA class I molecules are naturally associated with HLA class II molecules [7]. Indeed, a peptide carrying the relevant sequence of B27PD has been eluted from HLA-DR molecules. The HLA class II-allele(s) that presents this peptide to the T cells of our uveitis patients is currently under investigation. The crossreactive T cell responses, observed both in patients and animals, support the hypothesis that HLA-peptide-specific T cells might be responsible for autoaggressive retinal destruction through recognition of the retina-specific sequestered antigen. HLA-specific T cells should normally be eliminated in the thymus, or downregulated by mechanisms of peripheral tolerance. Infection, trauma or stress can increase the expression and turnover rate of MHC-molecules by release of cytokines [8] and thereby cause enhanced local presentation of class I peptides by appropriate class II molecules. This may stimulate some "forbidden" T cells which recognize self-MHC and are probably heteroclitic for the retinal autoantigen. Recognition of the S-Ag peptide presented by resident ocular cells (i.e. pigment epithelial cells) may lead to invasion of eye tissue by these activated T cells. Thereafter, a lack of adequate local immunological suppressor mechanisms might allow an efficient immune response to be elicited that results in autoimmune disease.

These data offer a possible mechanism of induction, as well as an explanation for tissue specificity of this autoimmune disease.

Acknowledgements

We thank Prof. O.-E. Lund for his promotion, Prof. R. Wank for HLA-typing, Dr. H.-P. Scheuber for access to the animal facilities, K. Thomassen for superior technical assistance and Dr. L.A. Mertin for critical reviewing of the manuscript. We especially thank Profs. D.J. Schendel and R. Wank for helpful discussions during the project. This work was supported by the Deutsche Forschungsgemeinschaft, the Friedrich-Baur-Foundation and the Münchener Medizinische Wochenschrift. Patent pending.

References

1   Brewerton, D.A., Caffrey, M., Nicholls, A. et al. Lancet 1973; 2: 994-996

2   Ohno, S., Asanuma, T., Sugiura, S., Wakisaka, A. et al. J. Am. Med. Assoc. 1978; 240: 529

3   Shinohara, T., Dietzschold, B., Craft, C.M., Wistow, G. et al. Proc. Natl. Acad. Sci. U.S.A. 1987; 84: 6975-6979

4   deSmet, M.D., Yamamoto, J.H., Mochizuki, M., Gery, I. et al. Am. J. Ophthalmol. 1990; 110: 135-142

5   Nussenblatt, R.B., Caspi, R.R., Mahdi, R., Chan, C.-C. et al. J. Immunol. 1990; 144: 1689-1695

6   Thurau, S.R., Chan, C.-C., Suh, E., Nussenblatt, R.B. J. Autoimmun. 1991; 4: 507-516

7   Chicz, R.M., Urban, R.G., Gorga, J.C., Vignali, D.A.A. et al. J.Exp.Med. 1993; 178: 27-47

8   David-Watine, B., Israel, A., Kourilsky, O. Immunol. Today 1990; 11: 286-292

© *1994 Elsevier Science B.V. All rights reserved.*
Advances in Ocular Immunology
R.B. Nussenblatt, S.M. Whitcup, R.R. Caspi and I. Gery, eds.

Expression of the complement regulatory proteins in the normal and diseased (EAI) rat eye.

N.S. Bora[a], N.H. Kabeer[a], M.C. Kim[a], S. Paryjas[a], J.P. Atkinson[b] and H.J. Kaplan.

[a]Department of Ophthalmology and Visual Sciences, [b]Department of Medicine, Washington University School of Medicine, 660 S. Euclid, St.Louis, MO 63110, USA.

INTRODUCTION

The complement system is an important component of humoral immune defenses. It provides a recognition and effector pathway which promotes the inflammatory response, assists in the processing of immune complexes and directly alters the membranes of microorganisms [1]. A critical step in the complement activation sequence in both the classical and alternative pathway is the formation of the C3 convertases which activate C3 resulting in the generation and deposition of the major opsonic fragments C3b and C4b on the cell membrane and promote the assembly of the membrane attack complex (MAC). It is essential that the formation and function of the convertases be carefully regulated so that the opsonic activity of C3b and the cytolytic activity of the membrane attack complex are directed against foreign and not to self tissue. Regulation of C3 activation is achieved by two membrane bound regulatory proteins, namely decay accelerating factor (DAF; CD55) and membrane cofactor protein (MCP; CD46). Regulation of the formation and activity of the membrane attack complex (MAC) is mediated by CD59 [2]. We have recently shown that MCP, DAF and CD59 are differentially expressed in the normal human eye [3]. The present study was undertaken to study their expression in the normal rat eye and to compare this with their expression in the rat eye with experimental autoimmune iritis (EAI). EAI is an animal model of anterior uveitis which we have recently developed in Lewis rats [4].

MATERIALS AND METHODS

a) Development of EAI:
    Male Lewis rats 6-8 weeks of age were used. EAI was induced by immunization with bovine melanin associated antigen (BMAA) isolated from iris and ciliary body [4]. Animals were sacrificed at the peak of inflammation and their eyes were harvested for the immunohistochemical analysis. Eyes were also harvested from the normal rats.

b) Antibodies and Immunohistochemistry:
    Antibodies against human MCP, DAF and CD59 were used. One mouse monoclonal antibody (mAb), 1A10, and one rabbit polyclonal antibody, DL 6.2, were used to identify DAF. Gb24, a mouse mAb, and one rabbit

polyclonal antibody were used to localize MCP. For CD59, two monoclonals, IF5 and A35, and one rabbit polyclonal antibody were used [3]. Immunohistochemistry was performed as described previously [3]. Control stains were performed with nonrelevant antibodies of the same immunoglobulin class, normal rabbit serum or by omission of the primary and/or secondary antibodies.

RESULTS

Control stains were negative. Table 1 summarizes the results. Using immunocytochemical techniques, we have observed a differential expression of MCP and DAF in the normal rat eye. Staining was observed only with the polyclonal antibodies (human); no cross-reaction was observed with the monoclonal antibodies. In the normal rat eye, constitutive expression of MCP and DAF was observed on corneal epithelium, corneal stroma, ciliary body, iris, choroid and the outer nuclear layer of retina. Corneal epithelium, ciliary body [Fig. 1] and iris were strongly stained while weak staining was observed in the corneal stroma, choroid and outer nuclear layer of retina (Table 1). Expression of MCP and DAF was upregulated in rat eye with EAI, though the expression pattern was similar to that observed in the normal eye (Table 1). Rods and cones stained strongly for MCP and DAF in the eye with EAI, while they were negative in the normal eye. CD59 antibodies (both polyclonal and monoclonal) did not stain the normal rat eye or the eye with EAI.

Table 1
MCP and DAF in the normal and rat eye with EAI.

| | MCP | | DAF | |
	Normal	EAI	Normal	EAI
Cornea				
Epithelium	2	4	2	4
Stroma	1	2	1	3
Ciliary Body	2	4	2	4
Iris	2	4	2	4
Choroid	1	3	1	4
Retina				
Ganglion cell layer	0	0	0	0
Inner plexiform layer	0	0	0	0
Inner nuclear layer	0	0	0	0
Outer plexiform layer	0	0	0	0
Outer nuclear layer	1	3	1	3
Rods and cones	0	3	0	3

Comparative staining intensities were graded as extremely intense (4) to negative (0).

85

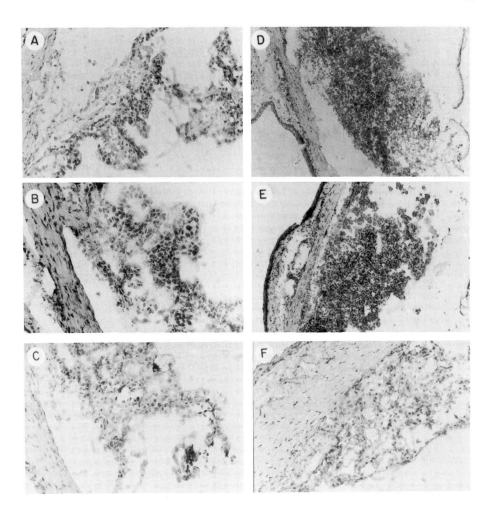

Figure 1. Expression of MCP, DAF, and CD59 in the ciliary body of normal
Lewis rat and Lewis rat with experimental autoimmune iritis. The normal
rat eye was examined immunohistochemcially for MCP (A), DAF (B) and
CD59 (C) using polyclonal antibodies against human proteins. Rat eye with
EAI was also stained for MCP (D), DAF (E) and CD59 (F). Original
magnification X 100.

DISCUSSION

With the use of immunohistochemical techniques, we have observed the differential expression of MCP and DAF in the normal rat eye. Both the proteins were strongly expressed on the corneal epithelium, iris and ciliary body while they were weakly expressed on the corneal stroma, choroid and outer nuclear layer of retina. Expression pattern of DAF in the normal rat eye was almost identical to that observed in the human eye except for the choroid [3]. However, high levels of MCP were present in the normal rat iris/CB which were negative in human eye [3]. Increased expression of MCP and DAF was observed on the ocular cells in experimental autoimmune iritis (EAI), though the expression pattern was almost similar to the normal eye. This upregulation was in part secondary to staining of invading inflammatory cells. Furthermore, in the animals with EAI there was acquisition of possibly new expression of MCP and DAF on the retina (rods and cones). Only the polyclonal antibodies against human MCP and DAF stained the rat eye. These results could be due to the cross reaction between some but not all immunogenic epitopes of human MCP and DAF and similar molecule(s) in the rat. Antibodies against human CD59 did not cross react with the rat antigen.

To the best of our knowledge, this is the first report describing the differential expression of MCP and DAF in the rat eye and their upregulation in EAI. Identification of MCP and DAF in the normal rat eye suggests that a regulatory system exists to protect these cells from destruction by complement activation and our results suggest that these molecules may play an important role in the pathogenesis of EAI.

FINANCIAL SUPPORT

This work was supported in part by grant from Research to Prevent Blindness, Inc., N.Y. and NIH grants 1R01-EY10543 and EY02687.

REFERENCES

1. Reid KBM. Activation and control of the complement system. Essays Biochem. 1986; 22:27-68.
2. Holers VM, Cole JL, Lublin DM, Seya T, Atkinson JP. Human C3b- and C4b-regulatory proteins: a new multigene family. Immunol Today.1985; 6:188-192.
3. Bora NS, Gobleman CL, Atkinson JP, Pepose JS and Kaplan, HJ. Differential expression of the complement regulatory proteins in the human eye. Invest Opth Vis Sci. 1993; 34:3579-3584.
4. Kabeer NH, Simpson SC, Gobleman CL, Kim MC, Tandhasetti MT, Kaplan HJ and Bora NS. Experimental Allergic Iritis (EAI), induction by immunization with bovine melanin associated antigen. Invest Ophth Vis Sci. 1994; 35:1481.

Advances in Ocular Immunology
R.B. Nussenblatt, S.M. Whitcup, R.R. Caspi and I. Gery, eds.

Experimental Autoimmune Iritis (EAI), Induction by Immunization with a Bovine Melanin Associated Antigen.

N. S. Bora, N. H. Kabeer, S. C. Simpson, M.C. Kim, M. T. Tandhasetti and H. J. Kaplan.

Department of Ophthalmology and Visual Sciences, Washington University School of Medicine, St. Louis, MO 63110, USA.

INTRODUCTION

Acute anterior uveitis (AAU) is a form of intraocular inflammation which includes both iritis and/or iridocyclitis. It is the most common form of uveitis and the inflammation occurs in either the iris or the ciliary body, with a spillover of vitreous inflammatory cells into the space behind the lens. Retinal involvement is not a component of anterior uveitis. Many investigators in the past have induced experimental autoimmune uveitis (EAU) in inbred rodents with various soluble retinal proteins. Unfortunately, EAU induced by soluble retinal proteins does not have the clinical characteristics of human AAU [1]. Recently, we have reported an animal model of anterior uveitis developed in Lewis rats using an insoluble antigen solely derived from bovine iris and ciliary body which resembles human AAU by its sudden onset, localization to anterior uvea and spontaneous resolution [2]. The present study was designed to partially identify the pathogenic antigen in EAI and to study its association with ocular melanin.

MATERIALS AND METHODS

Pathogen free male Lewis rats were purchased from Harlan Sprague Dawley, Indianapolis, IN.

(a)　Antibodies

Monoclonal antibodies against S-antigen, IRBP and Phosducin were kindly provided by Dr. Larry A. Donoso, Wills Eye Hospital, Philadelphia, PA. Monoclonal antibodies to rhodopsin were a gift of Dr. G. Adamus, R.S. Dow Neurological Sciences Institute Portland, OR.

(b)   Antigen preparation, immunization and assessment of EAI

Bovine melanin associated antigen (BMAA) was prepared as previously described [2]. In some experiments bovine skin was used as the source of the antigen. Animals were immunized with the 100 ul of stable emulsion prepared by mixing 100 ug of the antigen and the equal volume of CFA. Purified PTX (1 ug/animal) was used as an additional adjuvant. Control animals were injected with the mixture of CFA and PTX only. The animals were examined at days 7, 10, 12, 14, 16, 18, 20, 22, 24, 26, 28 and 30 post injection. Animals were sacrificed on these days, and their eyes were harvested for histological analysis to assess the development and severity of the inflammation.

(c)   Solubilization of BMAA and immunoblotting

BMAA was digested with Staphylococcus aureus V8 protease as described in the literature [3]. After digestion with these enzymes samples were centrifuged and the supernatant was extensively dialyzed against water, lyophilized, and redissolved in PBS. The soluble antigen was analysed on the SDS-PAGE. Proteins were transferred to nitrocellulose and these membranes were probed with the antibodies against S-Ag, IRBP, rhodopsin and phosducin. Bound antibody was traced by ^{125}I-protein A and were visualized by exposure of air dried nitrocellulose to Kodak X-OMAT AR films at -80º C.

RESULTS

In order to partially identify the pathogenic antigen in EAI, the insoluble BMAA was digested with the proteolytic enzyme V8 protease or Proteinase K and the soluble antigen was used to immunize Lewis rats. The Proteinase K digested soluble fraction was not pathogenic; however, all Lewis rats immunized with the V8 protease digested soluble antigen developed EAI [Table 1]. Disease severity and histopathological features were similar to that observed with insoluble BMAA. The possible presence of a pathogenic soluble retinal protein, namely S-Ag, IRBP, rhodopsin and phosducin in the soluble fraction obtained after V8 protease digestion was investigated by immunoblotting using monoclonal antibodies. Our results show the absence of S-Ag and IRBP, rhodopsin and phosducin in the soluble antigen fraction derived from the V8 protease digestion of BMAA (not shown). Association of the protein antigen with the ocular melanin was studied by isolating melanin containing the insoluble antigen from bovine skin. This antigen was used to immunize Lewis rats, and was not pathogenic [Table 1].

Table 1. Pathogenicity of soluble and skin derived BMAA in Lewis rats.

Antigen	Antigen Dose (ug)	Animals with EAI			Day of Onset
		Incidence	Mild	Severe	
Iris/CB BMAA	100	10/10	0	10	14+3
Proteinase K digested soluble fraction	100	0/10	0	0	--
V8 Protease digested soluble fraction	100	12/12	1/12	11/12	15.5+1.5
Skin BMAA	100	0/12	0	0	--

Incidence of EAI given as positive/total animals.
BMAA: Bovine melanin associated antigen.
* Mean + S.D.

DISCUSSION

Human acute anterior uveitis (AAU) is the most common form of intraocular inflammation. We have recently developed a clinically relevant animal model of anterior uveitis [2] and have named our model EAI-experimental autoimmune iritis. The present study reports the localization as well as partial identification of the putative uveitogenic antigen in EAI. In our system, the crude melanin associated insoluble antigen isolated from bovine skin was not pathogenic indicating thereby that the antigen is localized to the eye and is tissue specific. These findings are in contrast to those reported by Broekhuyse and coworkers. These workers have reported that bovine skin melanin is pathogenic [4]. Furthermore, our results show that the uveitogenic protein(s) can be solubilized and cleaved from melanin by proteolytic enzyme treatment. The soluble fraction obtained after V8 protease digestion has uveitogenic activity whereas that obtained after proteinase K treatment is not pathogenic. The uveitogenic activity associated with the V8 protease digested soluble fraction is probably not due to the presence of the known pathogenic soluble retinal proteins. Thus our results demonstrate that the uveitogenic antigen in EAI is a protein(s) associated with bovine melanin from the iris and ciliary body. Studies on the further characterization of the pathogenic antigen(s) are underway in our laboratory. They should help us to gain insights into the pathogenesis of this disease.

FINANCIAL SUPPORT

This work was supported in part by grant from Research to Prevent Blindness, Inc., N.Y. and NIH grants 1R01-EY10543 and EY02687.

REFERENCES

1.   Nussenblatt RB, Palestine AG. Uveitis: Fundamentals and Clinical Practice. Year Book Medical Publishers,Inc. 1989.
2.   Kabeer NH, Simpson SC, Gobleman CL, Kim MC, Tandhasetti MT, Kaplan HJ and Bora NS. Experimental Allergic Iritis (EAI), induction by immunization with bovine melanin associated antigen. Invest Ophth Vis Sci. 1994; 35:1481.
3.   Cleveland DW, Fischer SG, Kirschner MW and Laemmli UK. Peptide mapping by limited proteolysis in sodium dodecy sulfate and analysis by gel electophoresis. J Biol Chem. 1977; 252:11002-1106.
4.   Broekhuyse RM, Kuhlman ED and Winkens HJ. Experimental autoimmune anterior uveitis (EAAU): III. Induction by immunization with purified uveal and skin melanins. Exp Eye Res. 1993; 56:575-583.

Advances in Ocular Immunology
R.B. Nussenblatt, S.M. Whitcup, R.R. Caspi and I. Gery, eds.

Experimental Melanin-Protein Induced Uveitis ('EMIU', formerly 'EAAU'): Immunopathology, Susceptibility and Therapy

Chi-Chao Chan[1], Kourosh Dastgheib[1], Naofumi Hikita[1], R. Christopher Walton[1], Robert B. Nussenblatt[1], Rene M. Broekhuyse[2]

[1]Laboratory of Immunology, National Eye Institute, National Institutes of Health, Bethesda, MD, U.S.A. 20892

[2]Institute of Opthalmology, University of Nijmegen, Nijmegen, the Netherlands

Introduction

Purified bovine melanin protein (BMP) from the choroid and remnants of adherent retinal pigment epithelium (RPE) can induce an autoimmune uveitis in Lewis rats. Termed *experimental melanin-protein induced uveitis* ('EMIU', formerly 'EAAU'), the disease is characterized by bilateral, recurrent iridocyclitis and choroiditis.[1-5] This T cell mediated autoimmune uveitis serves as a useful model for non-infectious uveitis in humans.

Materials and methods

Animals

Different strains of rats including Lewis, Wistar-Furth, Fischer and Brown Norway, between 6 and 8 weeks of age (150-180 grams) and monkeys (Macaca Fascicularis and Macaca mulatta) were used in this study. ARVO guidelines regarding animal experimentation were followed.

Antigens

Sodium dodecyl sulfate (SDS) insoluble melanosome fraction (BMP) from bovine choroid and RPE was collected according to the method described by Broekhuyse and Kuhlmann.[3] Briefly, the choroid and adherent RPE were isolated from bovine eyes. The extracted sediment was washed and suspended in 2% SDS and heated at 75°C for 10 minutes. After centrifugation, purified BMP was washed, dried and stored. Fifty mg of the dry weight product corresponds to approximately 20 mg melanin protein.[4]

Immunization

Rats: Twenty-five µg BMP/0.03 ml PBS in Hunter's adjuvant (1:1 volume mixture) was injected into one footpad. At the same time 25 µg BMP and *Bordetella pertussis* (3×10^9 organisms) in PBS were injected intraperitoneally.[5]

Monkeys: Five hundred μg BMP in Hunter's adjuvant (1:1 volume mixture) was injected intracutaneously in the back as well as two to three μg of pertussis toxin. Five to nine weeks later, a booster of 250-300 μg BMP in incomplete Freund's adjuvant was administered at multiple skin sites.[2]

Treatment
Animals received daily administration of Dexamethasone (0.2 mg/kg/day), cyclosporin A (CsA 10 mg/kg/day), FK 506 (0.5 mg/kg/day), or the thromboxane synthetase inhibitor, CGS- 13080 (0.45 mg/kg/day), beginning on day 7 after immunization and continuing for two weeks when they were sacrificed. Eyes were collected for pathology as previously described.[5]

Results

Immunopathology
In the rats, bilateral ocular inflammation developed 8 days following immunization. The clinical presentation consisted of mild conjunctival congestion, keratic precipitates, irregular pupils with variable degrees of synechiae, as well as anterior chamber cells, flare and fibrin. A red reflex was present unless there was a marked hypopyon or hyphema. The clinical findingsworsened for 7 days then subsided gradually within one month. Recurrent uveitis occurred in some cases.

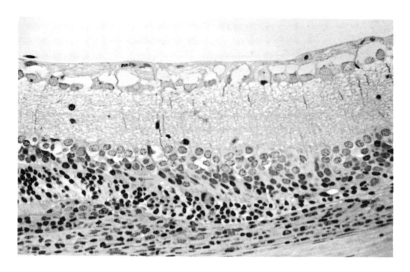

Figure 1. Chorioretinal scar is present in a rat with severe recurrent EMIU. (hematoxylin and eosin, x 400).

Histopathological examination disclosed mainly mononuclear cell infiltration in the anterior chamber, trabecular meshwork, iris, ciliary body, choroid and vitreous. Neutrophils, plasma cells, giant cells and occasional eosinophils were present. The main inflammatory cells were CD4+ T lymphocytes. Expression of adhesion molecules (CD 54, CD 11a) and major histocompatibility complex (MHC) class II antigens were detected on ocular resident cells prior to the recruitment of inflammatory cells. In some Lewis rats with severe, recurrent EMIU, there was retinal involvement with focal loss of photoreceptor cells and chorioretinal scar formation (Fig. 1). No inflammation was found in the skin, brain or inner ear. In the monkey, the findings were similar to that observed in the rat. However, a moderate number of CD20+ B cells in addition to T cells were noted in the choroid (Fig. 2).

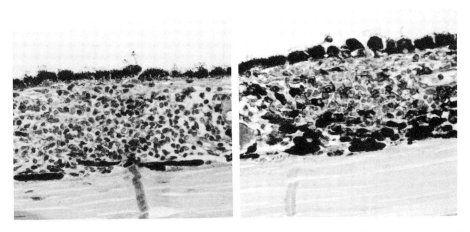

Figure 2. Left. Most infiltrating cells (arrows) in the choroid of a monkey with EMIU are CD3+ . Right. Some CD20+ Cells are also observed. (ABC, x 400).

Susceptibility

Rats with RT1 allele of l (Lewis, 20/20) or lvl (Fischer, 6/24) were susceptible to the development of EMIU. Wistar-Furth (0/20), with RT1 allele of u, and Brown Norway (0/20) with RT1 allele of n, in spite of dark pigmentation, failed to develop EMIU.

Therapy

Animals treated with CsA or FK 506 developed minimal or no EMIU. Corticosteroids and CGS-13080 also suppressed EMIU clinically and histopathologically.

Discussion

EMIU is an experimental autoimmune uveitis utilizing purified uveal melanin protein as the antigen.[1-5] Following immunization of BMP the disease develops in monkeys and several strains of rats. EMIU is a T lymphocyte mediated autoimmune disease that closely resembles several uveitic entities, such as sympathetic ophthalmia and Vogt-Koyanagi-Harada syndrome seen in humans.

Although the antigen of EMIU, BMP, originates from the pigmented melanosomes, the susceptibility does not depend on the amount of the pigmentation. Instead, the susceptibility of rats to EMIU, as in EAU is MHC restricted mainly by the genetic background, RT1 allele.[6, 7] This restriction further supports the role of MHC genes in the induction of autoimmune ocular diseases in rats.

Currently available immunosuppresants are effective in the down regulation of EMIU as previously documented for experimental autoimmune uveoretinitis (EAU).[8-11] CsA and FK 506 seem to have greater efficacy in suppressing the efferent phase of inflammation than corticosteroids and non-steroidal anti-inflammatory agents. Evaluation of the inhibitory effect on the recurrent stage of the disease is underway and may provide more practical solutions to the treatment of uveitis in humans.

References

1. Broekhuyse RM, Kuhlmann ED, Winkens HJ, Van Vugt AHM. Exp Eye Res 1991; 52:465-474.
2. Broekhuyse RM, Kuhlmann ED, Winkens HJ. Exp Eye Res 1992; 55:401-411.
3. Broekhuyse RM, Kuhlmann ED. Invest Ophthalmol Vis Sci 1993; 34:698-700.
4. Broekhuyse RM, Kuhlmann ED, Winkens HJ. Exp Eye Res 1993; 56:575-583.
5. Chan CC, Hikita N, Dastgheib K, Whitcup SM, et al. Ophthalmology (in press).
6. Gery I. In: Chandler JW, O'Connor GR, eds. Proceeding of the Third International Symposium on the Immunology and Immunopathology of the Eye. New York: Masson Publishing, 1984; 242-245.
7. Hirose S, Sasamoto Y, Ogasawara K, Narito T, et al. In: Usui M, Ohno S, Aoki K, eds. Ocular Immunology Today, Proceedings of the 5th International Symposium in the Immunology and Immunopathology of the Eye. Amsterdam-New York-Oxford: Excerpta Medica, 1990; 135 - 138.
8. Nussenblatt RB, Rodrigues MM, Salinas-Carmona MC, Gery I, et al. Arch Ophthalmol 1982; 100:1146-1149.
9. Kawashima H, Fujino Y, Mochizuki M. Invest Ophthalmol Vis Sci 1988; 29:1265-1271.
10. Mochizuki M, Nussenblatt RB, Kuwabara T, Gery I. Invest Ophthalmol Vis Sci 1985; 26:226-232.
11. Li Q, Lopez JS, Caspi RR, Roberge FG, et al. Exp Eye Res 1993; 57:601-608.

© 1994 Elsevier Science B.V. All rights reserved.
Advances in Ocular Immunology
R.B. Nussenblatt, S.M. Whitcup, R.R. Caspi and I. Gery, eds.

Sequential expression of ICAM-1, LFA-1, MHC-II molecules in the pathogenesis of Experimental Allergic Iritis (EAI).

M.C. Kim, N.S. Bora, N.H. Kabeer and H.J. Kaplan,

Department of Ophthalmology and Visual Sciences, Washington University School of Medicine, St. Louis, MO 63110, USA.

INTRODUCTION

Recently, we have reported an animal model of human anterior uveitis in Lewis rats which has been named as experimental autoimmune iritis (EAI) [1]. Our preliminary results indicate that EAI is a T cell (CD4+) mediated disease. It is possible that in EAI, a peripheral immunization of the BMAA mixed with adjuvants sets off a cascade of immune reactions, resulting in sensitization of autoreactive T effector cells and the targeting of these cells to the eye. The interaction between the antigen presenting cells (APC), T cells and the following transmigrations of lymphocytes across the blood-eye barrier are complicated processes involving MHC class II antigens as well as cell adhesion molecules such as ICAM-1 and LFA-1 (CD11a/CD18). Class II antigen of MHC (Ia in the rats) have an obligatory role in antigen presentation [2]. Expression of adhesion molecules is important for both leukocytes homing and migration through vascular endothelium [3]. Increased expression of these molecules appears to promote the migration of leukocytes to areas of inflammation. Endothelial cell surface ICAM-1 appears to contribute to the adhesion and transmigration of most leukocytes through an interaction with leukocyte adhesion molecules; LFA-1 which are expressed on neutrophils, monocytes, lymphocytes and NK cells [3]. Because these three proteins Ia, ICAM-1 and LFA-1 play an important role in immune and inflammatory response, we analyzed rat eyes during different stages of EAI for their expression using immunohistochemical techniques.

MATERIALS AND METHODS

(a)   Immunization and Evaluation of Disease
BMAA was prepared as previously described [1]. Male Lewis rats, 8 weeks old, were used. Experimental rats received 200 ug of the BMAA

emulsified (1:1) in Complete Freund's adjuvant (CFA) and Pertussis toxin (PTX; 1ug/animal). Control animals received CFA and PTX alone. Two rats were sacrificed and the eyes were harvested for the serial frozen sections at various days after immunization as follow: 6, 7, 8, 9, 10, 11, 13, 14, 19, 25 and 29. Clinically, the course of the disease was divided into four stages: early stage (day 8 and 9), onset (day 10 and 11), severe (day 12-14) and late stage (day 19-25).

(b)   Antibodies and Immunohistochemistry
Monoclonal antibodies were used in this study. Anti Ia (clone OX-6) were obtained from Accurate Chemical and Scientific Corp., New York, NY. The antibodies purchased from Harlan Bioproducts for Science, Indianapolis, IN were used to identify ICAM-1 (CD54, clone 1A29) and LFA-1 (CD11a, clone WT.1). Immunohistochemistry was performed using the standard technique. Control stains included staining with normal mouse ascites Ig, omission of the primary and/or secondary biotinylated antibodies.

RESULTS

Table 1 summarizes the results. Similar pattern of staining for ICAM-1, LFA-1 and Ia antigens was observed in normal and control eyes [Table 1]. Constitutive expression of ICAM-1 and MHC class II antigens was observed on iris, ciliary body and choroid [Table 1]. There was no staining in RPE, cornea (epithelium and stroma) or corneal endothelium and iris/ciliary body epithelium. There was a diffuse Ia+ cells in the areas adjacent to the episcleral veins, extending into the posterior margins of the cornea. The iris and the ciliary body showed occasional Ia+ cells. The choroid also stained for occasional Ia positive cells. No Ia+ cells were noted in the cornea, retina, retinal pigment epithelium, or in the iris/ciliary body epithelium. LFA-1 antibodies did not stain normal or the control eyes [Table 1].
Anti ICAM-1 antibody stained iris, ciliary body and choroid of the rats immunized with BMAA and the level of expression was similar to that observed in normal and control rats up to the early stage [Table 1]. Upregulation in the level of ICAM-1 was observed two days prior to the onset of the disease [Table 1]. LFA-1 positive cells increased on day 10 post immunization (onset) [Table 1]. An upregulation in the number of Ia positive cells was also observed on day 10 post immunization [Table 1]. Ia positive cells were mostly present in the iris, ciliary body and choroid. Expression of ICAM-1, LFA-1 and Ia molecules did not change with time in normal and control rats immunized with CFA and PTX alone.

TABLE 1. Sequential Expression of LFA-1, ICAM-1 and MHC Class II
Antigen (Ia) in EAI.

Antigen	Day Post Immunization	LFA-1		ICAM-1		MHC Class II(Ia)	
		Choroid	I/CB	Choroid	I/CB	Choroid	I/CB
BMAA							
	6	0	0	2	2	1	1
	7	0	0	2	2	1	1
	9	0	0	3	3	1	1
	10	1	1	3	3	1	1
	11	3	3	4	4	2	2
	12	3	3	4	4	3	3
	14	4	4	4	4	4	4
CFA/PTX	(6-14)	0	0	2	2	1	1
Normal Control	(6-14)	0	0	2	2	1	1

Comparative staining intensities were graded as extremely intense (4) to
negative (O) on an arbitrary five point scale (0 to +4).

DISCUSSION

This study demonstrates for the first time the sequential expression of
MHC class II antigens and cell adhesion molecules in EAI.   ICAM-1
expression was detected immunohistochemically in the normal and control rat
eyes. The location of the ICAM-1 molecules was limited to the iris/ciliary body
stromal tissues and the choroid. This is expected as the uveal tract consists of
highly vascularized capillary network for a nutritional support of neighboring
cells. The normal and the control rat eyes did not stain for LFA-1 in the
present study. However, in contrast to our observations Sakamoto et al. could
not detect ICAM-1 in the eyes of Lewis rats without inflammation [4]. In our
study we have also observed the constitutive expression of MHC class II (Ia)
antigens in the normal and control rat eyes. These results are in contrast to
those reported in the literature [5]. Expression of ICAM-1, LFA-1 and Ia
antigens was upregulated in the rat eyes with experimental autoimmune
iritis (EAI). Temporally, the increase in ICAM-1 expression precedes that of
LFA-1 and Ia. These observations suggest that the primary increase in
ICAM-1 expression in the target organ may be important in recruiting the

inflammatory cells to that organ. It is possible that during the early phase of EAI, an increase in ICAM-1 expression in the uveal tract may allow efficient adherence of immune cells to the vascular endothelia of the eye and will help in lymphocyte transmigration and inflammation. Selective blocking of ICAM-1 using monoclonal antibodies in vivo during this critical time period may be of use in therapeutically preventing EAI.

FINANCIAL SUPPORT

This work was supported in part by grant from Research to Prevent Blindness, Inc., N.Y. and NIH grants 1R01-EY10543 and EY02687.

REFERENCES

1. Kabeer NH, Simpson SC, Gobleman CL, Kim MC, Tandhasetti MT, Kaplan HJ and Bora NS. Experimental Allergic Iritis (EAI), induction by immunization with bovine melanin associated antigen. Invest Ophth Vis Sci. 1994; 35:1481.

2. Unanue ER, Beller DI and Lu CY. Antigen presentation: Comments on its regulation and mechanism. J Immunol. 1984; 132:1-5.

3. Marlin SD and Springer TA. Purified intracellular adhesion molecule-1 (ICAM-1) is a ligand for lymphocyte function associated antigen 1 (LFA-1). Cell 1987; 51:813-819.

4. Sakamoto T, Takahira KI, Sanui H, Kohno T and Imomata H. Intracellular adhesion molecule-1 on rat corneal endothelium in experimental uveitis. Exp Eye Res. 1993; 56:241-246.

5. Chan CC, Caspi RR, Ni M, Leake WC, Wiggert B, Chader GJ and Nussenblatt RB. Pathology of experimental autoimmune uveoretinitis in mice. J Autoimmun. 1990; 3:247-255.

© 1994 Elsevier Science B.V. All rights reserved.
Advances in Ocular Immunology
R.B. Nussenblatt, S.M. Whitcup, R.R. Caspi and I. Gery, eds.

Expression of Transforming Growth Factor β1 (TGFβ1) in Experimental Melanin Protein Induced Uveitis and Experimental Autoimmune Uveitis

Q. Li, K. Dastgheib, D. Luyo, C. Egwuagu, R.B. Nussenblatt, and C.-C. Chan

Laboratory of Immunology, National Eye Institute, Bethesda, MD

Introduction

TGFβ1 is a 25kd protein consisting of two identical subunit chains.[1] Although the main natural sources of TGFβ1 are platelets, placenta and kidney, almost all normal cells synthesize TGFβ and bear functional membrane-bound receptors for TGFβ1 and for members of TGFβ family. Being a multifunctional molecule, TGFβ1 can interact with other cytokines within the immune system and plays a role from the initiation of an immune response until its resolution.[2] Reports in laboratory animal models have confirmed that TGFβ1 plays an active part in autoimmune disorders such as experimental arthritis, and experimental allergic encephalomyelitis (EAE).[3,4] The role of TGFβ1 in experimental uveitic models, however, has not been reported.

Experimental melanin-protein induced uveitis[5] (EMIU) and experimental autoimmune uveitis[6] (EAU) are well-established animal models for uveitis and uveoretinitis in humans. It is of interesting to study whether there is expression of TGFβ1 in the eyes of rats with EAU or EMIU, and to further understand the potential of TGFβ1 in the prevention and treatment of these disorders.

Materials and Methods

Animals

Female Lewis rats weighing 200 grams each (6-8 weeks of age) were obtained from Charles River Raleigh, Raleigh N.C.. All were housed in environmentally controlled rooms with 12 hours of light and dark cycle and provided with food and water ad libium. All animals were treated according to the ARVO Resolution on the Use of Animals in Research.

Induction of EMIU and recurrence

Twenty-five µg bovine melanin protein (BMP) in Hunter's adjuvant (1:1 v/v) were injected into one footpad. At the same time 25µg BMP and Bordetella pertussis (3×10^9 organisms) in PBS were injected intraperitoneally. Recurrence of EMIU was induced in 100% of rats within two weeks by subcutaneous footpad injection of 5µg LPS 45 days after immunization. Eyes of EMIU rats were collected

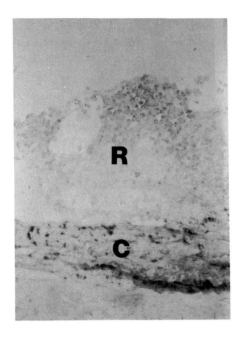
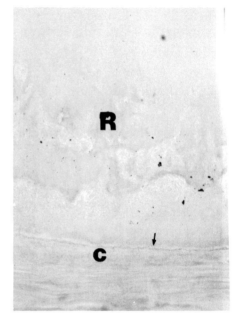

Figure 1. Retinal destruction and choroidal thickening of an EAU rat at day 40. The positive stain for the signal of TGFβ1 mRNA is located in the retina (R) and choroid (C). (x400)

Figure 2. A frozen section of an EMIU rat with mild recurrent choroiditis. The RPE cells (arrow) stains positively for TGFβ1. (R: retina, C: choroid, x400)

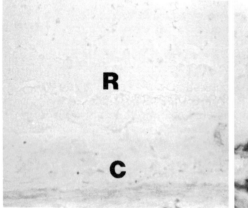
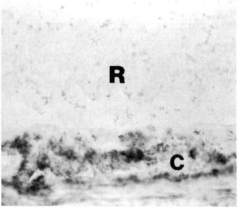

Figure 3. left: Severe case of recurrent EMIU, the thickeaned choroid shows no stain. right: Mild case of recurrent EMIU, showing a strong stain for the signal of TGFβ1 mRNA in the choroid. (R: retina, C: choroid, x400)

at different stages: remission (28 days), spontaneous recurrence (37-45 days), and one or two weeks after LPS booster (50 or 60 days).

Induction of EAU

EAU was induced in Lewis rats by footpad injection with 30μg of bovine S-Ag emulsified (1:1, v/v) in complete Freund's adjuvant (DIFCO, MI).[6] Eyes of EAU rats were collected at early, mid and late stages of EAU (10, 14, 21, 30, 40, and 50 days).

In situ Hybridization Histochemistry

The tissue handling and *in situ* hybridization was performed as described previously.[7] Rat TGFβ1 cDNA 985 bp HindIII and XbaI fragment was subcloned into the pBluescript II KS+ vector (Courtesy Drs Lalage Wakefield and Su Wen Qian, NCI, NIH). The plasmids were linearized at appropriate restriction sites prior to the transcription, and only discrete "runoff" transcripts were obtained. The restriction enzymes were XbaI for T3 in anti-sense RNA (negative probe) and HindIII for T7 in sense RNA (positive probe). RNA probes randomly labeled with dioxigenin-urindine-triphosphate by *in vitro* transcription using a DIG RNA Labeling Kit (Boehringer Mannheim Biochemica, IN).

Immunohistochemistry

Six μm-thick frozen sections were obtained. The presence of TGFβ1 molecule, recognized by polyclonal anti-TGFβ1 antibody, (R&D systems, MN) was assessed by staining with the avidin-biotin-peroxidase complex staining technique.[8] Chicken IgY was the control for the primary antibody.

Results

TGFβ1 mRNA was detected at the inflammatory sites of EMIU and scar tissue of EAU (Figure 1, 2). TGFβ1 and its mRNA were only detected in the remission (day 21) and quiescent stage (day 30) of EAU, the data were summarized in Table 1. TGFβ1 and its mRNA were detected in the remission of EMIU (day 28), and in the mild to moderate cases of recurrent EMIU (Table 2, Figure 3).

Table 1
TGFβ1 Expression in the Eyes of EAU Rats (positive rats/total rats)

Post-immunization	Day 10	Day14	Day21	Day30	Day40	Day50
mRNA	0/4	0/4	1/4	4/4	0/4	0/4
protein	0/4	0/4	0/4	1/4	0/4	0/4

Table 2
TGFβ1 Expression in the Eyes of EMIU Rats (positive rats/total rats)

Post-immunization Inflammation	Day28 none	Day37-45 moderate	Day50 severe	Day50 mild	Day60 severe	Day60 mild
mRNA	2/2	2/3	0/4	4/4	0/4	3/3
protein	1/2	1/3	1/4	2/4	1/4	0/3

Discussion

Although TGFβ1 and its mRNA are not detectable in the choroid of normal rats nor in the early stage (day 10 to day 14) of EAU, it is present in the period of remission and tissue repair (day 21 to day 30), suggesting that TGFβ1 may be involved in tissue repair in the eyes of EAU rats.

Our data for EMIU study demonstrate that TGFβ1 mRNA is found in each of the rats sacrificed at day 28, when ocular inflammation has subsided. TGFβ1 mRNA is also expressed in 2 of 3 rats with spontaneous recurrence, implying that this molecule may be involved in more than tissue repair. In the recurrent EMIU, TGFβ1 mRNA is expressed only in mild, not severe cases, suggesting that TGFβ1 may have a suppressive effect on the recurrence of EMIU.

In conclusion, our current study reveals that TGFβ1 may play an active role in tissue repair of EAU and EMIU; furthermore it may also have a suppressive effect on EMIU recurrence. The kinetic changes of TGFβ1 in EAU and EMIU processes provide valuable information on the immunoregulation of these two autoimmune ocular models.

References

1. Robert A.B. and Sporn M.B. In: Battey J.F., Arai K., Sporn M.B., Robert A.B., eds. New York: Springer-Verlag, 1990; 419-472.
2. Wahl S.M., McCartney-Francis N. and Mergenhagen S.E. Immun. Today, 1989; 10:258-261.
3. Brandes M.E., Allen J.B., Ogawa Y., and Wahl S.M. J. Clin. Invest., 1991; 87:1108-1113.
4. Racke M.K., Dhib-Jalbut S., Cannella B., Albert P.S., Raine C.S. and McFarlin D.E. J. Immunol., 1991; 146: 3012-3017.
5. Chan C.-C., Hikita N., Dastgheib K. et al. Ophthalmol. (in press).
6. Nussenblatt, R.B. Invest. Ophthalmol. Vis. Sci. 1990; 32: 3131-3141.
7. Chan C.-C., Li Q., Brezin A.P. et al. Ocul. Immun. Inflam. 1993; 1:71-77.
8. Hsu, S.M., Raine, L., Fanger, H. J. Histochem. Cytochem. 1981; 92:577-580.

Advances in Ocular Immunology
R.B. Nussenblatt, S.M. Whitcup, R.R. Caspi and I. Gery, eds.

A Spontaneous Model of Post-infectious, Immune Mediated Uveitis

Carolyn M. Kalsow[a] and Ann E. Dwyer[a,b]

[a] Department of Ophthalmology, University of Rochester School of Medicine and Dentistry, Rochester, New York, USA.

[b] Genesee Valley Equine Clinic, Scottsville, New York, USA.

Clinical investigation of uveitis is complex. Although an immunologic etiology is strongly suspected in some cases of uveitis, specific pathogenesis is not known. Ocular tissues are not readily available for study, particularly at the time of active or recent inflammation. Furthermore, prospective serological studies are not possible before symptoms develop, *i.e.*, individuals at risk are not readily identified or followed. It is also difficult to study these patients over an extended period.

The pioneering work of the laboratories of Wacker and Faure provided an experimental model of autoimmune uveitis induced by S-antigen purified from retina. There are now several models which use photoreceptor cell specific proteins, *e.g.* S-antigen, interphotoreceptor retinoid binding protein, rhodopsin, or peptides thereof. Animals systemically sensitized with these antigens in adjuvant consistently develop an experimental autoimmune uveoretinitis (EAU) and an experimental autoimmune pinealitis (EAP). Significant progress has been made in defining not only the antigens and specific epitopes but also the immune responses active in these models [1-3]. Studies of EAU and EAP have led to the initiation of clinical trials of induction of specific oral tolerance for immunotherapy of uveitis [4]. However, since these experimental uveitides are induced by systemic sensitization, the induction process interferes with study of systemic immune responses especially in relation to local (ocular) immune responses. The models also do not specifically address the immunopathogenesis of post-infectious uveitis.

Equine recurrent uveitis (ERU) can serve as a complementary model of uveitis, specifically of post-infectious uveitis. This is a spontaneous uveitis in which there is no artificial perturbation of the systemic immune response. ERU is similar to human uveitides in manifestations, incidence, lack of effective therapy and resulting loss of vision [5]. An equine practice population can present a more controlled study group than human patient populations. The early studies of ERU by Witmer provided initial evidence for intraocular antibody production in uveitis and established calculation of the ratio of aqueous to serum reactivity for confirmation of local antibody synthesis [6].

ERU can be a sequela to systemic leptospirosis. Although there are several etiologies for ERU, it is often associated with *Leptospira interrogans* infection. Post-leptospiral ERU was confirmed in a natural outbreak of leptospirosis on a small farm near Ithaca, New York. Five of 16 horses developed a febrile illness, leptospiral antibodies and recurrent uveitis [7]. The stablemates did not show systemic or ocular symptoms nor leptospiral antibodies. Post-leptospiral ERU has also been demonstrated in experimental leptospiral infections of Shetland ponies [8]. Furthermore, there are many studies worldwide correlating ERU and the presence of serum antibodies to several *L. interrogans* serovars especially *pomona* [9].

We have assessed the incidence and visual outcome of leptospiral associated uveitis in the Genesee River Valley (Manuscript in preparation). We retrospectively studied horses for uveitis, blindness and leptospiral seroreactivity. Over a 7 year period, 1.4% (130 horses) of the practice population was diagnosed as uveitic. A comparison of *L. pomona* seroreactivity of uveitic and nonuveitic horses confirmed an association of uveitis and leptospiral seroreactivity (Figure 1). An analysis of these uveitic horses revealed that seropositive, uveitic horses are at increased risk of losing vision in one or both eyes (Figure 2). A genetic influence in ERU was indicated by the incidence of uveitis and associated blindness in Appaloosas as compared to non-Appaloosas of the practice population. The Appaloosa breed was over represented in both seropositive and seronegative uveitic groups, and uveitic Appaloosas also had a higher rate of vision loss than non-Appaloosas (Figure 3).

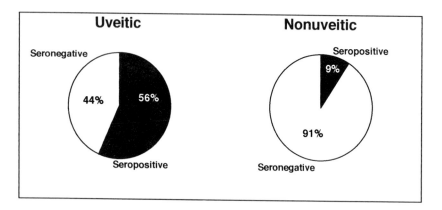

Figure 1. The association of *L. pomona* seroreactivity and uveitis was statistically significant and the odds ratio analysis showed that seropositive horses were 13.2 times more likely to have uveitis than seronegative horses.

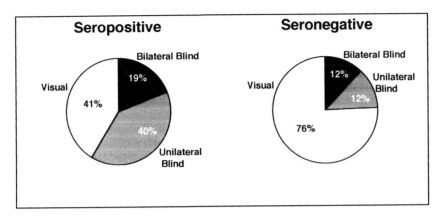

Figure 2. The association of *L. pomona* seroreactivity and blindness was statistically significant and the odds ratio analysis showed that seropositive horses were 4.4 times more likely to lose vision than seronegative, uveitic horses.

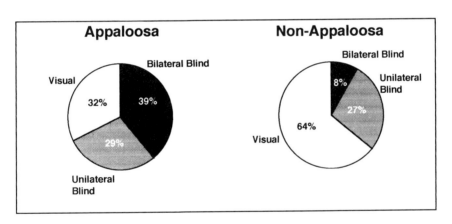

Figure 3. The association of Appaloosa breed and blindness was statistically significant and the odds ratio analysis showed that uveitic Appaloosas were 3.8 times more likely to lose vision than uveitic non-Appaloosas.

Post-leptospiral ERU is probably an immune mediated inflammation. The systemic infection usually responds to antibiotic therapy. However, immunosuppressives rather than antibiotics are required to quiet active episodes of uveitis [5]. Histologically there are many lymphocytes and plasma cells in affected eyes, particularly in the anterior uvea where the lymphocytes becomes organized into discrete lymphocytic nodules [10]. We have observed compartmentalization of T and B lymphocytes of these nodules into patterns suggestive of germinal centers [11]. We have also shown immunoglobulin deposition and MHC Class II antigen expression on resident and infiltrating cells of eye and pineal gland in ERU [12]. Pinealitis accompanying uveitis in a horse with documented post-leptospiral ERU validates the relevance of EAP in laboratory models and supports an immune associated pathogenesis for ERU [13]. Furthermore, sera and aqueous of some uveitic horses have anti-retinal antibodies [14,15].

On the basis of these observations we hypothesize that manifestations of ERU can be a result of leptospiral-immune system interaction. The uveitis could result from a direct immune response to leptospiral antigen in the eye. ERU may also be a manifestation of autoimmunity induced by cross reactivity of bacterial antigens that have epitopes similar to ocular antigens. Alternatively leptospiral infection could induce an immunomodulation that leads to breakdown of self tolerance resulting in autoimmunity.

ERU presents an opportunity to study uveitis and pinealitis that: a) is naturally occurring rather than laboratory induced, b) has an established link between bacterial infection and immune associated uveitis, c) allows identification and tracking of individuals at risk, and d) provides a more controlled setting than the study of human uveitides. As in ERU, these is evidence to support leptospiral etiology for specific cases of uveitis in humans [16]. Hence the results of the ERU studies could have direct application to human uveitis. Yet in the broader context, we project that delineating infectious/immune interaction in leptospiral ERU can impact understanding of the immunopathogenesis of other infectious/immune uveitides.

ACKNOWLEDGMENTS

This work was supported by NIH grant EY068666 (CMK), Amer. Soc. Vet. Ophthalmol. (AED) and an unrestricted grant from Research to Prevent Blindness, Inc. to the University of Rochester Department of Ophthalmology.

REFERENCES

1. Forrester JV. Eye 1992; 6: 433-446.
2. Wacker WB. Invest Ophthalmol Vis Sci 1991; 32: 3119-3128.
3. Nussenblatt RB. Invest Ophthalmol Vis Sci 1991; 32: 3131-3141.
4. Thompson HSG, Staines NA. Immunol Today 1990; 11: 396-399.
5. Schwink KL. Vet Clin North Amer [Equine Practice] 1992; 8: 557-574.
6. Witmer R. Amer J Ophthalmol 1954; 37: 243-253.
7. Roberts SJ. J Amer Vet Med Assoc 1958; 133: 189-195.
8. Williams RD, Morter RL, Freeman MJ, Lavignette AM. Invest Ophthalmol 1971; 10: 948-954.
9. Hines MT. Vet Clinics of N A [Large Animal Pract] 1984; 6: 501-512.
10. Jones TC. Amer J Vet Res 1942; 3: 45-71.
11. Kalsow CM, Turpin LC, Dwyer AE. Regional Immunol 1994 (In press).
12. Kalsow CM, Dwyer AE, Smith AW, Nifong TP. Curr Eye Res 1992; 11: 147-151.
13. Kalsow CM, Dwyer AE, Smith AW, Nifong TP. Brit J Ophthalmol 1993; 77: 46-48.
14. Hines MT, Halliwell REW. Prog Vet Comp Ophthalmol 1991; 1: 283-290.
15. Maxwell SA, Hurt D, Brightman AH, Takemoto D. Prog Vet & Comp Ophthalmol 1991; 1: 155-162.
16. Duke-Elder S, Perkins ES. In: Duke-Elder S, eds. System of Ophthalmol. London: Kimpton, 1966; 322-325.

© 1994 Elsevier Science B.V. All rights reserved.
Advances in Ocular Immunology
R.B. Nussenblatt, S.M. Whitcup, R.R. Caspi and I. Gery, eds.

Murine Model of Seasonal Allergic Conjunctivitis (SAC) to Ragweed.

Jesús Merayo-Lloves MD and C. Stephen Foster MD, FACS.

Hilles Immunology Laboratory and the Immunology Service, Massachusetts Eye and Ear Infirmary, Department of Ophthalmology, Harvard Medical School, Boston, MA, USA.

Introduction

SAC is one of the atopic phenomena that affects the ocular surface and is manifested by symptoms of itching and burning in response to a variety of ubiquitous air borne allergens and by mild clinical signs of chemosis and conjunctival redness [1]. In order to assess the therapeutic value of anti-allergic drugs and to study the pathophysiology of SAC, it is necessary to develop experimental animals models which mimic the human disease. Models previously described [2] do not closely resemble human disease and were developed in animals with immune systems not as well characterized as human and mice. We hypothesized that mice can develop an ocular allergic conjunctivitis after exposure to an airborne allergen via nasal and conjunctival mucosae, and we speculated that pro-allergic cytokines IL4, IL5, and IL6 could be used as adjuvants for enhancing the allergic reaction.

Material and methods

Animals. Ten weeks old female BALB/CJ, C57BL/6J, A/HeJ, SWR/J and CH3/HeJ mice (Jackson Laboratories. Bar Harbor, ME).

Immunization. Short ragweed, 1.25 mg, Ambrosia artemisiifolia, (Internationals Biologicals, Piedmont, OK) were delivered into the nostrils and into the conjunctival sac with an Eppendorf micropipette on days 1 to 5.

On day 8 mice were challenged in the conjunctival cul de sac with 1.25 mg of ragweed pollen powder.

Adjuvants. 150 U of recombinant murine interleukin 4 (mIl4), 25 U of mIl5 and 2500 U of mIl6 (Genzyme, Boston, MA.) in 0.01M PBS-0.5%BSA, pH 7.2 were admistered *IP* before each immunization.

Groups of animals.

Groups(*)	Immunization	Challenge	Adjuvant (IL-4,5,6)
Control	No	No	No
Challenge	No	Yes	No
Experimental	Yes	Yes	No
EXP+IL(#)	Yes	Yes	Yes

(*) At least five animals in each group.
(#) Experimental group treated with cytokines as adjuvants

Evaluation. <u>Clinical signs:</u> Five clinical signs (Conjunctival redness and chemosis, lid swelling and redness, and mucus secretion) were judged under an operating microscope. The evaluation was performed masked at 20 minutes after allergen challenge, scoring on a scale of 0-4+. <u>Histology:</u> Orbits were exenterated and specimens were processed for light microscopy; 2.5μ sections were stained with Hematoxylin-Eosin, Periodic Acid-Schiff reaction and Alkaline Giemsa. The slides were evaluated at 400x and cells were counted in 3 fields with a micrometer ocular grid.

Data analysis. The differences among the groups for each parameter were analyzed by an ANOVA followed by the Student-Newman-Keuls test.

Results

Clinical signs. All animals exposed to ragweed developed clinical signs (conjunctival redness and edema) of allergy, and there were statistically significant differences between the experimental and control groups. SWR/J mice developed the most important clinical signs and the most impressive differences after the challenge.

Clinical Signs: Conjunctival Edema

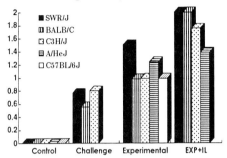

	Control	Challenge	Experimental	EXP+IL
SWR/J	0	0.75	1.50	2.0
	(0)	(0.45)	(0.52)	(0)
BALB/C	0	0.58	1.0	2.0
	(0)	(0.51)	(0)	(0.42)
C3H/J	0	0.91	1.0	1.75
	(0)	(0.28)	(0)	(0.46)
A/HeJ	0		1.37	1.4
	(0)		(0.51)	(0.54)
C57BL/6J	0		1.0	
	(0)		(0)	

Score of Conjunctival Edema: Mean (±SD)

Histology. Mice exposed and challenged with ragweed pollen developed an eosinophilic infiltration in the stroma closest to the epithelium, not found in the negative control and the challenge group. SWR/J strain develop the most impressive eosinophil response with significant differences with the other strains. No differences were found between the two experimental groups (treated with and without cytokines) and no significant differences were found in the number of mast cells and goblet cells.

Histology: Eosinophils/mm²

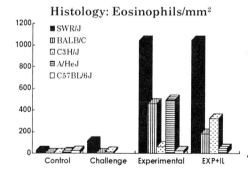

	Control	Challenge	Experimental	EXP+IL
SWR/J	7.1	36.6	397.3	363.8
	(9.7)	(81.8)	(316.2)	(382)
BALB/C	0	1.0	163.5	70.8
	(0)	(2.3)	(176.6)	(37.1)
C3H/J	0	3.5	20.7	114
	(0)	(7.9)	(28.4)	(82.3)
A/HeJ	4.7		179.2	14.2
	(11.6)		(56.4)	(31.8)
C57BL/6J	8.1		11.3	
	(15.4)		(17.8)	

Eosinophils /mm²: Mean (±SD)

Discussion

Mice developed clinical (conjunctival redness and edema) and histological (eosinophils) signs of SAC after exposure to an airborne allergen, ragweed pollen, and this findings are characteristic of human SAC [1]. The differences in the number of mast cells were not as striking possibly because they are totally degranulated and thus not visible by light microscopy [3]. No differences were found in the number of goblet cells, and it was reported that other mechanisms beside anaphylaxis are necessary for goblet cell degranulation [4]. The adjuvants at the dose and route used did not enhance the allergic response; no adjuvants were necessary to develop the conjunctival allergy. The most impressive response was obtained with female SWR/J mice. This murine model mimics human disease more closely than previously described animal models and can be valuable for further studies of the pathophysiology of SAC and for assays of antiallergic drugs.

Supported in part by Fondo de Investigación Sanitaria BAE 91/5005, PI 92/1111, PI 92/1277), Spain.

Reprint request: C. Stephen Foster, MD. Hilles Immunology Laboratory. Massachusetts Eye & Ear Infirmary. 243 Charles Street. Boston 02114.

References

1. Foster CS. Immunologic disorders of the conjunctiva, cornea and sclera. In: Albert DM, Jacobiec FA, eds. Principles and practice of ophthalmology. Vol I. Philadelphia: Saunders; 1994: 190-217.

2. Calonge M, Pastor JC, Herreras JM, González JL. Pharmacologic modulation of vascular permeability in ocular allergy in the rat. Invest Ophthalmol Vis Sci. 1990; 31: 176-180.

3. Allansmith R, Baird RS, Bloch KJ. Degranulation of ocular mast cells in rat undergoing systemic anaphylaxis. Invest Ophthalmol Vis Sci. 1980; 19: 1521-1254.

4. J Allergy Clin Immunol. 1985; 76: 200-206.

Advances in Ocular Immunology
R.B. Nussenblatt, S.M. Whitcup, R.R. Caspi and I. Gery, eds.

Corneal allograft rejection: Description of a new heterotopic murine model

A.R. de Toledo, M.A.M. Munarin and J.W. Chandler

Department of Ophthalmology and Visual Sciences, University of Illinois at Chicago, Chicago, IL, USA.

INTRODUCTION

Heterotopically transplanted corneas have been widely used to study various aspects of corneal allograft immunity in inbred strains of mice and rats. One of the main advantages to this approach is the ease with which the transplants can be performed. Orthotopical corneal transplantion in mice is quite difficult and the use of the subcutaneous pouch has proved to be a viable alternative. One of the limitations to these approaches are that the grafts are placed in a non-priviledge environment, which may be subjected to different physiological factors not present in the eye. Also, the sequential evaluations of the grafts is not feasible in subcutaneous abdominal pocket[1] and is impaired after 21 days in the subdermal thorax wall model[2] . With the subconjunctival heterotopic site, we tried to overcome the limitations of the previously described heterotopic sites in the mice and still take advantage of a technique that is easy to perform.

MATERIALS AND METHODS

Animals: Five to six week old C57BL/6 (H-2[b]) and BALB/c (H-2[d]) female mice were obtained from the Jackson laboratory (Benton Harbor, ME). Both strains served as donors and BALB/c mice were recipients in all cases. Animals were treated according to the ARVO resolution on the use of animals in research.

Transplant technique: Donor and recipient mice were anesthetized by intra-peritoneal injection of Ketamine hydrochloride 100 mg/Kg, and Xylazine 10 mg/Kg. Recipients mice also received topical Proparacaine 0.5% prior to conjunctival dissection. In order to facilitate the transplant procedure proptosis was induced by clamping a delicate hemostat to the lateral canthus. A small incision was made in the right eye starting at the midline perpendicular to the superior limbus with a micro-sharp knife. Subconjunctival dissection was carried out with a Vannas scissor towards the lateral canthus and a pocket was created to allow for the implantation of fresh excised corneal graft. Once the dissection was completed, donor mice were sacrificed by intra-peritoneal injection of sodium pentobarbital and corneal grafts measuring 1.5 mm in diameter were trephined and carefully positioned flat over the episclera with the endothelium facing down and allowed to heal by secondary intention. Bacitracin-neomycin-polymyxin ophthalmic ointment (E. Fougera) was applied once to both eyes immediately after the procedure. Syngeneic and allogeneic grafts recipients were sacrificed and had their eyes enucleated at 7, 11, 17 and 25 days and fixed in Tissue Tek OCT compound (Miles Laboratory) and snap-frozen in a dry ice/isopentane bath. Four micron sections were cut with a cryostat (IEC Minotome), placed on coated slides (Fisherbrand Superfrost Plus), and fixed for 15 seconds with room temperature acetone.

The slides were stored at -20°C until used. The section were stained by H&E and immunoperoxidase reaction.

<u>Hematoxylin and Eosin</u>: H & E stained sections were read in a masked fashion. A graft was recorded as not rejected if the graft contained no blood vessels or mononuclear cell infiltrates, was not edematous, and had intact epithelial and endothelial layers. In contrast, a graft was listed as rejected if it was vascularized, contained mononuclear cell infiltrates and the epithelial and endothelial cells were replaced by inflammatory cells.

<u>Immunoperoxidase reaction</u>: The slides were removed from the freezer, fixed in acetone (4°C) for 10 minutes, then allowed to air-dry at room temperature for 1 minute. The slides were washed twice for 15 minutes in 0.05 M Tris-saline pH 7.6, and incubated for 20 minutes with 50 μl of normal rabbit serum (NRS) diluted 1:5 in tris-saline containing 3% BSA, 0.25% gelatin, 5mM EDTA, and 0.025% NP-40 (BGEN). They were blotted dry and incubated with 50 μl of rat anti-mouse CD4 (L3T4), or rat anti-mouse CD8a (Ly-2), or rat-anti-mouse interferon-gamma. All primary monoclonal antibodies were obtained from Pharmigen and diluted 1:100 in BGEN. The slides were incubated either overnight at 4°C or for 1 hour at room temperature in a moisture chamber. Then the slides were washed in tris-saline for 10 minutes and then incubated with 50 μl of biotinylated rabbit anti-rat IgG (H and L, Vector Laboratories) diluted 1:150 in mouse skin extract. The slides were washed twice for 8 minutes in tris-saline, then incubated for 10 minutes in 3% H_2O_2 in methanol. They were then washed twice for 10 minutes in tris-saline and then incubated for 10 minutes with 50 μl of horseradish peroxidase strepavidin (Zymed Laboratories) diluted 1:100 in Tris-saline. The slides were washed twice for 20 minutes in Tris-saline, flooded with 3-amino-9-ethylcarbazol(AEC, Sigma) solution (1 ml of 4 mg/ml stock AEC in N, N-dimethylformamide, 14 ml 0.1 M sodium acetate buffer, pH 5.2, 150 μl 3% H_2O_2) and washed in distilled water for 2-3 minutes and counterstained with Meyer's hematoxylin (Sigma) for 3 minutes. Finally, the slides were overlaid with warm glycerin jelly (containing 8% gelatin, 50% glycerin) and coverslipped).

<u>Analysis</u>: The total number of positive stained cells were counted in an area of 1.04 mm² which included the graft and the surrounding tissue and were analyzed by analysis of variance.

RESULTS

Balb/cJ mice were selected as recipients based on preliminary studies, which demonstrated that the conjunctiva of C57BL/6J tended to be more friable upon manipulation and it has a certain luster which precluded ideal visualization of the grafts. Evaluation of the grafts was easily performed by mild proptosis of the globe. Although we have chosen to sacrifice the animals at each time point, sequential slit-lamp observation could be easily achieved. We have kept mice for over 90 days with no compromise in visualization of the graft. Table 1 shows the results of syngeneic and allogeneic grafts based on histological evaluation at four time periods. Most syngeneic grafts were clear at the time of sacrifice and it was common to see dilated conjunctival vessels surrounding, but not penetrating the grafts.

Table 1
Rejection of subconjunctival corneal grafts at four time periods.

Donor	Type of Evaluation	Days After Transplantation			
		7	11	17	25
Balb/cJ	H	0/5	0/8	0/8	1/7
C57Bl/6J	H	0/5	4/7	5/6	4/7

H = Histology; Balb/cJ were recipients in all experiments

Histologically, the donor corneal epithelium was intact and had a tendency to form a pseudo-cyst. The cysts were present from day seven and were lined by what we believe to be donor epithelial cells. At the lumen of the cyst a collection of exfoliated epithelial cells was observed in the majority of grafts that survived. The same was true for allogeneic grafts which did not experience rejection. The clinical manifestation of the pseudo-cyst was a bone-white looking material sitting on top of the graft which at times precluded reliable evaluation of the graft underneath.

Allogeneic grafts were associated with more intense vascularization of the conjunctiva particularly at days 11 and 17. Grafts that were experiencing rejection had an intense lymphocytic cellular infiltrate surrounding the graft and infiltrating the donor corneal stroma. The epithelium was either absent or quite disorganized with abundant vacuolated cells in all three epithelial cell layers. At 25 days, four out of seven allogeneic grafts survived (43%) and were indistinguishable from their syngeneic counterpart. An occasional OCT-fixed specimen was lost and the data in tables and the figures is based upon histological evaluation.

The sum of the mean number of CD4 and CD8 cells on syngeneic grafts were highest at seven days and steadily decreased thereafter. In the allogeneic transplanted mice, the sum of CD4 and CD8 cells peaked at 17 days and sharply decreased at 25 days (Fig.1). The difference between the sum of the mean number of cells in the syngeneic and allogeneic grafts was significant at 17 ($p < 0.0008$) and 25 ($p < 0.01$) days. CD8 cells accounted for the majority of positive stained cells at all four time points and comparing the total mean number of CD4 and CD8 cells over time the difference was significant at 17 ($p < 0.02$) and 25 ($p < 0.04$) days (Fig. 2).

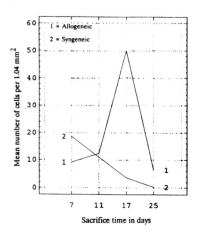

Figure 1. Total mean sum of CD4 and CD8 cells by type of transplant.

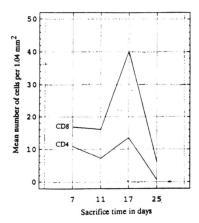

Figure 2. Total mean number of CD4 and CD8 cells over time.

114

The degree of cellular response of individual animals to the allogeneic graft challenge was variable as seen in (Fig. 3). Only three cells in this study stained positive for interferon gamma, which precludes any conclusions.

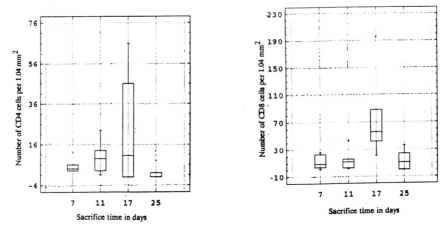

Figure 3. Variable cellular response by individual animals to allogeneic graft.

DISCUSSION

The strain of mice that we used has been widely studied in orthotopic and heterotopic corneal allograft rejection model and rejection rates of H-2, multiple minor H disparity has been well established by various studies[1-3]. The rate of rejection for allogeneic grafts at 11 and 17 days were similar to other published results. At 25 days, only 57% (4/7) rejected which is less than what has been previously reported. Due to the small number of animals in our study this issue has to be further addressed on a sequential study with larger sample size to verify if the pattern persist. The model also serve to demonstrate the dynamic of cells that migrates to the graft site. Both syngeneic and allogeneic grafts experience early invasion of CD4 and CD8 cells at day 7. On syngeneic grafts, the total number of stained cells gradually decreased over time probably due to insufficient signals to start the rejection process, while in allogeneic grafts the cell number continued to increase up to 17 days and then abruptly decreased. The model may prove to be beneficial in evaluating the effect of topical and systemic drugs in corneal allograft rejection.

This work was supported in part by NIH grant EY-07011 and an unrestricted grant from Research to Prevent Blindness, Inc.

REFERENCES

1   Ray-Keil, Chandler JW. Transplantation 1985; 39: 473-477.
2   Strelein JW, McCulley J, Niederkorn JY. Ivest Ophthalmol Vis Sci 1982; 23: 489-500.
3   Sonoda Y, Strelein JW. Transplantation 1992; 54: 694-704.

© 1994 Elsevier Science B.V. All rights reserved.
Advances in Ocular Immunology
R.B. Nussenblatt, S.M. Whitcup, R.R. Caspi and I. Gery, eds.   115

ALLOGENEIC GRAFT REJECTION IN A MURINE MODEL OF ORTHOTOPIC CORNEAL TRANSPLANTATION.

Choun-Ki Joo[1,4], Jay S. Pepose[1,2], Keith A. Laycock[1] and P. Michael Stuart[1,3].

Departments of Ophthalmology and Visual Sciences[1], Pathology[2], and Molecular Microbiology[3] , Washington University School of Medicine, 660 S. Euclid Avenue, St. Louis, MO 63110., Department of Ophthalmology, Catholic University Medical College, Seoul, Korea[4]

INTRODUCTION

Corneal transplantation can be divided into grafts that are placed into non-vascularized corneal beds and those that are placed into vascularized beds. In non-vascularized beds, the 5-year success rate is particularly impressive and may be as high as 90%. However in the latter case, the success rate can fall to 20 to 40% [1]. The murine cornea displays similar major histocompatibility (MHC) class I and II expression to that seen in human cornea as both demonstrate high levels of MHC class I antigen on epithelium and keratocytes and somewhat lower levels on corneal endothelium. Likewise, MHC class II$^+$ Langerhans cells in both human and murine corneas are located predominantly at the corneal limbus [2]. In the present study, we evaluated the pattern of allogeneic graft rejection in orthotopic corneal transplantation using mice which were mismatched at both major and minor histocompatibility antigens.

MATERIALS AND METHODS

Orthotopic Corneal Grafting

Female C57BL/6 (H-2^b) and BALB/c (H-2^d) mice, 7 to 10 weeks old, were purchased from the National Cancer Institute (Fredrick, MD). Mice were anesthetized by intraperitoneal injection of phenobarbital, 50 mg/kg. Donor corneal grafts were prepared by removing a central 2.0 mm corneal button from C57BL/6J mice (allogeneic graft) or from BALB/c mice (syngeneic graft) using an inner edged trephine and Vannas scissors (E2790, Storz, St. Louis, MO). The recipient corneal graft bed was prepared by removing a central 2.0 mm corneal button from BALB/c recipient mice using an outer edged trephine (SP7-50803, Storz, St. Louis, MO) and Vannas scissors. Once the graft bed was prepared, the donor corneal button was immediately applied to the graft bed and secured in place with 12 interrupted sutures (11-0 nylon, 70 μm diameter needle, Sharp-point; Vanguard, Houston, TX). Sutures were removed 7 days following surgery. At this time, recipient mice with signs of surgical complications such as hyphema, cataract, shallow or flat anterior chamber, or an opacity score of 4, were excluded from use in these studies.

Evaluation and Scoring of Orthotopic Cornea Transplants:

After transplantation, grafts were examined using a vertically oriented slit lamp biomicroscope at weekly intervals. At each time point, the corneal grafts were scored by two masked observers for opacity and neovascularization as described by Sonoda and Streilein [3]. In agreement with previous studies, we considered any corneal grafts with opacity score in excess of 2 to be undergoing a rejection reaction [3]. Mice with opacity score greater 2 eight weeks following the surgery were defined as having rejected the corneal graft, while those with opacity scores <2 at eight were defined as having accepted the corneal transplant.

RESULTS

Opacity scores for syngeneic and allogeneic grafts were indistinguishable at one week. Following one week, allogeneic C57BL/6 cornea grafts consistently displayed greater opacity scores than syngeneic BALB/c cornea grafts (Table 1). In allogeneic cornea grafts, a significant difference in opacity scores between those that accepted or rejected grafts was apparent by four weeks and these differences continued to the conclusion of the experiment (Table 1). The rate of corneal allograft rejection for this initial study was 42%, subsequent studies have demonstrated higher rejection rates that range from 55 to 65% (data not shown). It is interesting to note that corneal allografts, both those that are ultimately accepted and those that are rejected, demonstrate two general patterns of opacification during these studies.

TABLE 1: CLINICAL SCORE OF CORNEAL TRANSPLANTATION.

	Weeks					
	1	2	3	4	6	8
Opacity						
Allograft						
Rejected[1]	1.7+0.3	2.8+0.3	2.7+0.3	**2.7+0.3**[2]	3.0+0.2	3.5+0.3
Accepted[3]	1.7+0.2	2.6+0.3	2.4+0.2	2.0+0.2	1.3+0.2	0.9+0.2
Syngeneic graft[4]	1.4+0.4	1.3+0.4	0.8+0.6	0.5+0.3	0.3+0.3	0.7+0.4
Vascularity						
Allograft						
Rejected	3.3+0.3	5.7+0.3	6.6+0.4	6.1+0.4	6.7+0.3	6.9+0.3
Accepted	3.9+0.2	5.8+0.3	6.5+0.2	6.7+0.3	6.5+0.2	6.4+0.2
Syngeneic graft	5.0+0.3	4.5+0.5	4.4+0.5	5.1+0.5	5.1+0.5	5.4+0.2

[1]Rejected refers to those BALB/c mice whose C57BL/6 corneal grafts displayed an opacity score at 8 weeks that was >2, n= 17.

[2]Bold type refers to value that is significantly greater than accepted value, p<0.005.

[3]Accepted refers to those BALB/c mice whose C57BL/6 corneal grafts displayed an opacity score at 8 weeks that was <2, n= 24.

[4]Syngeneic graft refers to BALB/c mice engrafted with BALB/c corneas, n= 8.

Within both allograft groups, there were a significant number of mice that initially (within the first three weeks postengraftment) displayed opacity scores in excess of 2. This type of corneal opacity is probably due to an inflammatory response that may, or may not be a sign of allorecognition indicating that the corneal graft is experiencing a rejection episode. Following this early clouding of the cornea, those mice whose opacity scores are >2 at 8 weeks (82% of the rejected group) became progressively more cloudy, with the cornea becoming completely opaque (Group 3, Figure 1). Conversely, those mice whose corneas presented opacity scores <2 at 8 weeks (71% of the accepted group), became progressively less cloudy with time and were essentially clear by 8 weeks (Group 2, Figure 1). In addition to this pattern of opacity presented by mice which accept C57BL/6 corneal allografts, were those mice which never display an opacity score in excess of 2 at any time during these studies (29% of the accepted group), and thus never demonstrated any signs of inflammation (Group 1, Figure 1). The second opacity pattern displayed by those mice with opacity scores >2 at eight weeks (18% of the rejected group) was typified by opacity scores <2 until 4 weeks post engraftment, at which time the cornea rapidly became cloudy and remained cloudy until the termination of the experiment (Group 4, Figure 1). Examination of neovascularization indicated that at the time of suture removal (1 week following surgery),

the neovascularization scores ranged between 3 and 5 for both syngeneic and allogeneic grafts. Thereafter, the neovascularization score for both accepted and rejected C57BL/6 corneal allografts gradually increased until the end of the observation period. In contrast, BALB/c syngeneic corneal grafts did not demonstrate an increase in neovascularization following the first week of transplantation (Table 1). These data are in agreement with previous reports that accepted corneal grafts can display significant neovascularization.

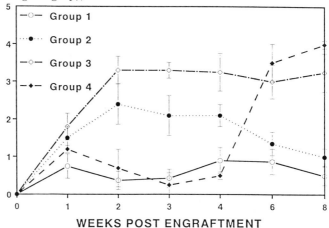

FIGURE 1. Graphic representation depicting the opacity scores of orthotopic allogeneic C57BL/6 corneal transplants into BALB/c mice. BALB/c mice, which were engrafted with C57BL/6 corneas, were divided into four groups based on the pattern of opacity scores observed. **Group 1** represents those BALB/c mice which never displayed an opacity score >2, n=7. **Group 2** are those BALB/c mice which initially had opacity scores >2, but later cleared up, n=17. **Group 3** represents those BALB/c mice which displayed opacity scores >2 within the first 3 weeks of the study and remained >2 throughout the study, n=14. **Group 4** are those BALB/c mice which remained clear through the fourth week of the study and then become cloudy (opacity scores >2) and remained so until the end of the study, n=3.

DISCUSSION

In these studies, BALB/c mice were recipients of either C57BL/6 allogeneic corneal grafts or BALB/c syngeneic corneal grafts. We chose these strains because previous studies [4], as well as our own, have shown that using C57BL/6 mice as graft recipients results in a 30-40% technical failure rate, as evidenced by hyphema, cataract, shallow or flat anterior chamber, or opacity score of 4 at the time of suture removal. In contrast, BALB/c recipients of C57BL/6 corneas presented a technical failure rate of 5-10%. In addition, BALB/c graft recipients displayed a more severe pattern of neovascularization than that seen with C57BL/6 graft recipients following corneal transplantation. It is interesting to note that clinical corneal transplants are sutured into either non-neovascularized or neovascularized recipient beds, with the latter carrying a higher risk of graft failure. Consequently, an animal model which displays a high degree of corneal neovascularization, such as seen when BALB/c mice are used as recipients of allogeneic corneal grafts, may mimic this important feature of "high risk" corneal transplantation.

The rejection rate (42%) in the present study was within the range previously reported by other investigators [3]. However subsequent experiments demonstrated a somewhat higher corneal allograft failure rate that ranges from 50 to 65%. As described earlier, most BALB/c mice engrafted with C57BL/6 corneas (83%) display some degree of corneal opacity during the 8 week observatation period. In contrast, only 20% of BALB/c mice engrafted with syngeneic BALB/c corneas displayed any corneal clouding. In many of the syngeneic corneal grafts, the opacity was restricted to the periphery of the transplant and may represent edema or non-specific inflammation in response to suture or surgical trauma. In the case of BALB/c mice engrafted with C57BL/6 corneas that are ultimately accepted by their hosts, we also observed an initial peripheral opacity near suture sites. However, this clouding of the cornea tended to be more severe and of longer duration (3-4 weeks compared with 1-2 weeks) with some involvement of the central regions of the cornea, in contrast to that observed for syngeneic corneal grafts. Because this pattern of corneal opacity in allogeneic transplants is distinct from that observed for syngeneic corneas, this suggests some form of allorecognition is taking place. Thus, the temporary opacity observed in BALB/c mice that ultimately accept C57BL/6 corneal allografts is likely a mild self limited rejection reaction that does not ultimately lead to graft failure.

References

1. Council on Scientific Affairs. Report of the Organ Transplant Panel: Corneal Transplantation. JAMA. 1988; 259:719-722.
2. Rodrigues MM, Rowden G, Hackett J, Bakos I. Inves Ophthal Vis Sci. 1981 21:759-765
3. Sonoda,Y. and J. W. Streilein. Transplantation. 1992; 54:694-704
4. He, Y., Ross, J., and Niederkorn, J. Y., Inves Ophthal Vis Sci. 1991; 32:2723-2728

Advances in Ocular Immunology
R.B. Nussenblatt, S.M. Whitcup, R.R. Caspi and I. Gery, eds.

T-CELL RECEPTOR ß-CHAIN VARIABLE GENE EXPRESSION AT THE SITE OF RPE CELL REJECTION IN THE RAT MODEL

L. Kohen,[a,b] G. Pararajasegaram,[a] John X. Qian,[a] S. Kohen,[a] P. Wiedemann,[b] S. J. Ryan[a] and N. A. Rao[a]

[a]Doheny Eye Institute and Department of Ophthalmology, University of Southern California School of Medicine, Los Angeles, California 90033, USA

[b]Department of Ophthalmology, University of Leipzig, 04103 Leipzig, Germany

INTRODUCTION

The underlying mechanism of rejection of transplanted retinal pigment epithelial (RPE) cells has not been studied in detail. We evaluated T-cell receptor (TCR) Vß expression at the site of rejection after RPE transplantation in a rat model of RPE rejection. TCR Vß expression was evaluated also in control eyes after RPE transplantation.

MATERIAL AND METHODS

Rat Model of RPE Rejection

The model used has been described elsewhere (1). Because transplantation of RPE in rats does not usually result in rejection(2), we sensitized the recipient rats with skin transplants two weeks prior to RPE transplantation(3). The skin donors are of the same strain as are the RPE donors. In a preliminary study using these skin transplantation-sensitized rats, transplanted RPE cells were rejected in all eyes within seven days after RPE transplantation.

Animals

Male inbred Lewis rats weighing 150-175 g (7-9 weeks old) were used as recipients or T-cell donors. The animals were divided into two groups. Group I (n=7): skin transplantation-sensitized, followed by RPE transplantation; Group II (n=7): RPE transplantation without prior sensitization (control group). The RPE and skin donors were 9-12-day-old Long Evans rats. In addition, five rats served as T-cell donors for PHA stimulation as control for the polymerase chain reaction (PCR) process.

Surgery

A 1-2 cm² segment of skin from a Long Evans rat was transplanted into the back of each Lewis rat of Group I. Skin was removed from the recipient and replaced by the donor skin, which was attached with 4.0 silk sutures. The transplanted skin was rejected within 9-11 days, indicating that sensitization had been achieved.

The separation of RPE was performed as described by Mayerson(4). In brief, following euthanasia, the eyes of Long Evans rats were enucleated and treated first with hyaluronidase and collagenase and then with trypsin to release the RPE sheets from their attachment. The RPE cells were cultured for 2-6 days prior to transplantation.

RPE cells (40,000-60,000/l) harvested from culture were transplanted into the subretinal space of the right eye of each sensitized Lewis rat (Group I) and of each naive rat (Group II) according to the technique described by Li and Turner (2). Following surgery, fundus examination revealed sub- and intraocular bleeding in two animals each from Groups I and II. These eyes were excluded from further study.

Enucleation

Seven days after RPE transplantation, the rats from Groups I and II were sacrificed and the RPE transplanted eye was enucleated for further study.

T-cell separation and activation

Mononuclear cells were obtained by Ficoll-Paque centrifugation of the peripheral blood from five rats. A total of 4×10^6 mononuclear cells from each rat were cultured in the presence of 2 µg/ml PHA-P for 48 hours and then harvested.

Reverse transcriptase PCR and gene amplification

The RNA of the whole eyes (Groups I and II) and of the T-cells was extracted by homogenation of the tissue or cells in RNAZol (Tel-Test, Friendswood, TX). cDNA synthesis and PCR amplification were carried out as described previously(5). Individual upstream rat TCR Vß sense sequence primers specific for TCR Vß families 1-20 were used for PCR and downstream C region primer(6) .

Southern blotting and hybridization were performed according to standard procedures(7). An ECL gene detection system (Amersham, Arlington Heights, IL) was used for ECL visualization.

RESULTS

Two eyes in each group were excluded from study because of intraocular bleeding.

Eyes of four of the five rats that underwent skin transplantation and the RPE transplantation (Group I) showed TCR Vß expression. Three of these eyes showed only limited expression of Vß 19, while the other eye expressed Vß 17 in addition to Vß 19.

In Group II, rats that were not sensitized prior to RPE transplantation, two of the five eyes showed TCR Vß 19 expression; no other TCR Vßs were expressed. The other three eyes showed no Vß expression.

When PHA-stimulated lymphocytes of Lewis rats were used as control for the PCR, they showed expression of all major Vß families.

DISCUSSION

There have been reports of restricted involvement of the TCR repertoire in the rejection of human kidney and cardiac allografts(8,9,10). In a rat (ACI to LEW) cardiac allograft rejection model, a limited repertoire of TCR Vß genes was observed; in the early stages (three days) of this rejection, the predominant expression was Vß 4(11).

In the present study, expression of TCR Vß 19 in four of five eyes in Group I indicate that there is restricted expression of TCR at the site of rejection.

In spite of the potential for nonspecific expression of TCR Vß due to the use of a non-inbred strain of rat as donors of skin and RPE, the Vß expression was very restricted. This restriction suggests that selective therapy, such as T-cell targeted immunotherapy, might prevent RPE transplantation rejection. Similar therapies have been successful in the prevention of some autoimmune diseases(12).

As mentioned at the outset, transplantation of RPE in non-sensitized rats does not cause a histologically obvious rejection. However, even though non-sensitized rats do not show histologic evidence of rejection following transplantation of RPE, TCR analysis demonstrated the presence of Vß 19 in two of five eyes in the present study. This might be an indication of histologically non-obvious rejection.

Further characterization of the mechanism of recognition of allograft antigen by TCR is required before selective treatment strategies to prevent rejection can be developed.

REFERENCES

1   Kohen L, Nishi M, Hall MO, Gabrielian K, et al. Invest Ophthalmol Vis Sci 1993; 34: 1095.

2   Li L, Turner JE. Exp Eye Res 1988; 47: 771-785.

3   Khodadoust AA, Silverstein AM. Invest Ophthalmol Vis Sci 1969; 8: 180-195.

4   Mayerson PL, Hall MO, Clark V, Abrams T. Invest Ophthalmol Vis Sci 1985; 26: 1599-1609.

5   Rao NA, Naidu YM, Bell R, Lindsey JW, et al. J Immunol 1993; 150: 5716-5721.

6   Gold DP, Vainiene M, Celnik B, Wiley S, et al. J Immunol 1992; 148: 1712-1717.

7   Maniatis T, Fritsch EF, Sambrook J. Molecular Cloning: A Laboratory Manual. New York: Cold Spring Harbor Laboratory Press, 1982.

8   Micelli MC, Finn OJ. J Immunol 1989; 142: 81-86.

9   Colvin B, Kurnick JT. Hum Immunol 1990; 28: 208.

10   Hand SL, Hall BL, Finn OJ. Hum Immunol 1990; 28: 82-95.

11   Shirwan H, Chi D, Makowka L, et al. J Immunol 1993; 151: 5228-5238.

12   Zaller DM, Osman G, Kanagawa O, Hood L. J Exp Med 1990; 171: 1943.

Advances in Ocular Immunology
R.B. Nussenblatt, S.M. Whitcup, R.R. Caspi and I. Gery, eds.

AN IMMUNOPATHOLOGICAL STUDY OF AUTOIMMUNE KERATITIS IN THE RAT THYMUS GRAFTED NUDE MOUSE MODEL

T. Asatani[1], R. Muramatsu[1], M. Usui[1] and O. Taguchi[2]

[1] Department of Ophthalmology, Tokyo Medical College Hospital, Tokyo, Japan

[2] Aichi Cancer Center Research Institute, Nagoya, Japan

INTRODUCTION

We have previously found that autoimmune diseases occur spontaneously in multiple organs, including the eye and lacrimal gland, in BALB/c nude mice that have received transplants of rat fetal thymus (TG nude mice) (1). In this murine model, dacryoadenitis and keratitis develop spontaneously. Analysis of this model may thus provide us understanding of the mechanism of autoimmune keratitis. In the present study, we observed the pathological changes of autoimmune keratitis in TG nude mice. In addition, we used immunohistochemical methods to search for the presence of autoantibodies to the cornea, and immunoblotting methods in attempting to identify the responsible corneal antigen in this murine model.

MATERIALS AND METHODS

Animals

Thymus grafted nude mice (TG nude mice): Fetal thymuses from 15-day-old F344 rats were transplanted beneath the renal capsules of 4-week-old BALB/c nude mice. Control mice: Lacrimal glands of normal BALB/c mice or normal BALB/c nude mice were removed to produce animals with keratoconjunctivitis sicca.

Pathology

Eyes of TG nude mice and control mice were enucleated and fixed in formalin. Samples were embedded in paraffin, sectioned, and stained with hematoxylin and eosin for pathological examination.

Detection of immune complex

The presence and localization of immunoglobulins and complement was determined by double staining method. Cryostat tissue sections of eyes of TG nude mice and control mice were fixed in acetone and incubated with a mixture of flourescein isothiocyanate (FITC)-conjugated anti-mouse IgG goat serum (diluted 1/100) (Cappel, Organon Teknika Corp., West Chester, PA), and rhodamine-conjugated anti-mouse complement goat serum (diluted 1/100) (Cappel, Organon Teknika Corp., West Chester, PA).

Detection of autoantibody

The presence of autoantibodies against antigens of normal murine cornea were determined immunohistochemically. Cryostat tissue sections of normal adult murine eyes were fixed in acetone and incubated with serum from TG nude mice with keratitis (diluted 1/40), followed by incubation with FITC-conjugated anti-mouse IgG goat serum (diluted 1/100)

Detection of cornea-specific antigens

Cornea-specific antigens of the normal murine cornea were identified using autoantibody of TG nude mice. Corneal buttons of normal BALB/c mice were homogenized in 0.01 mM Tris-HCl (pH 7.4) using a homogenizer. After centrifugation three times (first; 700 g for 10 min. second; 7,000 g for 10 min. third; 100,000 g for 60 min.), supernatants were collected and concentrated. These corneal extracts were separated by electrophoresis, and transferred to nitrocellulose membranes. Immunoblot analysis was carried out using a Vectastain ABC kit according to the manufacturer's protocol. Sera from TG nude mice with keratitis were used as the primary antibody for detection of cornea-specific antigens. Sera from normal BALB/c mice were used as the primary antibody for a negative control.

RESULTS

Clinical appearance

The transplanted rat thymuses did not get rejected, and showed normal development. In these mice, dacryoadenitis and keratitis developed spontaneously. Keratitis appeared in 20 percent of TG nude mice at 1 month, and in 70 percent of TG nude mice at 2 months, following rat thymus transplantation. Microscopic examination of these eyes showed irregular corneal surfaces, marked corneal neovascularization and stromal opacification (Fig. 1). The control mice, in contrast, showed only slight corneal neovascularization.

Pathology

Hematoxylin and eosin staining of the cornea from TG nude mice with keratitis revealed marked inflammation involving lymphocytic infiltration, stromal neovascularization and keratinized superficial epithelial cells (Fig. 2). No inflammatory cells were present in the corneas of control mice, although mild subepithelial neovascularization was observed.

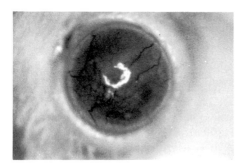

Fig. 1; Keratitis in TG nude mice
(anterior segment photo).

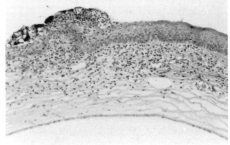

Fig. 2; Keratitis in TG nude mice
(hematoxylin and eosin staining).

Detection of immune complex

Deposition of IgG was localized in the subepithelial stroma along the basement membrane and in the anterior stroma in the inflammed corneas of TG nude mice. The strongest stainings were observed in the subepithelial stroma along the basement membrane. Deposition of complement in the cornea of TG nude mice with keratitis showed the same localization as with IgG (Fig. 3). In control animals, neither deposition of IgG nor complement were observed.

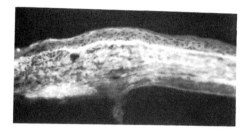 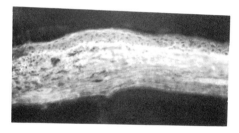

Fig.3; Deposition of IgG and complement (left; IgG localization using FITC. right; complement localization using rhodamine).

Detection of autoantibody

Sera from TG nude mice reacted with normal murine cornea in three patterns: in only the epithelial layer, in only the stromal layer, in both layers (Fig. 4). Sera from control mice did not react with normal murine cornea.

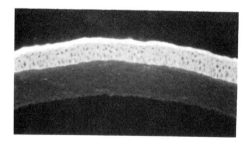 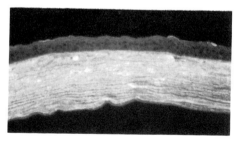

Fig. 4; Reactivity of sera from TG nude mice to normal murine cornea (left; autoantibody against epithelium. right; autoantibody against stroma).

Detection of cornea-specific antigens

Immunoblotting assay under non-reducing conditions showed that a soluble 185 kD protein from normal murine cornea was recognized by TG nude mouse serum that, by indirect immunofluorescence staining, had reacted in the epithelial layer only. With immunoblotting under reducing conditions, 42, 47, 49, and 50 kD proteins were recognized by the same serum. On the other hand, TG nude mouse serum that had reacted only in the stromal layer by indirect immunofluorescence identified no specific antigens in normal murine cornea (Fig. 5).

126

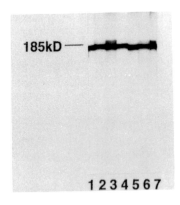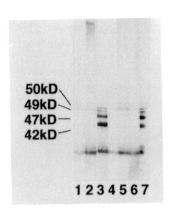

Fig. 5; Immunoblot analysis (left; non-reducing conditions. right; reducing conditions):
line 1; serum from normal BALB/c mouse. line 2; serum from lacrimal gland-excised BALB/c
mouse. lines 3, 7; serum from TG nude mouse that had reacted only with the epithelial layer.
lines 4, 5, 6; serum from TG nude mouse that had reacted only with the stromal layer.

DISCUSSION

We have previously described our TG nude mouse model for experimental autoimmune
disease, involving the transplantation of fetal rat thymuses in BALB/c nude mice originally
lacking in T cell function (1). The grafted thymuses seemingly undergo normal development
with production of lymphocytes, macrophages and dendritic cells. However, the thymic
epithelium in these animals is rat in origin, not mouse. The TG nude mouse spontaneousely
develops severe multi-organ autoimmune disease, including thyroiditis, gastritis, oophritis,
orchitis, prostatitis, uveoretinitis (2), dacryoadenitis and keratitis.

Light microscopic examination of eyes of TG nude mice with keratitis revealed
neovascularization and lymphocytic/neutrophilic infiltration in the corneal epithelium and
stroma. We hypothesized that autoantibodies to corneal antigen may be responsible for the
inflammation in this disease model. Thus we conducted further experiments, using
immunohistochemical and immunoblotting techniques, and were able to detect autoantibodies
against normal murine cornea, deposition of immune complex in the inflammed cornea, and
antigens in the normal murine corneal epithelium that are recognized by autoantibodies from the
TG nude mouse. These results strongly support the idea that keratitis in the TG nude mouse
depends on an autoimmune mechanism of disease, and thus may prove useful as an
experimental model for autoimmune forms of human corneal disease.

REFERENCES

1. Taguchi O, Takahashi T, Nishizuka Y. J Exp Med 1986; 164: 60-71.
2. Ichikawa T, Taguchi O, Takahashi T et al. Clin Exp Immunol 1991; 86: 112-117.

© 1994 Elsevier Science B.V. All rights reserved.
Advances in Ocular Immunology
R.B. Nussenblatt, S.M. Whitcup, R.R. Caspi and I. Gery, eds.

Transfer of the human lymphocytes from uveitis patients into severe combined immunodeficiency(SCID) mice.

Yoh-Ichi Kawano, Yuko Nishioka and Hiroki Sanui.

Department of Ophthalmology, School of Medicine, Kyushu University, 3-1-1 Maidashi, Higashi-ku, Fukuoka 812, JAPAN

INTRODUCTION

The CB.17 scid/scid(SCID) mouse strain lack both functional T and B cells[1]. These mice are permissive for survival and growth of transferred xenogeneic human peripheral blood leukocytes(PBL)[2-3]. It has been reported that PBL from patients of several autoimmune diseases produce autoantibodies of the same specificity in SCID mice. These recipients usually do not develop clinical disease although some histological lesions suggestive of autoimmunity were found[4-6].
The development of clinical and histological disease in SCID mice by the local transfer of T lymphocytes from CSF of multiple sclerosis patients was reported[7] and was attrributed to the recognition of mouse CNS antigen by human pathogenic cells in vivo. Thus, the SCID mice might be a tool to study organ specific autoimmune diseases of human.
We transferred PBL from patients of several types of endogenous uveitis into SCID mice in attempt to induce ocular disease in the recipient mice as an in vivo model of human uveitis.

MATERIALS AND METHODS

Animals
C.B.-17scid/scid mice were bred in the animal facility of Kyushu University in germ free conditions. 8 to 12 weeks old female mice were used for the experiments.
Isolation of peripheral blood leukocytes (PBL) from Uveitis patients.
40 ml of heparinized peripheral blood were collected from uveitis patients with active ocular inflammation before treatment. Mononuclear cell fraction was separated by gravity sedimentation method with Ficoll-Paque solution.
Systemic transfer of human PBL into SCID mice
As a systemic transfer experiment, 4×10^7 of human PBL from one patient were injected intraperitoneally into one SCID mouse. Eyes were examined clinically and enucleated 4 weeks after transfer for the

histological or immunohistochemical study. Sera of these recipients were collected for ELISA assay.

Local transfer of PBL into SCID mice

Mice were anesthesized with sodium pentobarbital. After paracentesis with 30G needle, 4×10^5 of PBL were injected intravitreally in a volume of $4\mu l$ under the operation microscope. The eyes with apparent lens injury or vitreous bleeding during this procedure were excluded from the experimental group. Enucleation for the histological or immunohistochemical study was done 7days after transfer . The numbers of mice and donor patients are summarized in table1.

Immunohistochemistry

Eyes were fixed and embedded in paraffin, and sections were stained with antibody against human CD45RO antigen(UCHL-1) by ABC(avidine-biotin horseradish peroxidase complex) method.

Enzyme linked immunosorbent assay

The concentration of human or mouse immunogloblin in SCID mice sera were measured by "sandwich" ELISA assay using goat anti human or mouse Ig(G+A+M) antibody(Cappel).

Table 1. The number of the donor patients and the mice used in this study

	No. of the patients	No. of the mice systemically transferred	No. of the eyes locally transferred
Behcet's disease	6	8	6
VKH*	6	9	6
Sarcoidosis	3	3	7
Acute anterior uveitis	2	2	5
Control(healthy donor)	3	3	5

*Vogt-Koyanagi-Harada syndrome

RESULTS AND DISCUSSION

In the systemic transfer experiments, the levels of human immunogloblins in all recipient SCID mice sera were considerably elevated (data not shown). Recipients of systemically transferred PBL did not show ocular changes, with the exception of one mouse, transferred with the PBL from the 40 years old Behct's disease patient whose PBL were collected when he suffered severe ocular attack with hypopyon formation in the anterior segment and large retinal exudate with optic nerve involvement in the ocular fundus. The left cornea of the recipient SCID mouse became cloudy by the clinical examination 21 days after the transfer . Histological examination of that eye showed

129

infiltration of inflammatory cells in the anterior segment(Fig. B) . The infiltrated cells in the anterior segment were polymorphonuclear leukocytes which were thought to be originated from mouse because they were different lineage from the transferred mononuclear cells[8]. Repeated experiments with PBL from the same donor caused no ocular change in SCID mice.

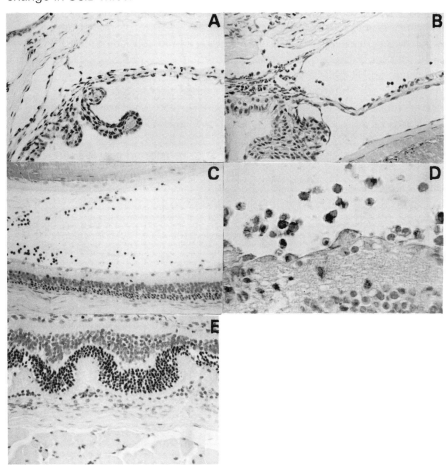

Figure. Microphotograph of anterior segment of the eye from SCID mouse transferred i.p. with the PBL from the healthydonor(A) and the inflamed eye of the mouse transferred i.p. with the PBL from the Behcet's disease patient(B).
Microphotographs of the eye locally transferred with the PBL from sarcoidosis patient(C) and its immunohistochemical staining with UCHL-1 antibody(D). Microphotographs of the eye locally transferred with the PBL from VKH patient(E).

The eyes locally transferred with the human PBL got inflamed 2 or 3 days after the injection by the clinical examination. Histological examination showed cellular infiltration in the vitreous cavity(Fig. C) and the anterior segment of the eye, with various degrees of the destruction of the retina. There were no significant differences in the clinical and histological findings between the recipients of the PBL from healthy donor and from uveitis patients. The infiltrating cells in the vitreous cavity consisted of polymorphonuclear cells and mononuclear cells, which were positive for UCHL-1 (Fig. D). The locally transferred human PBL probably caused host reaction mediated by residual cells in SCID mice such as NK cells and polymorphonuclear cells[9]. In addition, the human PBL could have reacted against mouse tissue. It was noteworthy that 2 eyes transferred with the PBL from VKH patients showed subretinal cellular infiltrates with choroidal thickening(Fig. E), a feature which was not seen in the eyes transferred with the PBL from healthy and other types of uveitis donors. As the choroid and RPE are usually affected in the eyes of VKH syndrome, there is a possibility that some pathogenic cells in the PBL of the patients accumulated around RPE and choroid in SCID mice. Further modification of experimental procedure, such as the suppression of non specific reaction between host and graft, might be necessary to clarify the disease specific change in the eye.

REFERENCES

1   Bosma GC, Custer RP, Bosma MJ. Nature 1983;310:523-530.
2   Moiser DE, Gulizia RJ, Baird SM, et al. Nature 1988;335:256-259
3   McCune JM, Namikawa R, Kaneshima H, Shultz LD, Lieberman M, Weissman IL. Science 1988;241:1632-1639.
4   Krams SM,Dorshkind K, Gershwin ME. J Exp Med 1989;170:1919-1930
5   Duchosal MA, McConahey PJ, Robinson CA, Dixon FJ. J Exp Med 1990; 172:985-988.
6   Machat L, Fukuma N, Leader K, et al. Clin Exp Immunol 1991;84:34-42.
7   Saeki Y, Mima T, Sakoda S, Fujimura H, Arita N, Nomura T, Kishimoto T. Proc Natl Acad Sci 1992;89:6157-6161.
8   Simpson E, Farrant J, Chandler P. Immunol Rev 1991;124:97-111.
9   Dorshkind K, Keller GM, Phillips RA, Miller RG, Bosma GC, et al. J Immunol 1984;132:1804-1808.

Advances in Ocular Immunology
R.B. Nussenblatt, S.M. Whitcup, R.R. Caspi and I. Gery, eds.

Transgenic rat and mouse models for studying the role of gamma interferon and MHC class II in intraocular diseases and autoimmunity

Charles E. Egwuagu[1], Jorge Sztein[3], Chi-Chao Chan[1], Rashid Mahdi[1], Robert B. Nussenblatt[1] and Ana B. Chepelinsky[2]

Laboratories of [1]Immunology and [2]Molecular and Developmental Biology; [3]Veterinary Research and Resources Section, National Eye Institute, National Institutes of Health, Bethesda, Maryland 20892, U.S.A.

Introduction

Gamma interferon (γIFN) is exclusively synthesized by activated T lymphocytes and natural killer (NK) cells [1]. It promotes growth and differentiation of leukocytes and plays a crucial role in the ontogenesis and phenomenology of the immune response [2]. It has potent immunomodulatory and antiproliferative effects on tumor cells [3]. Due to the pleiotropic effects of γIFN, it is becoming increasingly clear that this lymphokine may have functions that extend beyond its well recognized influence on cells of the immune system. Transgenic mice with ectopic expression of γIFN in pancreatic islet cells have been reported [4]. These mice developed insulin-dependent diabetes mellitus as a result of inflammatory destruction of the islets. Interpretation of these results is complicated by the possible synergism of γIFN with other lymphokines in the peripheral blood and by the inability to discriminate between effects due to the expression of the γIFN transgene from those due to secretion of the endogenous γIFN by T lymphocytes. We find the avascular lens to be ideally suited for studying the in vivo effects of γIFN on nonimmunological tissues and in particular during embryonic ocular development.

Results

We derived one FVB/N and one BALB/c transgenic mouse lines with expression of murine γIFN in the lens under the direction of the lens-specific αA-crystallin promoter [5,6]. The recombinant DNA construct used for generating the transgenic animals is shown in Figure 1. The FVB/N mouse strain is routinely used for the generation of transgenic mice due to the large pronucleus of its fertilized eggs, which facilitates the DNA microinjection. However, this strain has congenital retinal degeneration and as such it is not particularly suitable for studies involving the retina. The BALB/c mouse strain was chosen because it has a normal lens and retina, the genetics of its MHC locus is well defined and because it is resistant to the induction of experimental autoimmune uveoretinitis (EAU).

In both αA-Cry/γIFN transgenic mouse lines, ectopic expression of γIFN in the lens affected the growth of the whole eye, resulting in microphthalmia and blepharophimosis (Figure 2). Lens differentiation was severely affected [7] resulting in microphakia, impairment of lens fiber formation and cataract, thickening of the anterior lens capsule and rupture of the posterior capsule. Retardation of retinal differentiation into inner and outer neuroblastic layers was observed in the transgenic eyes [7]. Serous retinal detachment with presence of macrophages in the subretinal space, persistent hyperplastic primary vitreous,

αACry-γIFN

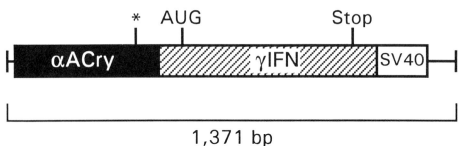

Figure 1: Diagram of the αA-Cry/γIFN DNA construct used for generating the transgenic mice and rats. It contains the murine γIFN coding sequence (hatched bar) under the control of the murine αA-crystallin promoter (solid bar). Empty bar: SV40 polyadenylation signal. *: initiation site of transcription. AUG: initiation codon. Stop: termination codon. See reference [7] for details.

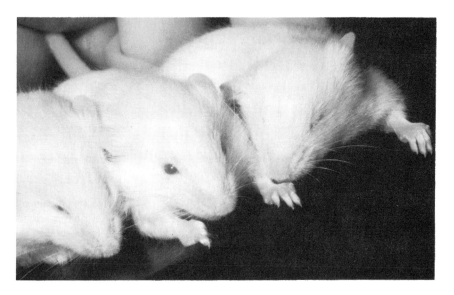

Figure 2. Eye phenotypes of αA-Cry/γIFN [BALB/c] (left), αA-Cry/γIFN [FVB/N] transgenic (right) and WT (center) mice.

corneal vascularization and absence of a normal anterior chamber was observed in the adult transgenic mice [8] (Figure 3).

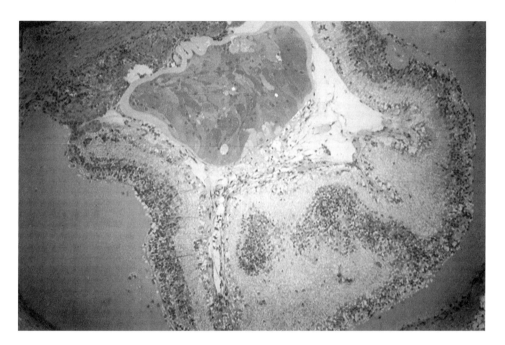

Figure 3: Photomicrograph of an αA-Cry/γIFN [FVB/N] adult transgenic mouse eye.

We also derived a transgenic Sprague Dawley rat line using the same murine αA-crystallin/γIFN construct shown in Figure 1. The transgenic rat eyes, similarly to those from the transgenic mice, present microphthalmia and microphakia with cataract formation. However, in contrast to the transgenic mice, the anterior chamber of the transgenic rat eye is well formed and the architecture of the retina is intact with focal retinal serous detachment. Because of the relatively better preserved ocular structure, the transgenic rat serves as a more suitable animal model for the study of autoimmune diseases.

MHC class II mRNA levels were significantly increased in the transgenic mouse eyes and MHC class II proteins were expressed in their cornea, iris, ciliary body, choroid, lens and RPE [8]. At the molecular level, expression of genes coding for γIFN-inducible transcription factors, interferon consensus sequence binding protein (ICSBP) [9] and interferon response factor 2 (IRF-2) [10], absent in the normal eye, were induced in the transgenic eyes. These results indicate that the ectopically expressed transgenic γIFN is biologically active in vivo.

Conclusions

In our initial studies of the αACry-γIFN transgenic mice and rats, we have focused on the effects of the transgene on lens and retinal morphogenesis and have started the molecular analysis of its effect on gene expression in the lens. The αA-Cry/γIFN transgenic rat is the first transgenic rat strain generated for vision research. This model is of particular interest as the rat is a well characterized species for EAU studies.

To fully understand the mechanism by which γIFN disrupts the developmental program of the eye, it would be useful to study the transcription factors induced by γIFN in the eye and how these factors synergise with or antagonize other cytokines (e.g. bFGF, PDGF, TGFβ) in cellular signalling during embryonic eye development.

Constitutive expression of γIFN, and its induction of MHC class II molecules in the eye, provides a useful model to study: 1) the linkage between aberrant MHC class II expression and predisposition to autoimmunity; 2) the role of γIFN in the treatment of inflammatory eye diseases and in ACAID (anterior chamber associated immune deviation); 3) cytokine signalling during embryonic eye development.

Taken together, the αA-cry/γIFN[FVB/N], αA-cry/γIFN[BALB/c] and αA-cry/γIFN [SD-Rat] transgenic animals represent a comprehensive transgenic model system for elucidating the in vivo effects of γIFN in the eye and for testing whether aberrant regulation and expression of MHC class II in a nonimmunological tissue such as the vertebrate lens would predispose mammals to autoimmune disease development.

References

1   Gray PW, Goeddel DV. Lymphokines. 1987; 13: 151-162.
2   Billiau A, Dijkmans R. Biochem. Pharmacol. 1990; 40: 1433-1439.
3   Sonnenfeld G, Mandel A, Merigan TC. Cell. Immunol. 1987; 40: 285-293.
4   Sarvetnick N, Liggitt D, Pitts SL, Hansen SE, Stewart TA. Cell 1988; 52: 773-782.
5   Chepelinsky AB, King CR, Zelenka PS, Piatigorsky J. Proc. Natl. Acad. Sci. U.S.A. 1985; 82: 2334-2338.
6   Overbeek PA, Chepelinsky AB, Khillan JS, Piatigorsky J, Westphal H. Proc. Natl. Acad. Sci. U.S.A. 1985; 82: 7815-7819.
7   Egwuagu CE, Sztein J, Chan C-C, Mahdi R, Nussenblatt RB, Chepelinsky AB. Dev. Biol. (in press)
8   Egwuagu CE, Sztein J, Chan C-C, Reid R, Mahdi R, Nussenblatt RB, Chepelinsky AB. Invest. Ophthalmol. Vis. Sci. 1994; 35: 332-341.
9   Driggers PH, Ennist DL, Gleason SL, Mak MS, Levi B-Z, Flanagan JR, Appella E, Ozato K. Proc. Natl. Acad. Sci. U.S.A. 1990; 87: 3743-3747.
10   Harada H, Willison K, Sakakibara J, Miyamoto M, Fujita T, Taniguchi T. Cell 1990; 63: 303-312.

Advances in Ocular Immunology
R.B. Nussenblatt, S.M. Whitcup, R.R. Caspi and I. Gery, eds.

MHC class I expression contributes to the development of cataract in transgenic mice with ectopic expression of IFN-γ

Kathrin Geiger and Nora Sarvetnick

The Scripps Research Institute, Department of Neuropharmacology, La Jolla, Ca 92037, U.S.A.

Introduction

The proinflammatory cytokine IFN-γ is capable of activating macrophages, natural killer cells (NK), B and T cells, and it induces the expression of MHC class I and class II molecules [1, 2]. In the immune privileged eye, IFN-γ may have a specific role, the cytokine it antagonizes a major constitutive immunosuppressant, transforming growth factor beta (TGF ß), which contributes to the maintenance of the intraocular immune privilege [3-5].

We are studying the influence of IFN-γ on the intraocular microenvironment *in vivo*, using a transgenic approach. By creating a transgenic mouse with expression of IFN-γ in the photoreceptor cells of the retina (rhoγ) we demonstrated that the cytokine altered the ocular morphology by inducing cellular infiltration of the whole eye, cataract and photoreceptor damage [6]. Furthermore, IFN-γ expression caused the disturbance of the blood-retina barrier, the loss of the intraocular immune privilege [Geiger, 1994 #661; Geiger et al. submitted for publication] and protected transgenic mice from intraocular infection with HSV-1 [7]. These rhoγ mice also developed expression of MHC class I and class II on cells of the retina which may be responsible for the observed retinal damage [6]. Interestingly, the lack of MHC class I or class II also elicited the disturbance of the intraocular immune privilege by allowing the development of a delayed type hypersensitivity reaction (DTH) [8, Geiger et al. submitted for publication].

To obtain further information about the relationship between transgenic expression of IFN-γ and the expression of MHC molecules, we now crossed rhoγ transgenic mice with mice deficient in MHC class I or class II. This approach allowed us to study the effect of IFN-γ induced expression of MHC molecules on the development of pathology in the eyes of rhoγ transgenic mice.

Material and methods

Mice : We used C57BL/6-derived b2m null mice, which do not express a functional MHC class I molecule, and I-Aß null mice, which are deficient in MHC class II expression. These mice were crossed with BALB/c derived rhoγ mice. The MHC deficient F2 offspring was then backcrossed to mice of the C57BL/6 background for at least 3 generations. Mice with MHC class I or class II deficiency, and mice in which these traits were combined with the rhoγ transgene, were studied by histology and immunohistochemistry at 4, 6-8, and 12 weeks of age. We examined at least 8 mice per group. All procedures adhered to the NIH guidelines. Transgene expression and knockout of MHC genes were confirmed by PCR of tail DNA (Lee at al. to be published elsewhere). MHC deficiency was additionally tested by immunocytochemistry with antibodies against MHC class I and II, CD4 (L3T4) and CD8 (LY2) cells.

Histology and immunocytochemistry : Both eyes and the brains of test mice were either fixed in 10% zinc formalin and embedded in paraffin, or snap frozen in OCT compound. Sections were stained with hematoxylin-eosin or periodic acid-Schiff (PAS). For immunocytochemistry, frozen serial sections, 6 μm thick, were fixed in cold acetone and then immunostained by using the indirect avidin-biotin-peroxidase complex method (Vector Laboratories). Primary antibodies were applied at a concentration of 5 μg/ml. [Polyclonal HSV-1 (Dako), monoclonal H-2, LY2, L3T4, NK, LFA-1, MAC-1 (Pharmingen), monoclonal Ia (Boehringer Mannheim)]. Diaminobenzidine (DAB) 0.05%, 0.04% nickel sulfate, 0.02% hydrogen peroxide or Vector VIP served as chromogen. The sections were counterstained in hematoxylin 2 g/L or in methyl green 1.4 %/ PBS.

Results and discussion

Lack of MHC class I or class II does not alter the retinal morphology in rhoγ mice.
Rhoγ mice developed cellular infiltration of the whole eye during their second week of life, and showed inflammatory changes to the age of 8-9 weeks. Simultaneously with the first appearance of inflammatory cells these animals exhibited shortening of the outer photoreceptor segments and cataract, due to hyperproliferation of the lens epithelium. Subsequently, the photoreceptor damage increased until the photoreceptors disappeared at the age of 8 to 9 weeks. The infiltrating cells included natural killer cells (NK), macrophages and lymphocytes. MHC class I expression was evident on the photoreceptors of the retina. Weak staining was seen on the lens epithelium. MHC class II expression was observed on the retinal pigment epithelium, the radial glia and astrocytes, and on some cells of the lens epithelium. Constitutive class II expression in the iris and the ciliary body was enhanced.

MHC class I deficient mice had no CD8 cells and MHC class II deficient mice had only low numbers of CD4 cells as confirmed by immunostaining on spleen sections [9-11]. IFN-γ expressing mice, deficient in either class I or class II expression showed the same amount of cellular infiltration of the eye as did the MHC expressing rhoγ mice. The infiltrating cells consisted of NK cells, macrophages and few lymphocytes. MHC class I deficient mice, and mice with additional expression of IFN-γ had slightly more NK cells than mice of the other groups. CD4 or CD8 cells were not evident in the eyes of any group. There were no significant differences in the morphology of cornea, uvea and retina. The time course of photoreceptor loss was similar. In MHC class II deficient mice, the amount of cataract formation was not altered. However, in MHC class I deficient mice with additional expression of IFN-γ, the extent of lens epithelium hyperproliferation and the amount of cataract formation appeared lower. Approximately 20% of the animals had no cataract (Fig.1 A-C).

These results confirm the notion that CD4 and CD8 cells are not involved in the generation of retinal pathology in rhoγ mice. Furthermore, IFN-γ expression induces retinal pathology without simultaneous expression of both MHC classes in the retina.

Thus, we cannot exclude, that the ectopic expression of either MHC class is capable of inducing the activation of retinal pigment epithelium cells, possibly leading to an active destruction of the photoreceptor outer segments. However, it is far more likely that the photoreceptor damage observed in rhoγ mice is initiated by direct toxic effects of IFN-γ, similar to the damage observed in transgenic expression of the diphtheria toxin under the same promoter [12]. Furthermore, it has been shown that IFN-γ can induce the production of nitric oxide in the retinal pigment epithelium [13], which may have a role in creating photoreceptor damage. It has been suggested that MHC class II expression might contribute to the development of tissue damage in several diseases [14, 15], or that MHC class I expression might protect cells from unspecific killing [16, 17]. However, we have so far no indication that these mechanisms might be active in our model. The cellular infiltration of the eye consists of relatively high numbers of macrophages and NK cells, and is possibly linked to the induction of several adhesion molecules by IFN-γ [6], which was not significantly influenced by the expression of MHC molecules.

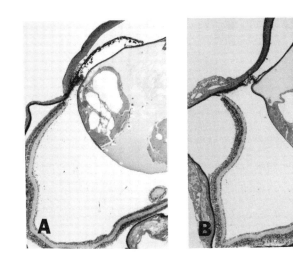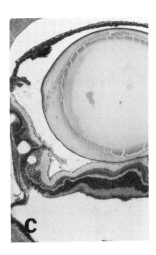

Figure 1.
Ocular pathology in rhoγ mice and MHC deficient mice with additional expression of IFN-γ at 4-5 weeks of age. PAS, magnification orig. x 4. A. Rhoγ mouse with moderate cellular infiltration, partial destruction of the photoreceptors and marked hyperproliferation of the lens epithelium. B. I-Aß null/ rhoγ mouse with the same amount of ocular pathology as the mouse in A. Note the lens epithelium hyperproliferation with vacuoles. C. ß2m null/ rhoγ mouse with similar changes of the retina as the mice in A. and B. Note the regular form and opacity of the lens with normal distribution of the lens epithelium cells.

138

In contrast, cataract formation apparently is linked to the expression of MHC class I in the eye which possibly contributes to stimulate the proliferation of the lens epithelium. The lens capsule is probably insufficient to prevent the exposure of the lens epithelium with IFN-γ present in the vitreous [6]. MHC class I or class II expression is not constitutive in the mouse lens, although the presence of MHC class I mRNA has been demonstrated in lens-derived cell lines [18], and it is likely that the observed class I expression in the lens is due to induction by IFN-γ. To date, it has been shown that IFN-γ can induce the expression of MHC class II in the lens of transgenic animals [19]. However, it is not likely that class II expression directly contributes to the development of cataract in this model, since class II deficient mice show the same amount of cataract formation.

We are dealing with a complicated *in vivo* system. Although we could elucidate the mechanisms of IFN-γ action in the eye only partially, our results allow us to exclude the participation of CD4 and CD8 cells in the development of retinal damage. However, MHC class I expression does influence the development of cataract in rhoγ mice.

SCRIPPS manuscript # 8740-NP, funded by NIH grant # MH 47680. Additional funding: Deutsche Forschungsgemeinschaft, Juvenile Diabetes Foundation.

References

1. Loh JE, Chang C-H, Fodor WL, et al. EMBO J 1992; 11: 1351-1363.
2. Kusuda M, Gaspari AA, Chan CC, et al. Invest Ophthalmol Vis Sci 1989; 30: 764-768.
3. Cousins SW, McCabe MM, Danielpour R, et al. Invest Ophthalmol Vis Sci 1991; 32: 2201-2211.
4. Streilein JW, Wilbanks GA, Taylor A, et al. Curr Eye Res 1992; 11: 41-47.
5. Streilein JW Curr Opin Immunol 1993; 5: 428-432.
6. Geiger K, Howes E, Gallina M, et al. Invest Ophthalmol Vis Sci 1994; 35: 2667-2681.
7. Geiger K, Howes EL, Sarvetnick N J. Virol. 1994; in press.
8. Hara Y, Okamoto S, Rouse B, et al. J Immunol 1993; 151: 5162-5171.
9. Zijlstra M, Li E, Saijadi F, et al. Nature 1989; 342: 435-439.
10. Gosgrove D, Gray D, Dierich A, et al. Cell 1991; 66: 1051-1066.
11. Grusby MJ, Johnson RS, Papaionnou VE, et al. Science 1991; 253: 1417-1420.
12. Lem J, Applebury ML, Falk JD, et al. Neuron 1991; 6: 201-210.
13. Goureau O, Lepoivre M, Courtois Y Biochem Biophys Res Commun 1992; 186: 854-859.
14. Lang RA, Metcalf D, Cuthbertson RA, et al. Cell 1987; 51: 675-687.
15. Lee MS,Sarvetnick N Curr Opin Immunol 1992; 4: 723-727.
16. Karre K Sem Immunol 1993; 5: 127-145.
17. Walev I, Kunkel J, Schwaeble W, et al. Arch Virol 1992; 126: 303-311.
18. Shaughnessy M,Wistow G Curr Eye Res 1992; 11: 175-181.
19. Egwuagu CE, Sztein J, Chan CC, et al. Invest Ophthalmol Vis Sci 1994; 35: 332-341.

Advances in Ocular Immunology
R.B. Nussenblatt, S.M. Whitcup, R.R. Caspi and I. Gery, eds.

Analysis of peripheral tolerance to autologous antigens expressed in an immunologically privileged site

James C. Lai[1,3], Eric F. Wawrousek[2], R. Steven Lee[2], Chi-Chao Chan[1], Scott M. Whitcup[1], Igal Gery[1].

Laboratories of [1]Immunology and [2]Molecular and Developmental Biology, National Eye Institute, NIH, Bethesda, MD 20892, USA and [3]Howard Hughes Medical Institute.

INTRODUCTION

The immune system must learn to tolerate self-antigens that are not expressed in the thymus. Autoreactive cells which escape intrathymic mechanisms of self-tolerization migrate into the periphery where they can be tolerized through poorly understood mechanisms. Transgenic (TG) animals have been used extensively to examine the processes involved in peripheral tolerance because the use of tissue-specific promoters allows the expression of any particular protein in specific organs. These experimental systems have shown that tolerance develops against foreign antigens expressed in extra-thymic organs which are exposed to the immune system, such as the liver and pancreas (1). However, it is unclear whether tolerance can develop to antigens sequestered from the immune system. To examine whether expression of a foreign antigen in an immunologically privileged site results in tolerance development, we examined 2 different TG mice which express chloramphenicol acetyltransferase (CAT), or hen egg lysozyme (HEL) in the lens, an encapsulated organ devoid of any lymphoid tissue.

MATERIALS AND METHODS

Transgenic Mice
CAT mice-TG mice expressing CAT under the control of the lens-specific murine αA-crystallin promoter were kindly provided by C. Sax (LMDB, NEI).

HEL mice-The coding portion of HEL plasmids pMTH and KLK (kindly provided by C. Goodnow, Stanford University) were placed under the transcriptional control of the murine αA-crystallin promoter to generate constructs PRL1 and PRL2, respectively. The transgenes were excised from the plasmids and injected into FVB/N single cell embryos to generate TG mice which express respectively, a soluble (S-HEL) form (PRL1, 1 line) and a membrane bound (M-HEL) form of HEL (PRL2, 4 lines). Potential founders were screened for the presence of the transgene by Southern blot analysis. Positive offspring of the transgenic founders were identified by a standard PCR assay using HEL primers.

Confirmation of transgene expression
Strict lens-specific expression of CAT was confirmed by a bi-phase CAT assay as performed in (2). Particle concentration fluorescence immunoassay (PCFIA),

as described in (3), confirmed the presence of HEL in eye extracts but was unable to detect HEL in the sera or thymi of the TG mice.

Immunizations
Mice were immunized s.c. into the base of the tail and hind thighs with either 20 μg CAT or 25 μg HEL, in 0.2 ml emulsion with complete Freund's adjuvant (1:1).

Assessment of Immune Responses
Immune responses were measured 2 weeks after immunization. Lymphocyte proliferation assays were set up in triplicate in 96 well flat bottom plates. Splenocytes (3×10^5 cells/well) were cultured in a final volume of 0.2 ml RPMI-1640 medium supplemented with HL-1 (Ventrex Laboratories, Portland, ME), 2-ME (5×10^{-5} M), penicillin (100 U/ml) and streptomycin (100 μg/ml). Cells were incubated with CAT or HEL for 72 hours at 37°C with 5% CO_2 and the cultures were then pulsed for 16 hours with ^{3}H-thymidine, 0.5μCi/10μl/well. Results are expressed as stimulation indices. To measure humoral responses, serum antibody levels against HEL or CAT were quantitated by direct ELISA (4).

RESULTS

Histology
Eyes of CAT TG mice were unaffected by transgene expression; there was a lack of lens disruption or ocular inflammation (Fig. 1). Whereas the eyes were also unaffected in the S-HEl mice and in 2 lines of M-HEL mice with low transgene copy numbers, lens fiber and capsule disruption were observed in the 2 higher copy lines (Fig. 2). No ocular inflammation though, was observed in any lines of M-HEL mice, even after immunization with HEL.

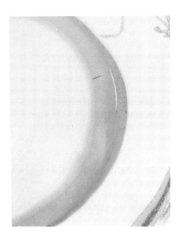

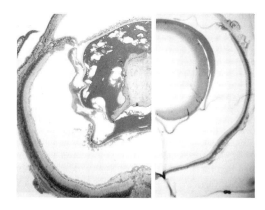

Fig. 1 No abnormalities were found in eyes of CAT TG mice (H & E, x50)

Fig. 2 Eyes from HEL TG mice showed abnormal lens in the high copy lines (left) and normal structure in the low copy lines (right). (H & E; left x50, right x25)

HEL but not CAT mice develop tolerance

A minimal level of cellular tolerance and no humoral tolerance was found in CAT mice (Fig. 3). In contrast, all lines of HEL, both M-HEL and S-HEL mice, developed both cellular and humoral tolerance to HEL. Results from tolerance tests in S-HEL animals are shown in Fig. 4. Similar findings of both complete cellular and humoral tolerance were observed in all 4 M-HEL lines (not shown).

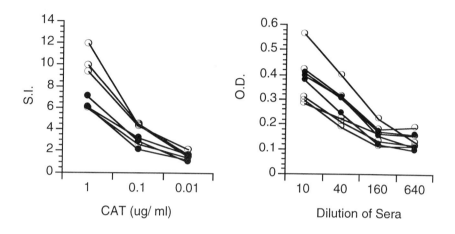

Fig 3. Cellular (left) and humoral (right) responses to CAT in individual wild type (WT) (O) and TG (●) mice. (SI= mean cpm in cultures with antigen / mean cpm in control cultures without stimulant)

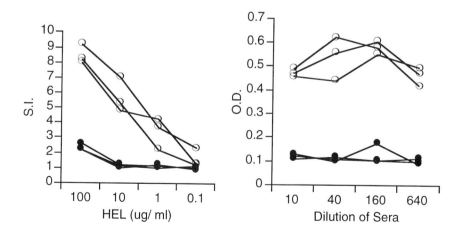

Fig 4. Cellular (left) and humoral (right) responses to HEL in WT (O) and S-HEL TG (●) mice.

142

DISCUSSION

While minimal or no tolerance developed in CAT mice, a state of complete cellular and humoral tolerance existed in mice expressing either the membrane or soluble forms of HEL. The state of tolerance in the HEL mice was further depicted by the lack of inflammation in their eyes following immunization with HEL. Severe inflammation could be induced, however, in eyes of mice with ruptured lens by adoptive transfer of lymphocytes from WT mice sensitized against HEL (data not shown).

There are two possible explanations for the observed tolerance. First, HEL could leak from the eye into the circulation. This mechanism would be expected to play a more important role in tolerance induction in TG mice secreting HEL (S-HEL) than in mice expressing a membrane bound form of HEL (M-HEL). Second, HEL could be expressed in extra-ocular organs, particularly in the thymus, where clonal elimination can take place. Although PCFIA did not detect HEL in the thymus or serum of these mice, the possibility of a very low expression of HEL in the thymus, at a level below that of sensitivity of PCFIA, is currently being tested by RT-PCR. If it is determined that HEL is expressed extra-ocularly, this TG model may be useful for the determination of levels of self-antigen expression necessary for tolerance induction.

CONCLUSIONS

This study shows for the first time that tolerance may develop to antigens expressed in the lens, an encapsulated organ which is sequestered from the immune system. The results suggest that the immune privileges of the lens may not be as complete as previously believed.

ACKNOWLEDGEMENTS

The authors thank Dr. Sandra Smith-Gill, Dr. Chris Sax, and Ms. Barbara Vistica for their assistance in performing, respectively, the particle concentration fluorescence immunoassay, the analysis of the CAT mice and the direct ELISAs.

REFERENCES

1   Hanahan D. Annu. Rev. Cell Biol. 1990; 6:493-537.

2   Sax CM, Ilagan JG, Piatigorsky. Nucleid Acids Res. 1993; 21(11): 2633-2640.

3   Newman MA, Mainhart CR, Mallett CP, Lavoie TB, Smith-Gill SJ. J. Immunol 1992; 149:3260-3272.

4   Mochizuki M, Kuwabara T, McAllister C, Nussenblatt RB, Gery I. Invest. Ophthalmol. Vis. Sci. 1985; 26: 1-9.

© 1994 Elsevier Science B.V. All rights reserved.
Advances in Ocular Immunology
R.B. Nussenblatt, S.M. Whitcup, R.R. Caspi and I. Gery, eds.

PROGRESSIVE INFLAMMATORY DISEASE AND NEOVASCULARIZATION IN THE EYES OF INTERLEUKIN-1β TRANSGENIC MICE.

E.F. Wawrousek[a], J.C. Lai[b,c], I. Gery[b] and C.C. Chan[b]

[a]Laboratory of Molecular and Developmental Biology and [b]Laboratory of Immunology, National Eye Institute, 9000 Rockville Pike, Bethesda, MD 20892, USA and [c]Howard Hughes Medical Institute.

INTRODUCTION

Interleukin 1(IL-1) is a potent cytokine exhibiting pleiotropic effects in inflammatory processes. Intraocular injection of IL-1 preparations has been shown to induce ocular inflammation in both rabbits[1,2,3,4] and rats[5]. IL-1 levels have also been found to be elevated in some humans suffering from intraocular inflammations[6] suggesting that this cytokine plays an important role in inducing and/or propagating ocular inflammation. Both human IL-1α and β have been shown to be angiogenic factors when slowly released into rabbit cornea[7], although IL-1α appears to be significantly more potent in this system. All of the animal models used to study the effect of IL-1 on ocular inflammation depend on physical administration of the cytokine resulting in a spike of cytokine concentration followed by a gradual decrease. We have generated a transgenic mouse model in which IL-1β is continuously expressed and secreted from lens cells and induces a chronic ocular inflammation accompanied by neovascularization of many ocular tissues. This transgenic model will be a valuable tool for studying chronic ocular inflammation.

MATERIALS AND METHODS

Construction of IL-1β vector
The human IL-1β expression cassette, containing sequences encoding the human tissue plasminogen activator secretion signal peptide fused in frame to the coding region of mature human IL-1β and the bovine growth hormone polyadenylation signal, was excised with KpnI and Eco47III from plasmid TPAIL-1β mature[8]. This fragment was put downstream of the murine αA-crystallin promoter to form pEW34. The transgene was excised from the plasmid by digestion with SalI and NotI and gel purified in preparation for pronuclear microinjection.

Creation of Transgenic Mice
Standard methods were used to generate transgenic mice by injecting the transgene DNA (4 μg/ml) into a pronucleus of single celled mouse embryos of the FVB/N strain. Mouse lines were established by mating founder animals to normal FVB/N mice. For this study, transgenic FVB/N mice were mated to normal DBA2 mice and the resulting FVB/N x DBA2 F_1 hybrid mice were examined.

DNA, RNA and Protein Analysis
Standard methods were used to perform Southern and Northern analysis. Levels of hIL-1β were measured by ELISA using the High Sensitivity Interleukin-1β ELISA Kit from Cistron Biotechnology (Pine Brook, NJ). Protein concentration was measured with the BCA Protein Assay Kit from Pierce (Rockford, IL).

144

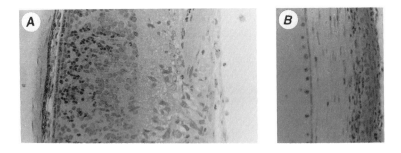

Figure 1.   A, Retina (20X); B, Cornea (20X) of a 16 day old transgenic mouse. Retinitis, loss of photoreceptors, and preretinal neovascularization are evident in A. Keratitis and corneal neovascularization can be seen in B.

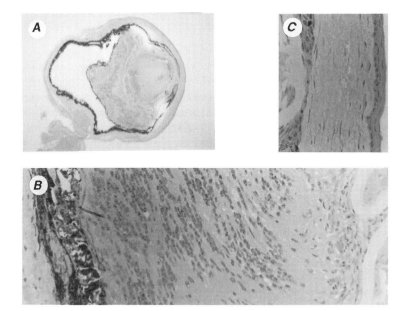

Figure 2.   A, Eye (2X); B, Retina (10X); C, Cornea (20X) of a 19 week old transgenic mouse. The eye is phthisical with inflammatory cells and neovascularization throughout.

Systemic Effects on IL-1 Mediated Responses
Mice were injected with lipopolysaccharide (40μg/gbw i.p.) and observed at 18 hour intervals with one additional early observation at 6 hours post injection and ending at 72 hours post injection. At each time point mice were rated as healthy, ill or dead.

Thymi were removed from freshly euthanized N and T mice and their cells were tested for enhanced response to phytohemagglutinin in the presence of IL-1[9].

RESULTS

Production and Analysis of Transgenic Mice
Repeated microinjection of the transgene resulted in only one surviving F_0 founder mouse containing the transgene. Several F_0 mice which died shortly after birth also harbored the transgene, suggesting that expression of this transgene can be deleterious and indeed lethal to the animal. Southern blot analysis of DNA from mice in the one surviving line demonstrated the presence of a single complete copy of the transgene. Northern Blot analysis of RNA from tissues of these mice revealed expression of the transgene only in the eyes. The RNA was detected by Northern analysis with 0.5 μg of total eye RNA, but not in other tissues with 20 μg of total RNA. Presence of the hIL-1β protein in the eyes of these mice was confirmed by ELISA performed on eye extracts. In all mice tested, hIL-1β levels were greater than 2,000 pg/mg protein; the level of ocular hIL-1β varied with the age of the mice. Using the same ELISA reagents, levels of hIL-1β in plasma samples were below detection limits (2.0 pg/ml) of the assay.

Histology
Examination of histological sections of eyes from transgenic mice (T) and normal (N) littermates at ages ranging from embryonic day 11.5 to adulthood (186 days old) revealed a progressive inflammation and neovascularization of ocular tissues culminating in phthisis bulbi. The first detectable difference between eyes of T and N littermates was at 4 days of age when inflammatory infiltrate cells appeared to be actively recruited into the optic cup area of T mice. By 9 days of age, vitritis,retinitis and pre-retinal and corneal neovascularization were detected in T mice. By day 16, retinitis had caused a disruption of retinal architecture with partial loss of photoreceptors (figure 1A) and keratitis was evident and corneal neovascularization had progressed (figure 1B). At day 26, the lens epithelium had migrated posteriorly and cataract was evident. Neovascularization was evident throughout the retina and photoreceptor loss was complete. The inflammation and neovascularization continued to increase, destroying much of the ocular tissue. In the adult T mice (~19 weeks old) the eyes were phthisical (figure 2A) and exhibited inflammation and neovascularization (figure 2B and C). Normal littermates showed no signs of ocular inflammation, neovascularization or cataract.

Immunohistochemical and histological analysis of eye sections from T and N littermates revealed the infiltrate to be composed predominantly of macrophages with some lymphocyte and PMN involvement.

Systemic Effects
Although hIL-1β expression appeared to be restricted to the eye, with no detectable hIL-1β in the circulating plasma, the T mice exhibited systemic effects. When T and N littermates were injected with lipopolysaccharide at 40 μg per gram body weight, all (n=16) of the N mice became ill within 6 hours and 88% died from the ensuing shock reaction within 72 hours of injection. Conversely, only one of the T

mice (n=11) became ill within 6 hours and only 27% of the mice had died by the end of the 72 hour observation period suggesting that chronic expression of hIL-1β in the eye afforded protection against LPS induced (IL-1 mediated) shock. When thymocytes isolated from T mice were stimulated *in vitro* with IL-1, their proliferative response was consistently less than those of the N mice at each age tested, strengthening the probability that these mice become systemically tolerized to the effects of IL-1.

DISCUSSION

The transgenic mouse model we have generated by continuously expressing human IL-1β in lens cells exhibits many of the characteristics expected in a localized IL-1 response. IL-1 induces an inflammatory response characterized by leukocyte infiltration and increased vascular permeability when injected intraocularly in rabbits[1,2,3,4] and rats[5]. Similarly, this transgenic mouse line exhibits an ocular inflammation with massive infiltration of leukocytes. IL-1 is also a potent angiogenic factor and has been shown to induce neovascularization in rabbit cornea[7]. Neovascularization was also observed in our transgenic mice, beginning in the cornea and preretina, progressing to the entire retina and eventually to all tissues in the phthisical adult eye.

In addition to the localized inflammatory reaction to constant hIL-1β secretion, a systemic partial unresponsiveness to IL-1 was also detected in these transgenic mice. It is presently unclear how this systemic effect is established, but it is probable that continuous exposure to IL-1 induces the partial unresponsiveness to this cytokine.

This new transgenic model will provide a new tool for studying the processes involved in chronic ocular inflammation and will help elucidate the mechanisms by which a local inflammation can mediate systemic immunomodulatory effects.

REFERENCES

1   Bhattacherjee P, Henderson B. Curr Eye Res 1987; 6:929-934.
2   Rosenbaum JT, Samples JR, Hefeneider SH, Howes LH Jr. Arch Ophthalmol 1987; 105:1117-1120.
3   Fleisher LN, Ferrell JB, McGahan MC. Invest Ophthalmol Vis Sci 1992; 33:2120-2127.
4   Kulkarni PS, Mancino M. Exp Eye Res 1993; 56:275-279.
5   Ferrick MR, Thurau SR, Oppenheim MH, et al. Invest Ophthalmol Vis Sci 1991; 32:1534-1539.
6   Franks WA, Limb GA, Stanford MR, et al. Curr Eye Res 1992; 11:187-191.
7   BenEzra D, Hemo I, Maftzir G. Arch Ophthalmol 1990; 108:573-576.
8   Krasney PA, Young PR. Cytokine 1992; 4:134-143.
9   Gery I, Davies P, Derr J, Krett N,Barranger JA. Cell Immunol 1981; 64:293-303.

Advances in Ocular Immunology
R.B. Nussenblatt, S.M. Whitcup, R.R. Caspi and I. Gery, eds.

Immunological recognition of transgene encoded MHC class I alloantigen in the lens.

Jerold G. Woodward[1*], W. David Martin[1], Julia L. Stevens[2], and Rita M. Egan[3]. Departments of [1]Microbiology and Immunology, [2]Ophthalmology, and [3]Medicine, University of Kentucky School of Medicine, Lexington, KY 40536-0084. *Corresponding author.

Abstract

Transgenic mice expressing the MHC class I antigen, H-2D^d, specifically in the lens were utilized to determine whether alloreactive, D^d specific T cells were capable of recognizing a cell-bound alloantigen sequestered behind the lens capsule. Our results indicate that the lens capsule is an effective barrier to lymphocyte infiltration and is capable of preventing recognition of a potent alloantigen.

The immune privileged nature of the eye is well established. Allografts introduced into the anterior chamber enjoy prolonged survival time [1], while other antigens injected into the anterior chamber stimulate a much different response than when administered to a non-privileged site [2]. This "immune deviation" is generally manifested as a reduction in cell-mediated immunity and an increase in humoral immunity [1,2]. Thus, immune privilege in the eye is not simply due to a decrease in overall immune responsiveness within the microenvironment of the eye, although there is also evidence that cell mediated immunity is impaired in the anterior chamber [3]. Rather, it appears that immunological recognition of antigens does indeed take place within the eye, but that there are complex mechanisms governing the type of response that occurs.

In spite of the fact that cell mediated immune responses are impaired within the eye, autoimmune uveitis mediated by T cells is a significant problem, implying that breakdowns in self-tolerance mechanisms can and do occur [4]. Transgenic mice have proven extremely useful for the understanding of immunological tolerance toward self antigens [5,6,7,8]. While these studies have shed considerable light on our understanding of peripheral tolerance, their results may not be directly applicable to tolerance toward self antigens within immune privileged sites.

In order to examine this issue, we have produced transgenic mice expressing the MHC class I gene, H-2D[d], in the lens of the eye under the control of the αA-crystallin promoter. Seven lines of mice were produced that contain between one and 22 copies of the transgene and are described in detail elsewhere [9]. All mice express the D[d] protein in the lens but not in any other tissue including the thymus. Two phenotypes of transgenic mice were observed. In mice with a low to intermediate copy number of integrated transgene, the eyes and lenses were normal with the exception of punctate cataracts detectable by slit-lamp exam. In the high copy number mice, the eyes were microphthalmic and had small, abnormally developed lenses with severe cataracts. In addition, lens capsule rupture was a prominent feature [9].

Given that these mice had a foreign alloantigen (H-2D^d) expressed in their lenses (the founder mice were H-2(b x k)F$_1$ and backcrossed to the b haplotype), we examined the eyes for inflammation by slit lamp as well as histology. No evidence was found for an inflammatory response to the D^d alloantigen except in the high copy number mice coincident with lens capsule rupture [9]. This led us to postulate that alloantigen expressed in the intact lenses of the low copy number mice was completely sequestered by the lens capsule and therefore unavailable for T cell recognition [9]. This view was strengthened by our observations that these transgenic mice were capable of generating D^d specific CTL *in vitro* (Martin et al., unpublished observations). In order to test the strength of this sequestration, we immunized low copy number transgenic mice two times with H-2D^d bearing Balb/c spleen cells or Balb/c tail skin grafts, and then observed the mice for signs of inflammation. Eyes of selected mice were also examined by histology. In no case did we observe any inflammation in the eyes of these transgenic mice. This result suggested either that the low copy transgenic mice were tolerant to the transgene, or that the D^d alloantigen was totally sequestered. To examine this issue more directly, we produced a D^d specific CTL line that was highly lytic toward D^d bearing target cells *in vitro*. When these cells were administered into the anterior chamber of the eye, we saw no evidence of recognition or destruction of lens material as long as the lens capsule integrity was preserved. These results indicate that the lens capsule forms a lymphocyte-impermeable barrier which completely prevents immune infiltration. While these results imply that cell-associated D^d is completely sequestered within the lens, thus preventing its direct recognition by CD8+ T cells, it is likely that breakdown products of D^d protein diffuses out of the lens capsule, where it could be handled as a "typical" protein antigen. Future experiments will determine whether this form of the D^d protein is recognized or induces tolerance in these mice.

Acknowledgement

This work was funded by NEI grant EY0963.

References

1. Streilein, J. W. Curr Opin Immunol 1993;5:428.

2. Niederkorn, J. Y. Adv. Immunol. 1990;48:191.

3. Cousins, S. W., Trattler, W. B. and Streilein, J. W. Curr. Eye Res. 1991;10:287.

4. Linssen, A., Rothova, A., Valkenburg, H. A., Dekker, S. A., Luyendijk, L., Kijlstra, A. and Feltkamp, T. Invest Ophthalmol Vis Sci 1991;32:2568.

5. Miller, J. Immunol Cell Biol 1992;70:49.

6. Burkly, L. C., Lo, D., Kanagawa, O., Brinster, R. and Flavell, R. Nature 1989;342:564.

7. Lo, D., Burkly, L. C., Widera, G., Cowing, C., Flavell, R. A., Palmiter, R. D. and Brinster, R. L. Cell 1988;53:159.

8. Miller, J. F. A. P., Morahan, G., Allison, J. and Hoffmann, M. Immunol Rev 1991;122:103.

9. Martin, W. D., Egan, R. M., Stevens, J. L. and Woodward, J. G. 1994;Submitted for publication.

© 1994 Elsevier Science B.V. All rights reserved.
Advances in Ocular Immunology
R.B. Nussenblatt, S.M. Whitcup, R.R. Caspi and I. Gery, eds.

Isolation and Characterization of the Mouse Ornithine Aminotransferase Gene for Gene Targeting by Homologous Recombination

Noriko Esumi and Moncef Jendoubi

Laboratory of Immunology, National Eye Institute, National Institutes of Health, Bethesda, MD 20892-1858, USA

Introduction

Gyrate atrophy (GA) of the choroid and retina is an autosomal recessive eye disorder involving a progressive loss of vision due to chorioretinal degeneration [1,2]. A variety of ornithine-δ-aminotransferase (OAT) gene mutations have been reported in GA patients and suspected to associate with this ocular disease [3]. However, the precise mechanism by which the OAT deficiency and hyperornithinemia lead to the chorioretinal degeneration remains unknown. To elucidate the pathophysiological role of OAT, we are attempting to create OAT deficient mice by gene targeting via embryonic stem (ES) cells. Toward this ultimate goal, we isolated murine OAT gene to construct OAT targeting replacement vector.

Materials and methods

Isolation of mouse OAT functional gene

The 129 mouse genomic library, OLA 129-λGEM-12, was kindly provided by Dr. Anton Berns (Cancer Institute, Netherlands). This library was screened with a nearly full length rat OAT cDNA probe [4] labeled with ^{32}P-dCTP by random oligonucleotide priming. Screening procedures were performed using standard protocols [5].

Polymerase chain reaction (PCR) analysis

To determine the structure of positive genomic clones, PCR was performed with primers from each exon based on mouse cDNA sequence (Genebank, X64837) to amplify each exon and intron [6,7]. Standard reaction conditions were used [5].

Sequencing

The promising Clone 11 was subcloned into BlueScript vector (Stratagene, La Jolla, CA) and designated pBSmOAT6. This plasmid was sequenced by dideoxy nucleotide chain termination method of Sanger [8] using ^{35}S-dATP and the CircumVent Thermal Cycle Dideoxy DNA Sequencing Kit (New England Biolabs, Beverly, MA).

Construction of targeting vector

The mouse genomic fragment in pBSmOAT6 was 16 kb in length and used nearly entirely to make a targeting vector. Neomycin resistance gene (Neo^r) was purified from pMC1neo PolyA [9] kindly provided by Dr. Mario Capecchi and inserted at Sca I site of exon 4 to disrupt the OAT gene. Herpes simplex virus thymidine kinase (HSV-TK) gene was purified from TGV-TK$_2$ (M Jendoubi, unpublished) originated from pIC19R/MC1-TK [10] provided by Dr. Mario Capecchi and added at the 3' end of the OAT fragment in targeting construct. Standard procedures were used in all subcloning and constructing process [5].

Results and Discussion

Isolation and characterization of mouse OAT gene

By genomic library screening, sixteen clones were isolated from 6 x 10^6 phage plaques. All clones were analyzed by PCR, and the results were compared with the PCR amplification pattern with mouse genomic DNA as a template. Among 16 clones, Clone 11 seemed to encode the functional OAT gene containing 5' flanking region and coding region up to exon 5 (Fig. 1).

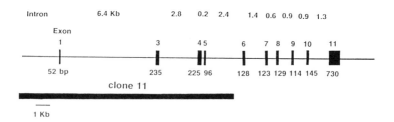

Figure 1. Structure of Clone 11 and the functional mouse OAT gene. Clone 11 is indicated as a solid horizontal bar. Exons are indicated as solid boxes.

Since OAT gene has been reported to have at least several pseudogenes and related sequences in human and rat genome [11-14], it is highly suspected that mouse genome also has at least several related sequences. Therefore, sequencing of Clone 11 was performed to confirm that this clone encoded the functional OAT gene. Sequence of total 444 bases from exon 3, 4, and 5 was comparable to the sequence of the mouse OAT cDNA.

Construction of targeting vector

A targeting vector was constructed according to a positive-negative selection strategy [10]. Using 16 kb fragment in pBSmOAT6, exon 4 was disrupted by insertion of Neo[r] gene at Sca I site for positive selection by G418. Two targeting vectors were made in which Neo[r] gene was introduced in forward and opposite direction as referred to the coding strand of OAT gene. HSV-TK gene was added at the 3' end of the genomic fragment for negative selection by Gancyclovir. The length of homologous region was 14 kb upstream from Neo[r] and 2.2 kb downstream from Neo[r] (Fig. 2). This construct is designed for three favorable features that genomic fragment used is isogenic to ES cell (129 strain of mice) [15], that a positive-negative selection can be used for identifying clones after electroporation into ES cells [10], and that a long homologous region is expected to yield a high frequency of homologous recombination events [9].

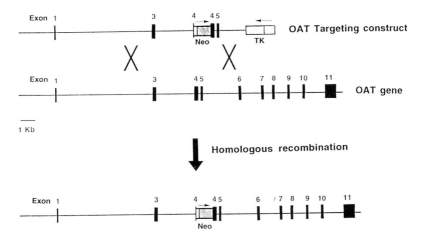

Figure 2. The targeting vector to disrupt the OAT gene in ES cells. The hypothetical crossovers between the endogenous OAT allele and the targeting construct are indicated by the crossed lines. The direction of Neo[r] and HSV-TK is indicated by the arrow 5'→3' above the gene.

154

References

1. Ramesh V, Gusella JF, Shih VE. Mol Biol Med 1991; 8;81-93.
2. Kaiser-Kupfer M, Caruso RC, Valle V. Arch Ophthalmol 1991; 109:1539-1548.
3. Brody LC, Mitchell GA, Obie C, Michaud J, Steel G, Fontaine G, Robert MF, Sipila I, Kaiser-Kupfer M, Valle D. JBC 1992; 267:3302-3307.
4. Mueckler MM, Pitot HC. JBC 1985; 260: 12993-12997.
5. Sambrook J, Fritsch EF, Maniatis T. Molecular Cloning: A Laboratory Manual, 2nd ed. 1989, Cold Spring Harbor Laboratory Press.
6. Saiki RK, Gelfand DH, Stoffel S, Scharf SJ, Higuchi R, Horn GT, Mullis KB, Erlich HA. Science 1988; 239: 487-491.
7. Friedman KD, Rosen NL, Newman PJ, Montgomery RR. Nucl Acids Res 1988; 16: 8718.
8. Sanger F, Nicklen S, Coulson AR. Proc Natl Acad Sci USA 1977; 74: 5463-5467.
9. Thomas KR, Capecchi MR. Cell 1987; 51: 503-512.
10. Mansour SL, Thomas KR, Capecchi MR. Nature 1988; 336: 348-352.
11. Mitchell GA, Looney JE, Brody LC, Steel G, Suchanek M, Engelhardt JF, Willard HF, Valle D. JBC 1988; 263: 14288-14295.
12. Shull JD, Pennington KL, Pitot HC, Boryca VS, Schulte BL. BBA 1992; 1132: 214-218.
13. Zintz CB, Inana G. Exp Eye Res 1990; 50: 759-770.
14. Shull JD, Pennington KL, George SM, Kilibarda KA. Gene 1991; 104: 203-209.
15. Van Deursen J, Wieringa B. Nucl Acids Res 1992; 20: 3815-3820.

© 1994 Elsevier Science B.V. All rights reserved.
Advances in Ocular Immunology
R.B. Nussenblatt, S.M. Whitcup, R.R. Caspi and I. Gery, eds.

Retinal survival in transgenic mice expressing human ornithine ∂-aminotransferase

Moncef Jendoubi

Laboratory of Immunology, National Eye Institute. National Institute of Health, Bethesda
MD 20892.

Introduction

Certain inbred strains of mice, such as FVB/N, present a progressive retinal degeneration
beginning a few days after birth and becoming complete a few months later (1-3). Retinal
degeneration in these mice has been associated at least in part with a deficiency in a
phosphodiesterase (PDE) activity, which leads to the accumulation of cyclic GMP in
affected retina degenerative (rd) photoreceptors (4, 5). We postulated that other gene
products such as OAT, which is associated with retinal degeneration in human may be
involved. Thus, persistent expression of human OAT (hOAT) in retinal degenerated mice
could have a role in the development of retinal cell layers. To study the physiological
relevance of OAT *in vivo* and to determine whether its expression could rescue the retinal
cell layers from degeneration, we produced two transgenic lines (OATtg), expressing the
human OAT gene in strains of mice normally exhibiting a progressive retinal degeneration.
Here we show that transgenic mice expressing human ornithine ∂-aminotransferase exhibit
less severe retinal degeneration than control mice litter mates.

Material and Methods.

Production of transgenic mice. Human OAT cDNA was cloned under the
transcriptional element of Moloney murine leukemia retrovirus long terminal repeat (LTR-
MoMuLV), and the construct was injected into zygotes of FVB/N mice strain genetic
background (6, 7).

Biochemical analysis of transgenic mice. Cells were prepared from different
tissues (Fig. 1. retina, muscle, heart, kidney and liver; lanes A, B, C, D and E
respectively) from both transgenic mice and control litter mates, and lysed in 500 mM
NaCl, 50 mM Tris pH 7.5, 1% NP40. 30 µg of protein extracts from each sample was
subjected to sodium dodecyl-sulfate polyacrylamide gel electrophoresis (SDS/PAGE) and
stained with coomassie blue or transferred to nylon filters for immunoblot analysis (8).

Histopathology

Enucleated eyes were prefixed in 4% phosphate-buffered glutaraldyde for one hour, post
fixed in 10% formaldehyde overnight, dehydrated, and embedded in methacrylate. Four

μm thick sections were cut horizontally along the pupillary-optic nerve plane of the eye and were stained with hematoxylin-eosin. Sections were evaluated and micro-photographs were taken at a magnification of 400 X.

Results

Biochemical analysis. OATtg mice were born normal. The expression of the transgene was assessed primarily by Northern blot analysis, and then in several tissues using immunoblot analysis using specific antibodies raised against human OAT (data not shown). When the protein extracts were separeted on SDS-polyacrylamide gel electrophoresis and stained with coomassie blue, we saw either the presence of new polypeptides and/or an enhancement of several others at all range of molecular weights only in the OATtg tissue protein extracts as compared to those of their litter mates (Fig.1).

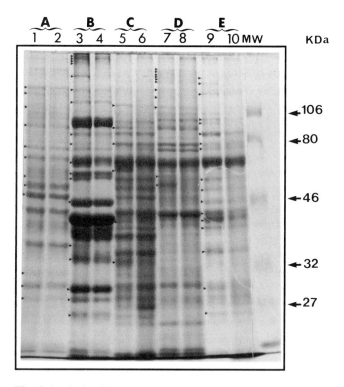

Fig. 1 Analysis of protein extracts from retina, muscle, heart, kidney and liver; lanes A, B, C, D and E respectively. Number 1, 3, 5, 7, and 9 correspond to OATtg extracts, while 2, 4, 6, 8 and 10 correspond to extracts from control tissues. The arrows point to the new and/or enhanced polypeptides in OATtg tissues extracts.

Histopathology. To determine whether the expression of hOAT would have any consequence on the retinal cell layer development, we examined histopathologically OATtg and the control litter mates on several siblings derived from both founders at different time points. At birth, no significant differences of the retinal structure, mainly the inner and outer neuroblast layers, between wild type and OATtg mice were observed. On the contrary, OATtg retina showed better preserved inner and outer segments of the photoreceptors (IS/OS), with larger numbers of intact nuclei both in the outer and inner nuclear layers (ONL and INL) (Fig. 2).

After two months, retina in the control litter mates showed complete degeneration and atrophy with total loss of all photoreceptor cells, including the nuclei and the IS/OS.

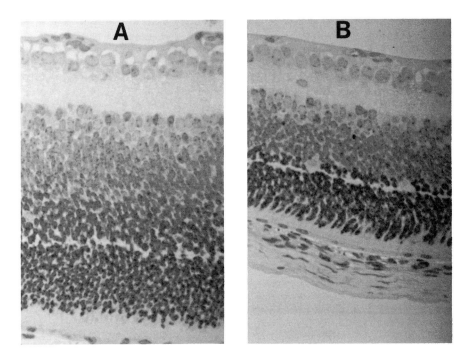

Fig. 2. A and B correspond to the histological analysis of the retina from OATtg and control litter mates respectively.

158

Discussion

Although the physiological role of OAT and how it contributes to retinal cell growth whether directly or indirectly remains to be understood, the present study provides strong evidence that OAT plays a critical role in rescuing neural cell lines in the retina. Also by virtue of its role like a growth-factor represents a valuable model that may aid studies of the pathogenesis and treatment of human retinal degeneration.

Acknowledgments. I would like to thank Dr. Chi-Chao Chan for the histopathology and Curtis Barrett for his technical assistance.

References

1. Agarwal, N. et al. *J. Neuroscience* **10,** 3275-3285 (1990).
2. Tansley, K. *J. Hered.* **45,**123-127 (1954).
3. Sidman, R. L. & Green, M. C. *J. Hered.* **56,** 23-29 (1965).
4. Bowes, C. et al. *Nature* **347,** 677-680 (1990).
5. Charbonneau, H. et al. *Proc. Natl. Acad. Sci. U. S A.* **87,** 288-292 (1990).
6. Hogan, B., Constantini, F. & Lacy, E. *Manipulating the Mouse Embryos*: *A Laboratory Manual* (Cold Spring Harbor Laboratory Press, New York). (1986).
7. Lang, R. A., et al. *Cell* **51,** 675-686 (1987).
8. Lacorazza, H. D., et al. *Human Gene Ther.* in press

© 1994 Elsevier Science B.V. All rights reserved.
Advances in Ocular Immunology
R.B. Nussenblatt, S.M. Whitcup, R.R. Caspi and I. Gery, eds.

ORNITHINE-δ-AMINOTRANSFERASE GENE TRANSFER TO CHO DEFICIENT CELLS BY RETROVIRUS TRANSDUCTION

H. Daniel Lacorazza and Moncef Jendoubi

Laboratory of Immunology, National Eye Institute, National Institutes of Health, Bethesda MD, 20892

Introduction

Ornithine-δ-aminotransferase (OAT) is a nuclear-encoded mitochondrial matrix enzyme which catalyzes the reversible interconversion of ornithine and α-ketoglutarate to glutamate semialdehyde and glutamate. It has been shown that Gyrate atrophy (GA) patients have a high concentration of ornithine in their body fluids. This hyperornithinemia was associated with the absence of OAT enzymatic activity.

With the final goal of applying a genetic therapy to GA patients and correcting the OAT enzyme deficiency by supplying a functional gene, we established an *in vitro* model system in which we attempted to correct the enzymatic deficiency in an OAT deficient cell line, as a first step toward a somatic gene therapy.

Materials and methods

Production of recombinant retrovirus vectors.
LPOSN (Fig. 1a) correspond to a retroviral construct where the human OAT (hOAT) cDNA coding region was cloned under the transcriptional control of phosphoglycerate kinase (PGK) promoter. The PG13-GALV packaging cell line was transfected with this construct and the supernatant was used to transduce a deficient cell line C9.

Cell lines.
In this work we used the packaging cell line PG13-GALV, which was obtained from the American Tissue Culture Collection (ATCC, CRL-10686) and the OAT deficient cell line C9, from Dr. J.M. Phang (NCI/NIH, Frederick).

OAT enzymatic assay.
Cell lysates were used to measure radiochemically OAT enzymatic activity[1], following the procedure described by Brody et al.[2].

160

Immunodetection of OAT protein in transduced cell lines.
Total proteins were subjected to SDS-PAGE, and transferred onto nitrocellulose filter. The immunostaining was performed with an OAT specific rabbit polyclonal antibody raised against a 19 aminoacid peptide (KTVQGPPTSDDIFEREYKY).

Southern and Northern blot analyses.
We followed standard procedures[3]. The EcoRI/HindIII hOAT fragment containing the whole coding region was used as probe.

Results

Stable Genomic Integration of OAT provirus into transduced C9 cells.
Genomic DNA from wild type and transduced C9 cells was digested with EcoRV/PstI (EV/P), EcoRI/HindIII (E/H) and EcoRV (EV), and analyzed by Southern blot (Fig 1b). The size of the fragments generated with the different restriction enzymes correspond to the expected pattern of the hOAT provirus integrated into the C9 genome.

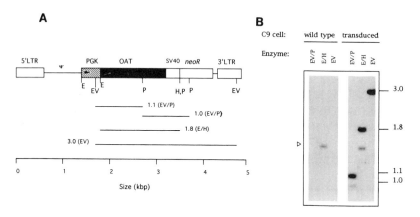

Figure 1: A- Structure of hOAT recombinant retrovirus
B- Southern blot analysis of C9 cells.

Correction of OAT deficiency in C9 transduced cell line.
To further assess the expression of integrated hOAT sequences, we analyzed the production of the OAT mRNA. The results showed strong hybridization on a 5.0-kbp and a weaker one on a 3.6-kbp transcript

(Fig. 2B, lane 2). The native hOAT transcript from human fibroblasts showed the corresponding size, 2.1-kbp (Fig. 2B, lane 3). The hOAT transcripts in the transduced C9 cell line were in greater abundance as compared to the endogenous hOAT mRNA in the normal human fibroblasts as clearly shown in Fig. 2B (lanes 2 and 3, respectively), taking into account that the lanes contain the same amount of total RNA as confirmed by hybridization with a β-actin probe (Fig. 2C).

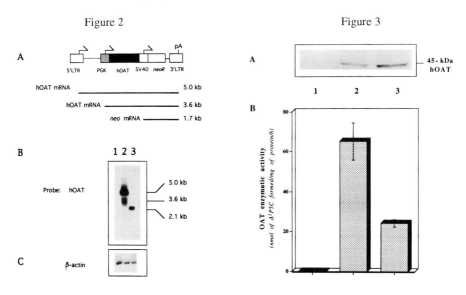

Figure 2   Figure 3

Expression of hOAT in C9 wild type (lane 1), C9 transduced (lane 2) and human fibroblast (lane 3).

Figure 2: Diagram showing the transcription pattern of LPOSN vector (A). Northern blot analysis hybridized with hOAT (B) and β-actin (C) probes.

Figure 3: Western blot analysis (A) and OAT enzyme activity (B).

In order to test if the mRNA transcript from the proviral insert was being appropriately translated and processed into a mature protein, we performed a Western blot analysis. As shown in Fig. 3A (lane 1), no significant immunological reaction was observed in C9 wild type extract, while in transduced cells a strong reaction was seen on one polypeptide (Fig. 3A, lane 2), which comigrates with an apparent molecular weight of 45-kDa with that detected in human fibroblasts (Fig. 3A, lane 3).

Cell lysates were analyzed for the presence of an active OAT. The results are shown in Fig. 3B. The deficient cell line had almost no OAT enzymatic activity, whereas the transduced C9⁺ cells produced at least a 3-fold increase of OAT activity as compared to human fibroblasts. These results show that the LPOSN provirus is capable of expressing high levels of functional hOAT enzyme that represents at least 10-fold higher than the OAT residual activity in deficient cells.

Discussion

Ornithine δ-aminotransferase deficiency is associated with hyperornithinemia and degeneration of the choroid and retina, suggesting that the accumulation of ornithine may produce a toxic effect on the eye tissue[4,5].

The introduction of a normal OAT gene into somatic cells of GA patients may turn the hyperornithinemia to normal level, and lead consequently to an improvement in visual function. Given this hypotheses, we designed a OAT retrovirus vector that would provide optimal gene expression in an OAT deficient cell line.

In conclusion, our results demonstrate that the retrovirus-mediated transfer of hOAT results in a stable integration of the transferred gene without rearrangement into the transduced cells genome. In addition, we have shown that the gene was transcribed, translated and processed into a protein recognized by a specific hOAT antibody, and able to metabolize the ornithine its natural substrate.

There are currently more than 40 approved human gene therapy protocols, however to date none of these trials involves ocular diseases. Our data provide the basic knowledge necessary to focus on the appropriate human cells as a target tissue for a future gene therapy trial in GA genetic disease.

References

1- Valle, D., Kaiser-Kupfer, M.I. & Del Valle, L.A. *Proc. Natl. Acad. Sci. U.S.A.* 1977; **74**: 5159-5161.
2- Brody, L.C., Mitchell, G.A., Obie, C., Michaud, J., Steel, G., Fontaine, G. et al. *J. Biol. Chem.* 1992; **267**: 3302-3307.
3- Maniatis, T., Fritsch, E.F. & Sambrook, T. In *Molecular Cloning: A Laboratory Manual,* Cold Spring Harbor Laboratory, Cold Spring Harbor, NY, 1982.
4- Kuwabara, T., Ishikawa, I. & Kaiser-Kupfer, M.I. *Ophthalmology* 1981; **88**: 331-334.
5- Valle, D. & Simell, O. In *The Metabolic basis of inherited disease,* (Schriver, C.R., A.L. Beaudet, W.S. Sly, and D. Valle eds) 6th ed., pp. 599-627, 1989.

Advances in Ocular Immunology
R.B. Nussenblatt, S.M. Whitcup, R.R. Caspi and I. Gery, eds.

Gene Targeting of Invariant Chain Gene by Homologous Recombination as a Tool to Study Immunoregulation in Autoimmune Diseases.

J. Luis Rivero and Moncef Jendoubi

Laboratory of Immunology, National Eye Institute, National Institutes of Health, Bethesda, MD 20892, U.S.A.

Introduction

Experimental autoimmune uveoretinitis (EAU) in rodents is a T cell-mediated autoimmune response particularly, against the photoreceptors of the neural retinal cells and can serve as a model for human uveitis. The role of MHC and non-MHC genes have been strongly associated with EAU in rats and mice[1-3]. To further study, the MHC class II participation in mice animal model, we decided to generate deficient mice for the invariant chain gene (Ii). This glycoprotein, combines with MHC class II heterodimers from the beginning of their synthesis in the endoplasmic reticulum, travels through the Golgi apparatus, and end up in endosomal compartments where it is either proteolytically cleaved or degraded. The absence of Ii has been shown to affect the transport of class II molecules, resulting in a poor antigen presentation[4-6].

Materials and Methods

Targeting Vector

A replacement vector has been designed to introduce a mutation in Ii murine gene, where neomycin phosphotransferase gene was inserted in the middle of the second exon. Two fragments of 0.3 Bgl II-Sac I and 9.2 Kb Sac I-EcoR I were added up stream and down stream of the neomycin gene respectively. Furthermore, two copies of herpes simplex virus thymidine kinase (HSV-tk), that allow the negative selection[7] ,were cloned at the end of the targeting vector. The targeting fragment used for the electroporation was excised from the back bone vector by digestion with Not I, dialyzed against TE (Tris/HCl 10 mM pH 7.5, EDTA 1 mM), precipitated with ethanol, resuspended in an appropriate buffer at a concentration of 1 mg/ml.

164

Electroporation

Embryonic stem cells (D3, from 129/Sv strain) were fed two and a half hours prior to electroporation. Cells were trypsinized, washed with DMEM and resuspended in HBS (Hepes 25 mM, NaCl 134 mM, 5 mM KCl, Na_2PO_4 0.7 mM, pH 7.1) at $2x10^7$ cells/ml. The same volume of HBS containing 100 μg/ml of targeting vector was added to the cell suspension, incubated ten minutes on ice. The electroporation was carried out using a 600 BTX electroporator with the following conditions: Volts: 250, μFaradays: 300, Resistant: R8.

Transfected cells were left at room temperature for ten minutes and seeded at a concentration of $5x10^6$ cells/10 cm petri dish. Twenty four hours later the cells were selected using G418 (200 μg active substance/ml) and gancyclovir (2μM).

Blastocyst Injection

Blastocysts, 3.5 days old, were collected by flushing the uterus of super ovulated C57BL/6 females. Mutated cells in the li gene were injected into blastocysts prior to their transfer to pseudopregnant B6D2 F1 foster mothers.

A   B

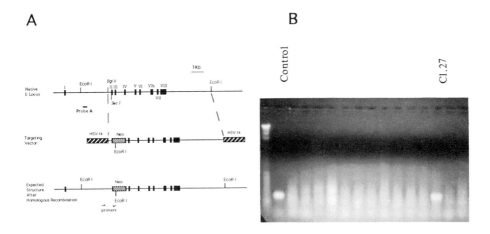

Fig.1: **A**: Correspond to the structure of li murine gene, the replacement targeting vector and the expected targeted structure.
B: Correspond to the PCR analysis of the different DNA samples from the double resistant clones

Results and Discussion

A total of 8×10^7 D3 cells were electroporated with the targeting vector (Fig. 1A) and selected with G418 and gancyclovir for ten days. Double-resistant clones were picked up individually and expanded in 24 well plate. DNA was isolated from each clone and analyzed by PCR for homologous recombination events: 3 out of 130 double-resistant clones scored positive (Fig. 1B).These three targeted clones were further expanded and injected into blastocyst, and the embryos were later transferred into the foster mothers. Offspring carrying the mutated Ii gene were identified by their chimeric coat color. Chimerics mice coming from one of the clones, 27, gave germ line transmission as shown by the coat color and confirmed by Southern blotting (Fig. 2A and 2B). Heterozygous and homozygous mice were born normal and they grow up without showing any obvious abnormality.

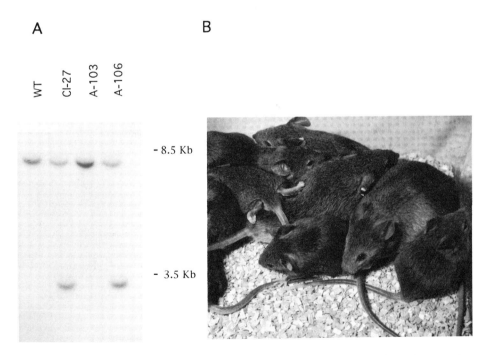

Fig. 2. **A**: correspond to the Southern blot analysis of DNA samples from both the targeted clones and mutated mice. **B**: represents a litter of deficient mice for the invariant chain gene.

References

1. Gery I. In: Chandler JW, O'connor GR, eds. Proceeding of the Third International Symposium on the Immunology and Immunopathology of the Eye. New York: Masson Publishing, 1984; 242-245

2. Hirose S, Sasamoto Y, Ogasawara K, Narito T, et al. In: Usui M, Ohno S, Aoki K, eds. Ocular Immunology Today, Proceeding of the Fith International Symposium on the Immunology and Immunopathology of the Eye. Amsterdam-New York-Oxford: Excerta Medica, 1990; 135-138.

3. Caspi RR, Grubbs BG, Chan C-C, Chader GJ and Wiggert B.   J. Immunol. 1992, 148, 2384-2389.

4. Viville S, Neefjes J, Lotteau V, Dierich A, Lemeur M, Ploegh H, Benoist C and Mathis D.   Cell 1993, 72, 635-648.

5. Bikoff EK, Huang L-Y, Episkopou V, van Meerwijk J, Germain RN and Robertson EJ.   J. Exp. Med. 1993, 177, 1699-1712.

6. Elliott EA, Drake JR, Amigorena S, Elsemore J, Webster P, Mellman I and Favell R.   J. Exp. Med. 1994, 179, 681-694.

7. Mansour SL, Thomas KR and Capecchi MR.   Nature 1988, 336, 348-351

1. Ocular Immunology and Inflammation
b. ACAID and related processes

Advances in Ocular Immunology
R.B. Nussenblatt, S.M. Whitcup, R.R. Caspi and I. Gery, eds.

On the role of extracellular, antigen-specific T cell proteins in immune deviation elicited by intracameral soluble protein antigens.

R.E. Cone[1], Y. Wang[1], J. O'Rourke[1] M. Kosiewicz[2], S. Okamoto[2], J.W. Streilein[2]

[1]Dept. of Pathology, Vision-Immunology Center, UConn Health Center, Farmington, CT, USA. [2]Schepens Eye Res. Inst., Boston, MA, USA.

Correspondence Address:

Dr. R.E. Cone
Dept. of Pathology,
University of Connecticut Health Center,
Farmington, CT 06030-3105 USA

Abstract

Extracellular antigen specific T cell proteins which share epitopes with T cell receptor α and β chains [TABM] are produced in serum after systemic immunization with soluble proteins and adjuvant. These proteins are also provided in serum after intracameral [IC] injection of trinitrophenylated spleen cells followed by sensitization with picrylchloride. To determine whether IC injection of soluble protein antigens would induce a similar serum TABM response, splenectomized and sham-operated mice sensitized to ovalbumin [OVA] received an IC injection of OVA. Serum was obtained 48 hr and 7 days after injection and TABM levels were quantitated by ELISA-based antigen binding using antisera specific for TABM. Splenectomized, OVA-immune mice that received an IC injection of OVA produced OVA-specific serum TABM within 2 days, but TABM were not detected in the sera of sham-operated mice. Naive mice receiving an IC injection of OVA or BSA did not produce serum TABM <u>unless</u> a systemic challenge followed IC injection. We infer that IC injection can deliver a strong systemic signal to stimulate TABM production in pre-sensitized mice. This suggests that TABM may play an immunoregulatory role when ACAID is imposed on previously sensitized mice.

Introduction

Intracameral [IC] injection of soluble or particulate antigens induces suppression of delayed-type hypersensitivity [DTH], and the production of IgG2a antibody specific for the antigen [1]. This systemic effect, Anterior Chamber Associated Immune Deviation [ACAID], appears to be due to cellular and/or humoral factors derived from the anterior chamber. These elements are believed to create a local immunosuppressive environment and induce systemically immunoregulatory [suppressor] T lymphocytes able to maintain a prolonged antigen-specific suppression of DTH. For example, transforming growth factor -β [TGF-β] present in aqueous humor induces F4/80+ peritoneal macrophages to resemble eye-derived macrophages present in blood in transferring an ACAID-like response to naive mice [2,3].

Intracameral [IC] injection of mice with spleen cells derivatized with trinitrophenol [TNP] induces TNP-specific ACAID [4] and, after epicutaneous sensitization, also induces an increase in serum of T lymphocyte-derived, extracellular proteins [TABM] specific for TNP [5]. TABM specific for the immunizing antigen also increase in serum when mice are injected systemically with high doses of soluble antigens and adjuvants [6,7]. These soluble antigen-specific TABM may be related to TNP-specific proteins detected in serum [TsIF] after the IC injection of TNP-spleen cells which impose ACAID on immune T cells [8] since both TABM and TsIF bear T cell receptor [TcR] $C\alpha$ and/or $C\beta$ epitopes [6,7,9].

Because the IC injection of TNP-spleen cells and epicutaneous sensitization induces a rise in serum TABM specific for TNP, we wished to determine whether an ACAID-inducing IC injection of soluble protein alone into sensitized mice would induce a similar rise in serum of TABM specific for the injected antigen. We used a polyclonal antiserum raised against monoclonal antigen-specific polypeptides [which induce the activation of suppressor T cells 10,11] to quantitate serum TABM specific for OVA after the intracameral injection of OVA into both naive mice and mice presensitized to OVA. We observed that the IC injection of OVA into sensitized mice induced a rapid rise of OVA-specific TABM which did not occur when naive mice received an IC injection of OVA. The results suggest that detectable TABM production is induced by IC injection in presensitized animals when sufficient TABM producing cells are present. This further suggests that these TABM participate in the activation of suppressor T cells whose numbers may have been expanded by the presensitization.

Results

Titration of OVA-Specific TABM in sera of AC-injected Mice.

To detect and quantitate Ovalbumin [OVA]-specific TABM in the sera of OVA sensitized mice, splenectomized and sham-splenectomized mice received a subcutaneous injection of OVA and Freund's complete adjuvant [FCA] and 7 days later an IC injection of OVA. Serum was collected 48 hr or 7 days after IC injection and dilutions of pooled serum were added to microtiter wells coated with OVA or bovine serum albumin [BSA]. Bound TABM were detected with a polyclonal antiserum specific for TABM [10] in ELISA-based antigen binding [6,7,10]. As shown in Fig. 1, pooled serum taken from OVA-sensitized mice 2 days after receiving an IC injection of OVA contained a higher titer of TABM binding OVA [but not BSA] than naive mice. In addition, this serum did not contain more trinitrophenol [TNP] binding TABM than sera from naive mice and splenectomized mice receiving an IC injection of BSA did not contain levels of OVA-binding TABM higher than naive mice [data not shown].

To define further the effect of IC injection of OVA on TABM production, the sera of splenectomized or sham-splenectomized mice that received an IC or subconjunctival injection [SC] of OVA two or seven days previously were assayed for OVA-binding TABM as shown in Fig. 1. To simplify data interpretation the O.D. obtained with a like dilution of pooled naive serum was subtracted from that obtained with a dilution of immune serum. As shown in Fig. 2A, sera obtained 2 days after splenectomized, sensitized mice received an IC injection of OVA [Group

1] contained significantly higher amounts of OVA-binding TABM than sera of splenectomized mice receiving no IC injection of OVA or an SC injection of OVA [Groups 3 and 2 respectively]. Moreover, no increase in TABM was detected in the sera of sham-splenectomized mice [Groups 4-6]. Similar results were obtained at other dilutions of pooled serum [data not shown]. Seven days after IC injection [Fig. 2B] OVA-specific TABM diminished in the sera of splenectomized mice but were still significantly greater than OVA-specific TABM found in the sera of sensitized mice which received an SC injection of OVA or no ocular injection of OVA.

The above observations indicate that IC injection of OVA alone into mice presensitized to OVA induces a rapid rise in OVA-specific TABM. To determine whether a single injection of soluble protein antigen into naive mice also induces a rise in TABM specific for the antigen, mice received an IC injection of BSA or OVA alone or received BSA and were challenged 7 days later by subcutaneous injection of BSA and Freund's complete adjuvant. As shown in Fig. 3, naive, splenectomized mice injected IC with BSA had a very small increment in BSA-binding TABM, while no increase in OVA binding TABM was observed. IC injection of naive, splenectomized mice with OVA did not increase OVA or BSA -specific serum TABM. In contrast, naive mice which received an IC injection of BSA and 7 days later an injection of BSA + FCA had significant titer of BSA-binding TABM two days after the challenge injection.

Discussion

IC injection of TNP-spleen cells into naive mice promotes the appearance in serum of TNP-specific TABM detectable by ELISA-based antigen binding subsequent to epicutaneous sensitization with picrylchloride [5]. Our results in this study using soluble antigens are consistent with those obtained with IC injection of TNP spleen cells into naive mice and demonstrate that the introduction of either antigen type into the anterior chamber exerts a profound influence on serum TABM production. However, IC injection of TNP-spleen cells alone into naive mice did not induce a detectable rise in serum TABM, while IC injection of OVA into OVA-sensitized mice induced a rapid appearance of TABM in serum which was not sustained. The rapid, evanescent rise in serum TABM after IC injection specific for the immunizing antigen is similar to a rise in serum TABM observed in sensitized mice receiving an intravenous, desensitizing dose of antigen [12].

The rise in serum TABM in sensitized mice after IC injection was detected only in the sera of splenectomized mice, suggesting that the spleen either inhibits TABM production or "filters" TABM from serum. The effect of splenectomy on the detection of serum TABM resembles the absence of detectable antigen-specific TsIF in the sera of mice which received an IC injection of TNP-spleen cells [8]. Because IC injection of antigen alone induces a rise in serum TABM specific for the antigen only in sensitized mice it is possible that the prior sensitization expands clones of TABM-producing cells which are activated by subsequent IC injection. In naive mice, IC injection may prime TABM producing cells which are activated by subsequent sensitization and/or challenge. Thus, if TABM production is primed, a subsequent exposure to antigen may have the same effect as IC injection into sensitized mice.

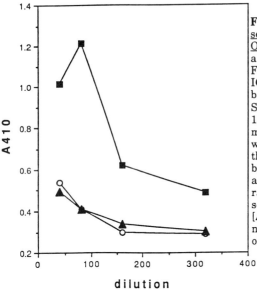

Figure 1: <u>Titration of OVA-specific TABM in serum from OVA-sensitized mice injected IC with OVA.</u> One week after splenectomy mice received a subcutaneous injection of 100 ug OVA in Freund's complete adjuvant and 7 days later an IC injection of 3ul CVA [16.7mg/ml in Hank's balanced salt solution]. and were bled 48 hr later. Sera were pooled, frozen at -70°C for storage and 100 ul of diluted serum from immune or naive mice was added to microtiter tray wells coated with 10 ug/well OVA or BSA. After 1.5 hr at 37°C the trays were washed and bound TABM detected by the addition of rabbit anti-TABM antiserum and alkaline phosphatase-conjugated goat anti-rabbit IgG. [■] Binding to OVA by TABM in serum from mice receiving IC injection of OVA [▲] Binding to OVA by TABM in serum from naive mice [○] binding to BSA by TABM in serum of mice receiving IC injection of OVA.

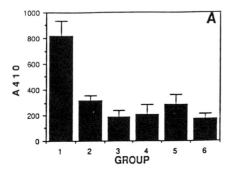

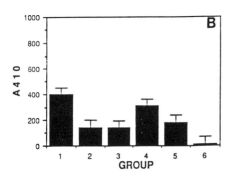

Figure 2: <u>IC injection of OVA into OVA sensitized, asplenic mice induces a rise in OVA-specific TABM.</u> OVA-sensitized, asplenic and sham-operated mice [see Fig. 1] received an IC or subconjunctival [SC] injection of OVA and serum obtained 48 hr [A] or seven days [B] after injection was assayed for OVA-specific TABM. Data represents the means ± SE [15 replicates of 5 experiments] of the O.D. obtained with 100 ul of a 1:160 dilution of serum minus the O.D. obtained with naive serum. Group 1: Splenectomized [SPX], OVA sensitized, IC injection of OVA. 2: SPX, OVA sensitized, SC injection of OVA, 3: SPX, OVA sensitized. 4: sham-operated [SO], OVA sensitized, IC injection of OVA. 5: SO, OVA sensitized, SC injection of OVA. 6: SO, OVA sensitized.

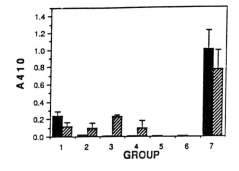

Figure 3: TABM production in naive mice receiving an IC injection of BSA or OVA.
Naive splenectomized [SPX] and sham-splenectomized [SO] mice received an IC or SC injection of BSA and 48 hr after injection sera were obtained, pooled and assayed for BSA or OVA-binding TABM. Data is the mean ± SE of five replicates of 100 ul 1:20 [solid] or 1:80 [hatched] dilution of serum binding to 25 ug/well BSA, 10 ug/well OVA. Group 1: SPX IC injection of BSA. 2: SPX, SC injection of BSA binding BSA. 3: SO + IC injection of BSA binding BSA. 4: SO + SC injection of BSA binding BSA. 5: SPX + IC injection of OVA binding OVA. 6: SPX, SC injection of OVA binding OVA. 7: BSA binding by serum from SPX mice that received an IC injection of BSA, 7 days later a subcutaneous injection of BSA in Freund's complete adjuvant and were bled 48 hr later.

The role of TABM in ACAID is not yet defined, however we note that the anti-TABM antiserum we used was made against a monoclonal protein that induced the activation of suppressor T lymphocytes [10,11]. Thus, it is possible that these serum TABM, like TsIF [8,13], act in concert with antigen to induce a proliferation and/or activation of suppressor T cells. The possibility that TABM may participate in ACAID is further supported by our observation that cyclophosphamide inhibited ACAID and serum TABM production promoted by an IC injection, while immunoglobulin production was not affected [14]. However, the IC injection of naive mice did not induce TABM production detectable by ELISA-based antigen binding during 7 days following injection. A single IC injection of antigen into naive mice may thus signal an early sequence of events which could result in the suppression of DTH while TABM producing cells are proliferating. The subsequent production of TABM could then induce and/or activate suppressor T cells distal to the early immunosuppressive signal. TABM in non-immune animals may thus maintain ACAID by amplifying the induction of suppressor T cells. On the other hand, if T cell populations have already expanded in response to a previous immunization, TABM may activate directly the suppressor cell population and thereby induce ACAID.

The physical nature of TABM and the mechanisms by which they may influence cell-mediated immune responses remains unelucidated. TABM are not B lymphocyte-derived immunoglobulins although, like immunoglobulins, they bind specifically to non-processed antigens (albeit with lower avidity than immunoglobulins [7]. A limited amino acid sequence of the variable region of two distinct monoclonal TABM shows a significant similarity to TcR Vα [15]. This finding, and the observation that serum TABM are recognized by monoclonal antibodies to TcR Cα [6,7] suggest that TABM are a soluble analogue of the TcR. Beyond this, the connection between the anterior chamber and peripheral TABM-inducing cells is unknown, although preliminary experiments suggest that TGFβ-treated peritoneal macrophages may induce TABM production. If confirmed, these recent observations would suggest that anterior chamber-derived macrophages activate suppressor T cells in the spleen directly, or perhaps indirectly, by the induction of TABM-producing T lymphocytes.

174

Acknowledgment

This work was supported by a University of Connecticut Health Center Faculty Research Grant, and Connecticut Lions Research Foundation and EY05678 to JWS. We are grateful to Ms. C. Mitchell for her assistance in the preparation of this manuscript.

References

1. Streilein, J.W. FASEB J. 1987. 1:199-205
2. Streilein, J.W., Wilbanks, G.A., Taylor, A. and Cousins, S. Cur.. Eye. Res. 1992. 11:41-47.
3. Wilbanks, G.A., Mammolenti, M. and Streilein, J.W. Eur. J. Immunol. 1992. 14:165-173.
4. Waldrep, J.C. and Kaplan, H. J. J. Immunol 1983. 131:2746-2750.
5. Hadjikouti, C., O'Rourke, J. and Cone, R.E. Inv. Opthamol Vis Sci. 1993. 34:1411 [Abstr. 3493].
6. Urbanski, M.M. and Cone, R.E. J. Immunol. 1992. 148:2840.
7. Urbanski M.M. and Cone, R.E. Cell Immunol. 1993. 153:131-141
8. Ferguson, T.A., Hayashi, J.D. and Kaplan, H.J. J. Immunol 1989. 143:831-826.
9. Kahn, M., Lima, S., Herndon, J.M., Kaplan, H. J., and Ferguson T. .A. Inv. Opthamol. Vis Sci 1993 34:803 (Abstr. 1003).
10. Cone, R.E., Weischedel, A-K., Kristie, J. and Urbanski, M. Mol. Immunol. 1992. 299:689-696.
11. Chue, B., Ferguson, J.A., Beaman, K.D., Rosenmann, S.J., Cone, R.E., Flood, P. and Greene, D.R. Cell Immunol 1989. 118: 30-40.
12. Cone, R.E., Gerardi, D.A., Davidoff, J., Kobayashi, K. and Cohen, S. 1987. 138: 234--239.
13. Ferguson, T.A., Beaman, K.D. and Iverson, G.M. 1983. J. Immunol. 167:3163-2172.
14. Cone, R.E., Wang, Y., and O'Rourke, J. Inv. Opthamol Vis Sci. 1994 25:1687 (Abstr. 2205)
15. Cone, R.E. and Marchalonis, J. J. Immunol. Invest. 1993. 22:541-552..

© 1994 Elsevier Science B.V. All rights reserved.
Advances in Ocular Immunology
R.B. Nussenblatt, S.M. Whitcup, R.R. Caspi and I. Gery, eds.

Suppression of Graft Rejection in Keraoepithelioplasty (KEP) Model by Anterior Chamber Injection of Donor Lymphocytes

Yoshiyuki Hara[1], Yu-Feng Yao[2], Yoshitsugu Inoue[3], and Yasuo Tano[2]

[1]Department of Ophthalmology, Sumitomo Hospital, 5-2-2, Nakanoshima, Kita-ku, Osaka, 530 Japan

[2]Department of Ophthalmology, Osaka University Medical School, 2-2, Yamada-oka, Suita-city, 565 Japan

[3]Department of Ophthalmology, Otemae Hospital, 1-5-34, Otemae, Chuo-ku, Osaka, 540 Japan

INTRODUCTION

Eyes are considered to be an immunological privilege site for a long period. Now it is termed as anterior chamber associated-immune deviation (ACAID), with the characterization of impaired delayed hypersensitivity (DH) in the recipient with inoculated antigens into the anterior chamber (AC). Recently, She et al. reported that prior AC injection of donor-type lymphocytes into the recipient eye promoted corneal graft survival in a rat penetrating keratoplasty model. More recently, Sonoda and Streilein assessed the ability of DH expression in mice that had received penetrating corneal transplants, and found that the unrejected allogenic cornea at its orthotopic site altered the immune reactivity of the recipient animal such that it did not develop graft-antigen specific DH responses.

As described in these reports, it is clear that ACAID is induced by two different routes: one is the corneal graft itself, that constitutively formed the recipient anterior chamber and shed foreign antigens into the aqueous humor; the other route was via donor-type lymphocytes inoculation to the recipient anterior chamber prior to grafting. Considering these two different induction of ACAID, using penetrating keratoplasty model to evaluate AC injection of donor lymphocytes on suppression of graft rejection is not suitable, since it is impossible to distinguish whether ACAID induced by the graft itself or by AC injected donor lymphocytes, we therefore developed a new model of keratoepithelioplasty in inbred rats, in which lenticules from the donor cornea are placed around the limbus of the recipient cornea. Since the recipient AC is not interfered with by the corneal graft, this model enables precisely analyzing the effect of AC injection of donor-type antigens on graft survival. Our results indicate that ACAID-related suppression of allograft rejection correlates with the recipient's decreased DH reaction specific to the donor-type antigen.

MATERIALS AND METHODS

Animals.
Female rats of Fisher 344 (RT1vl) and DA (RT1a) inbred strains (8 week old, weighing 120-150 mg) were purchased from Nippon Clea Co. Ltd (Tokyo, Japan). Except for the syngeneic grafts, Fisher rats served as recipients, DA rats as donors.

All animals were treated according to the Association for Research in Vision and Ophthalmology resolution on the use of animals in research; all procedures were carried out under sodium pentobarbital anesthesia or ketamine and xylazine mixtures as anesthetics.

Splenocytes preparation and Intracameral injections.

Spleen cells were harvested from DA rats. Before injection, the cells were counted and adjusted to 3×10^8 /ml. The methods of AC injection described by She et al. were used, with slight modification.

Surgical procedures of KEP.

The cornea of the sacrificed donor animal was excised along the limbus. The endothelium was scraped with a cotton swab, and the epithelial surface turned up to prevent epithelial damage. The cornea was then cut into four 2 mm x 3 mm lenticules, which were stored in RPMI 1640 medium until use.

The corneas of both eyes of the recipient were then prepared. First, 360° peritomy was performed at 2 mm from the corneoscleral limbus to remove the conjunctiva; then the corneal epithelium was scraped off by a Greafe's knife, with care taken to ensure complete removal. The four epithelial-stromal lenticules were then placed around the corneoscleral limbus and sewn at the limbus, with two or three interrupted 10-0 nylon sutures for each lenticule. At the end of the procedure, erythromycin antibiotic ointment was placed into the conjunctival sac of the operated eyes.

Postoperative care and inspection.

The grafted eyes were instilled with antibiotic ointment once daily for 3 days postoperatively, to prevent infection. The sutures were not removed postoperatively. The eyes were inspected every two days for the first two weeks and twice weekly afterwards, for a total of 30 day. The cornea was stained with 0.5% methylene blue to observe re-epithelialization and subsequent graft rejection under the stereomicroscope. After complete recovery of the epithelium, the cornea was scored according to the epithelial edema, imflammatory opacity, epithelial defect and neovascularization to assess graft rejection. Histological evaluation of the enucleated eyes at various time intervals was also made in other groups of animals.

DH assay on AC injection of donor lymphocytes.

DH assay in rat was similar to that described by others.

RESULTS

Graft survival in different experimental panels.

The purpose of our first series of experiments was to test whether AC injection of donor-type lymphocytes to the recipient eye prior to corneal grafting could suppress subsequent corneal allograft rejection in the KEP model. To accomplish this, we divided the graft-recipient Fisher rats into 3 groups; excepting the syngeneic graft group of 3 animals, the other 2 groups included 8 animals each. At 7 days prior to corneal grafting, each recipient received AC injection of 3×10^6 DA lymphocytes in 10 μl PBS (DAL group) or PBS only (positive control group) in the right eye; 7 days later, both eyes received grafts of lenticules of DA rat corneas. Another group of Fisher rats received grafts of syngeneic Fisher corneal lenticules without any AC injection prior to corneal grafting as negative control. Postoperative biomicroscopic observation revealed that epithelialization commenced in the grafted cornea, with gradual migration from the lenticules to the central cornea. 5 days after grafting, the corneal surface was totally re-epithelialized.

After re-epithelialization, the recovered epithelium in positive control group tended to become edematous and break down within 10 days, followed by prominent vascular proliferation into the lenticules and the host cornea. These changes reached a peak by day 15, marking a maximal mean score of 8.8. By day 15, 32% of those eyes (5/16) suffered corneal hemorrhage. In 88% (14/16), the ocular surface began to be replaced by highly vascularized tissues, finally resulting in scarred corneas to varied extent.

By contrast, in the DAL group, slight epithelial edema or small area of epithelial defect was observed within 10 postoperative days in only 37% of the eyes (6/16). Mild vascularization occurred in the lenticules and occasionally in the central cornea, gradually receding after day 20 . The area of epithelial defect also healed, the corneal surface remaining smooth. This effect was observed in both grafted eyes. The results strongly imply that AC injection of donor-type lymphocytes caused systemic suppression of graft rejection, rather than local suppression.

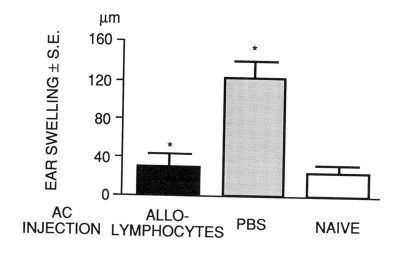

Figure 1. DH responses in Fisher rats. Ear swelling responses were measured at 24 hours with a micrometer. Mean values ± mean standard error for ear swelling responses are presented; * indicates values significantly different from positive control (p < 0.01).

Effect of AC allogeneic lymphocyte injection on DH response

Panels of Fisher rats received AC injection of 10^6 DA lymphocytes in 10 μl PBS or PBS only. Seven days later, these animals were immunized subcutaneously by 10^8 DA lymphocytes in 0.5 ml CFA. Seven days thereafter, the ears in these groups and another group of naive animals were challenged by intrapinnal injection of 10^6 DA lymphocytes in 10 μl PBS. Panels of Fisher rats received AC injection of 10^6 DA lymphocytes in 10 μl PBS or PBS only. Seven days later, these animals were immunized subcutaneously by 10^8 DA lymphocytes in 0.5 ml CFA. Seven days thereafter, the ears in these groups and another group of naive animals were challenged by intrapinnal injection of 10^6 DA lymphocytes in 10 μl PBS. Results, presented in the figure, indicate that the Fisher rats pretreated with AC injection of DA lymphocytes (group A) displayed significantly lower values of ear swelling than did the positive controls (group B; $p < 0.01$).

DISCUSSION

To precisely study whether intracameral injection of donor-type antigens into the recipient eye is capable of inducing ACAID and suppressing graft rejection, we developed a new model of KEP in rats. The surgical procedures were relatively simplified and the graft rejection was well characterized in this KEP model. In addition, as the recipient anterior chamber is not interfered with or shedded into by the corneal graft, this model is considered much more suitable for studying the influence of ACAID on corneal graft rejection. In this model, vigorous allograft rejection occurred at high incidence (88%: 14/16) in the positive control group. Edema of grafted lenticules-derived epithelium or epithelial defect and vascularization are hallmarks of this particular reaction. In contrast, when donor-type lymphocytes were injected intracamerally prior to KEP, only 37% of the eyes presented signs of allograft reaction. Although the clinical scores in these eyes were higher than those in syngeneic grafts (negative controls), they were significantly lower than those in positive controls. Moreover, clinical manifestations were much less pronounced even in symptomatic animals.

Our study has shown that animals receiving AC injection of donor-type lymphocytes demonstrated significantly minimal development of DH, the DH activity observed in each group of animals according well to the incidence and intensity of graft rejection. Presumably, the donor-type antigen intracamerally presented to the recipient prior to KEP induced immune deviation of impaired DH reaction, leads graft survival .

Recently, we have successfully to use KEP techniques in more immunogenetically determined species of mice, and the phenomena of AC injection of donor-type lymphocytes suppressing epithelial rejection in murine KEP model will be described in other place.

Address for correspondence; Yoshiyuki Hara, M.D. Department of Ophthalmology, Sumitomo Hospital, 5-2-2, Nakanoshima, Kita-ku, Osaka, 530 Japan.

Advances in Ocular Immunology
R.B. Nussenblatt, S.M. Whitcup, R.R. Caspi and I. Gery, eds.

ESTABLISHMENT OF A TH2 CELL LINE SPECIFIC FOR IRBP-DERIVED PEPTIDE AND ITS ROLE IN IMMUNOLOGICAL SUPPRESSION

T. Kezuka[1], M. Takeuchi[1], H. Yokoi[1], J. Sakai[1], M. Usui[1] and J. Mizuguchi[2]

[1]Department of Ophthalmology, Tokyo Medical College Hospital, Tokyo, Japan

[2]Department of Immunology, Tokyo Medical College, Tokyo, Japan

INTRODUCTION

EAU is an organ-specific intraocular inflammatory disease. It is mediated by CD4 T cells and is induced by IRBP or S-Ag. Recently, several T cell immunogenic determinants in the IRBP molecule have been identified in Lewis rats [1-2]. The synthesized peptide, P518-529 (TA12), was found to be an immunogenic determinant in Lewis rats by our group (data to be published). In the present study, we investigated whether or not TA12 acts as a T cell immunogenic determinant region of the IRBP molecule in B10.A congenic mice as well.

MATERIAL AND METHODS

1. Antigen
Bovine IRBP was purified using the methods described by Redmond [3]. Peptides, shown in Table 1, were synthesized with the Applied Biosystems Inc. Model 430A peptide synthesizer, using tBOC chemistry [4]. The sequences were derived from that of bovine IRBP.

Table 1 Amino acid sequence of synthetic peptide.

Peptide	Amino acid sequence
P518-529	SHRTATAAEELA

2. Animals and Immunization
Female B10.A mice were injected with an emulsion of 100 μg IRBP, or 5 μM synthetic peptide, in CFA containing 2.5 mg/ml *Mycobacterium tuberculosis* H37RA (Difco). The emulsion was injected into the hind footpads. An additional adjuvant, *Bordetella pertussis* bacteria was injected intraperitoneally, 10^{10} organisms/mouse, concurrently with the immunizations.

3. Experimental design
The animals were sacrificed on day 28 after the footpad injections. The eyes were enucleated and fixed in Bouin's solution. Sections of the sample were then embedded in paraffin and stained with hematoxylin and eosin for histological study.

4. Lymphocyte proliferation assay
The proliferation assay was performed with RPMI 1640 medium containing 10% FCS, and 5×10^{-5} M 2-ME in 96-well plates. 2×10^5 lymph node cells of IRBP-immunized B10.A

mice were dispensed into each well, followed by diluted Ag (IRBP or TA12). Cultures were incubated for 90 hours at 37°C in 5% CO_2 with a pulse of [^{3}H] TdR (0.5μ Ci /10 μ l/well) given 16 h prior to harvesting, and the incorporated counts were assessed. Thymidine uptake in cpm was expressed as a stimulation index: Stimulation index = cpm with stimulus / cpm with medium.

5. Establishment and maintenance of TA12 specific T cell line

A T cell line specific to TA12 was established from lymph node cells of TA12-immunized B10.A mice. Single cell suspensions at a density of 5×10^6 cells/well were cultured with TA12 (1 μ M) in 2 ml of conditioned medium in 24-well culture plates, along with syngeneic irradiated spleen cells (2000 rad) at 5×10^6 cells/well. After incubation for 7 days, 1 ml of supernatant was removed from each well and replaced with 1 ml of conditioned medium enriched with recombinant IL-2 at 20 U/ml. Following incubation for 4 days, the cells were collected, washed three times, and recultured at 2×10^5 cells/ml in 2 ml of conditioned medium with the peptide at 0.1 μ M along with syngenic irradiated spleen cells at 1×10^6. After incubation for 7 days, 1 ml of supernatant was removed from each well and replaced with 1 ml of conditioned medium with IL-2 (20 U/ml) and incubated for 4 days. With the cells at 2×10^5/well and syngenic irradiated spleen cells at 1×10^6/well, the cycle of stimulation with the peptide (0.1 μ M) and expansion with IL-2 was repeated.

6. Cytokine production assay

The P518-529 specific T cell line was assayed for IL-2, IFN-γ, IL-4 and IL-10 production. The cell line was incubated with TA12 of a concentration of 1 μ M. Culture supernatants were removed from each well 48 hours after the initiation of culturing, and cytokine (IL-2, IFN-γ, IL-4, IL-10) production was assayed by ELISA.

The ELISA protocol used was as follows. 1) Dilute purified anti-cytokine capture mAb to 5 μ g/ml in coating buffer (0.1 M NaHCO3, pH 8.2). Add 50 μ l to well of an enhanced protein binding ELISA plate. 2) Cover plate and incubate overnight at 4 °C. 3) Wash with PBS / Tween and block with Block Ace at 200 μ l per well. 4) Incubate at 37 °C for 2 hours and wash. 5) Add standards and samples at 100 μ l per well (diluted in PBS / 10% serum). 6) Incubate overnight at 4 °C and wash. 7) Dilute biotinylated anti-cytokine detecting mAb to 2 μ l /ml in PBS / 10% serum. 8) Incubate at room temperature for 1 hour and wash. 9) Dilute avidin, biotinylated-peroxidase to manufacturer's recommendation in PBS / 10% serum. Add 100 μ l per well. 10) Incubate at room temperature for 30 minutes and wash. 11) Add 10 mg of o-phenylenediamine and 10 μ l of H2O2 per 10 ml of citrate-phosphate buffer. Add 100 μ l per well and allow to develop at room temperature. Color reaction can be stopped by adding 50 μ l of 4 N H2SO4. 12) Read plate at OD 490 nm.

7. Adoptive transfer of TA12-specific T cell lines

Cells were transferred intraperitoneally into naive recipient B10.A mice in three groups as follows: (1) 5×10^6 cells from the TA12-specific T cell line, (2) 4×10^7 spleen cells from mice with IRBP-induced EAU, and (3) both TA12-specific cells and EAU mouse spleen cells at the concentrations as above. The mice were sacrificed 2 weeks later and eyes were examined histologically.

RESULTS

We have previously shown that EAU was induced in rats by immunization with the synthetic peptide TA12 of IRBP. In the present study, we investigated whether mice also develop EAU with TA12 immunization. None of the B10.A mice (0/7) displayed signs of EAU with TA12 stimulation, although IRBP induced the disease in 50% of the mice (5/10) by pathological criteria (Table 2). TA12 stimulated proliferative responses in IRBP-primed lymph node T cells, suggesting that a clone reactive to TA12 is present in the T cell repertoire of B10.A mice. To analyze the character of T cells reactive to TA12 or IRBP, specific T cell lines were established. As shown in Figure 1, T cell proliferation was obtained by TA12 in a dose-dependent manner in the presence of irradiated spleen cells as the antigen presenting cells. The TA12-specific T cell line produced both IL-4 and IL-10, while the IRBP-specific T cell line generated both IL-2 and IFN-γ ; thus the former may be designated as being of the Th2 type, with the latter being of the Th1 type [5-9]. Finally, we investigated whether TA12-specific T cells prevented the onset of EAU induced by the transfer of IRBP-primed spleen cells into unprimed mice. Our data showed that IRBP-primed spleen cells were capable of inducing cells in unprimed mice, whereas the induction of EAU was completely blocked by co-transfer of TA12-specific T cells. These results indicate that Th2 type cells play a pivotal role in the regulation of IRBP-mediated EAU.

Table 2   Incidence of EAU in B10.A mice

	Incidence of EAU
Incidence of EAU in IRBP-immunized mice	5/10
Incidence of EAU in TA12-immunized mice	0/7

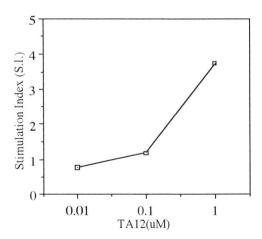

Fig 1   Proliferation assay of TA12 cell line

Table 3 Cytokine assay of TA12- and IRBP- specific T cell lines

	TA12-specific T cell line	IRBP-specific T cell line
IL-2 (ng/ml)	<0.1	0.3
IFN-γ (U/ml)	<1	78
IL-4 (ng/ml)	6.25	<0.1
IL-10 (ng/ml)	4	<0.1

DISCUSSION

We showed in these experiments that the TA12 peptide of IRBP prevents the onset of IRBP-mediated EAU in B10.A mice. This finding appears to fit the Th1/Th2 paradigm proposed by Mosmann & Coffman [5]. The TA12-specific T cell line (CD4$^+$) produced IL-4 and IL-10 (Th2 type), while the IRBP-specific T cell line (CD4$^+$) produced IL-2 and IFN-γ (Th2 type). Th1 cells may be involved in the inflammation caused by IRBP injection, which is then suppressed by Th2 cells induced by TA12 injection. Thus TA12 peptide injection, which favors Th2 cell expansion, is effective as a treatment of the local autoimmune disease EAU.

REFERENCE

1 Sanui H, Redmond TM, Kotake S, Wiggert B, et al. J Exp Med 1989; 169: 1947
2 Kotake S, Wiggert B, Redmond TM, Borst DE, et al. Cellular Immunol 1990; 126: 331-342.
3 Redmond TM, Wiggert B, Robey FA, Nguyen N, et al. Biochemistry 1985; 24: 787
4 Houghtem RA. Proc Natl Acad Sci USA 1985; 82: 5131
5 Mosmann TR, Coffman RL. Ann Rev Immunol 1989; 7: 145-173
6 Mossmann TR, Moore KW. Immunol Today 1991; 12: A49
7 Cher DJ, Mossmann TR. J immunol 1987; 138: 3688
8 Snapper CM, Finkelman FD, Paul WE. Immunol Rev 1988; 102: 51
9 Saoudi A, Kuhn J, Huygen K, DeKozak Y, et al. Eur J Immunol 1993; 23: 3096-3103.

Advances in Ocular Immunology
R.B. Nussenblatt, S.M. Whitcup, R.R. Caspi and I. Gery, eds.

Characterization of the effector and regulatory cells in ACAID

M. M. Kosiewicz and J. W. Streilein

Schepens Eye Research Institute and Department of Ophthalmology, Harvard Medical School, 20 Staniford St., Boston, MA, USA

INTRODUCTION

Injection of antigen into the anterior chamber of the eye induces a deviation in the systemic immune response referred to as anterior chamber associated immune deviation (ACAID). ACAID is characterized by the antigen-specific inhibition of delayed hypersensitivity (DH; 1). The inhibition of DH is mediated by two populations of spleen cells, a CD4 cell that inhibits the induction of DH and a CD8 cell that inhibits the expression of DH (2). We have recently reported that ACAID can be induced in previously primed mice; the spleens of these mice contain the CD8 cell that inhibits the expression of DH (3). The suppressor cells that are involved in the ACAID response have not been well-characterized and the mechanism(s) by which these cells effect suppression of DH is still unknown. We are in the early stages of characterizing these cells and we report our preliminary findings in this manuscript.

MATERIALS AND METHODS

Animals. Female BALB/c mice (6-8 wk) were purchased from Taconic Farms (NY) and were maintained under the guidelines stipulated by the ARVO Resolution on the use of animals in research.

Antigen. Ovalbumin (OVA) and bovine serum albumin (BSA; Sigma, St. Louis) were used in the following experiments.

Exposure to antigen. Anterior chamber (AC) inoculations were performed as described previously (1). OVA (50 µg) was injected into the right eye. The control for the AC injection consisted of a injection of antigen into the subconjunctival space (SCon). Mice were sensitized by subcutaneous (SC) injection of 100 µg of antigen emulsified in complete Freund's adjuvant.

Preparation of cells for adoptive transfer assays. CD4 or CD8 spleen cells were depleted as previously described (1). For the adoptive transfer assay, 50-100 x 10^6 CD4 spleen cells were injected into the tail vein in 100 µl. The ears of mice were then challenged with OVA (200 µg) 24 hr later. Ear swelling was measured 24 and 48 hr after ear challenge. The use of the local adoptive transfer assay (LAT) for the detection of efferent suppressor cells has been described previously (3). Briefly, 2 x 10^6 responder cells from the lymph nodes (LN) of naive or SC immunized mice were mixed with 5 x 10^5 CD8 regulatory spleen cells and antigen (200 µg) and injected into the ear pinnae of naive mice. The LAT was also used to detect effector CD4 cells directly. For this experiment, 2 x 10^6 CD4 cells were injected into the ear pinnae of naive mice. For the LAT assays, ear swelling was measured 24 and 48 hr later.

Assay for delayed hypersensitivity. Mice were challenged with 200 µg of antigen. Ear swelling was 24 and 48 hr later by micrometer. Data is presented as mean±SEM.

Proliferation assay. Spleen cells at 5 x 10^5 cells/well were cultured with 400 μg/ml OVA for 48 hr. Cells were pulsed with [^{3}H] thymidine (0.5 μCi/well) and 24 hr later, harvested and counted on a liquid scintillation counter. Data are presented as mean Δ cpm = (cpm of stimulated lymphocytes) - (cpm of unstimulated lymphocytes) ± SD.

Statistics. Analysis of variance and the Scheffe test were used to analyze the data. Means at $p<0.05$ were considered significantly different.

RESULTS

The CD8 efferent suppressor cells in ACAID are antigen-specific. In the LAT assay, efferent suppressor cells are detected by their ability to inhibit the expression of DH by primed LN cells after they have been co-transferred into the ear pinnae of naive recipients. For this experiment, responder cells were generated from naive LN or the draining LN of mice that had been primed with either OVA or BSA 7 days earlier. OVA-primed cells were mixed with CD8 regulator cells from mice that had received the following treatments: (1) no treatment (positive control); (2) an OVA inoculation into the AC 7 days earlier (AC; ACAID control); or (3) a SC immunization with OVA followed by an OVA inoculation into the AC 7 days later, then sacrifice at day 14 (SC-AC; experimental group). BSA-primed cells were mixed with CD8 cells from mice that had received the following treatments: (1) no treatment (positive control); (2) SC-AC (antigen specificity control). These mixtures of cells were injected into the ears of naive mice along with OVA and BSA. The CD8 cells from both SC-AC (84±25) and AC (93±12) treated animals were able to significantly inhibit the DH response of OVA-primed responder cells compared to the positive control (177±8). However, the CD8 cells from SC-AC (226±27) treated animals could not inhibit the DH response of BSA-primed responder cells when compared to the positive control for BSA (202±26). Naive responder cells were mixed with naive CD8 spleen cells for the negative control (65±18). We conclude that the CD8 cells which inhibit the expression of DH in animals that receive an AC inoculation either before or after priming are antigen-specific.

AC injection of antigen does not permanently inactivate CD4 cells. Two types of assays were used to test for the responsiveness of CD4 cells found in ACAID. The LAT assay was used to determine whether the CD4 cells found in ACAID could express DH when transferred into a naive recipient. In this assay, CD4-enriched spleen cells from mice with the following treatments were injected with OVA into the ear pinnae of naive mice: (1) a SC immunization with OVA followed 7 days later by SCon inoculation of OVA, then sacrifice at day 14 (SC-SCon; positive control); (2) an OVA inoculation into the AC, followed by a SC immunization with OVA 7 days later, then sacrifice at day 14 (AC-SC); (3) SC-AC (primed ACAID). There was no statistical difference in the ability of CD4 cells to transfer DH between AC-SC (138±20) or SC-AC (172±9) mice and the positive control SC-SCon (170±7). Negative controls received intrapinnae injections of naive cells (85±9). We conclude that the CD4 cells from ACAID animals can express DH in the absence of the CD8 efferent suppressor cells.

In order to determine whether the CD4 cells from ACAID mice are able to home to the site of ear challenge, CD4 spleen cells were adoptively transferred into naive recipients and DH was measured. For this assay, CD4 spleen cells from SC-SCon, AC-SC and SC-AC treated mice were injected into the tail vein of naive mice. Ears were challenged with OVA 24 hr later. The results are similar to that found with the LAT assay. The DH response of CD4 cells from mice of the AC-SC (71±9) and SC-AC (86±8) treated groups was not significantly different from the positive control, SC-Scon (85±14). Mice that had received naive cells only served as negative controls (17±13). We conclude that the ability of the CD4 cells to home to the site of ear challenge is apparently not permanently downregulated by the regulatory cells found in ACAID.

Proliferative responses involving ACAID spleen cells. The first experiment was designed to determine whether unfractionated spleen cells from ACAID animals can proliferate in response to antigen in vitro. Unfractionated spleen cells from naive, SC-SCon, AC, AC-SC, or SC-AC-treated mice were cultured with OVA for three days. Spleen cells from AC mice (1231±242) showed statistically significant (but minimal) proliferation compared to negative controls (591±47), but not compared to the positive controls, SC-SCon (4592±367). However, the spleen cells from both AC-SC (5536±608) and SC-AC (4945±216) mice exhibited a proliferative response similar to that found with SC-SCon cells. We conclude that the spleen cells from mice receiving an AC injection before or after priming can proliferate in response to the sensitizing antigen; spleen cells from mice receiving AC injection alone exhibit very low proliferative capacity.

In the next experiment, the capacity of CD4 cells from the spleens of ACAID mice were tested for their ability to proliferate in response to antigen. The CD4 cells from naive, SC-SCon, AC-SC and SC-AC mice were cultured for 3 days with OVA. The CD4 cells from both AC-SC (13954±1846) and SC-AC (11298±901) mice exhibited a proliferative response that was comparable to that found with CD4 cells from the positive control, SC-SCon (11226±746). Naive spleen cells served as negative controls (2498±320). We conclude that the CD4 cells from the spleens of ACAID animals exhibit a strong antigen-driven proliferative response in vitro.

Since the spleens of ACAID animals contain suppressor cells, we designed the next experiment to determine whether ACAID spleen cells can inhibit the proliferative response of LN cells from conventionally primed mice. Naive spleen cells (positive control) or AC spleen cells (experimental group) were mixed with OVA-primed LN cells and cultured for three days. There was no significant difference in the proliferative response of primed LN cells that had been cultured with either naive spleen cells (13836±1456), or AC spleen cells (16468±1095). Naive spleen cells cultured with naive LN cells served as negative controls (4157±611). We conclude that the suppressor cells found in the spleens of ACAID animals are not able to suppress an in vitro proliferative response.

DISCUSSION

In the present series of experiments we describe some of the characteristics of the effector and regulatory cells that are found in the spleens of mice with ACAID. We have shown that regardless of whether mice receive the AC injection before or after priming, their spleens contain CD8+ efferent suppressor cells that are antigen-specific. It is likely that these cells play a very important role in the downregulation of the on-going immune response and are, therefore, a potent mediator of ACAID in primed mice. However, the mechanism by which this suppression is effected is not yet known. For example, it is not known whether this is an active process requiring the direct and continued presence of the suppressor cell, or whether the suppressor cells inactivate the effector cells which then remain permanently hyporesponsive. Using two different systems with hapten-modified lymphoid cells as the tolerizing agents, Miller et al (4, 5) have reported that: 1) LN cells from tolerant mice possessing afferent suppressor cells cannot transfer contact hypersensitivity (CH) to naive recipients; and 2) LN cells from tolerant mice possessing efferent suppressors can transfer CH. Based on these data, we predicted that the afferent suppressor cells found in the spleens of mice that had received an AC injection of soluble antigen before priming would inhibit the induction of DH-mediating cells. These cells would then be unable to transfer DH to naive recipients. On the other hand, we predicted that mice that had received an AC injection of soluble antigen after priming would have sensitized cells whose responsiveness would be subsequently inhibited by the efferent suppressor cells. The question in the latter case would then be, does the inhibition of the expression of DH in ACAID require the continued presence of the efferent suppressor cell or is the effector cell permanently inactivated after transient contact with the efferent suppressor cell? Surprisingly, CD4 cells from ACAID mice, regardless of the timing of priming relative to AC injection, are capable of transferring DH to naive recipients. This may mean that the CD8 efferent suppressors, at least for soluble antigen, are the primary mediators of ACAID regardless of the timing of AC injection. The inability of the afferent suppressors to inhibit the induction of the immune response is further suggested by the antigen-driven proliferative response found in spleen cells, specifically CD4 cells, from ACAID mice. The efferent suppressor cells in ACAID apparently cannot permanently inhibit OVA-specific CD4 cells from either expressing the cytokines required to mediate DH or homing to the site of the immune response by, for example, downregulating adhesion molecules that are required for extravasculation. Further, our preliminary data suggest that these efferent suppressor cells cannot inhibit the antigen-driven proliferative response of primed LN cells.

We are currently attempting to isolate and clone both the regulatory and effector cells found in ACAID. Once these goals have been accomplished, we can begin a more refined and specific analysis of the regulatory cells that mediate ACAID.

REFERENCES

1 Mizuno K, Clark AF, Streilein JW. *Invest Ophthal Vis Sci* 1989 :30 :1112-1119.
2 Wilbanks GA, Streilein JW. *Immunol* 1990 :71 :383-389.
3 Kosiewicz MM, Okamoto S, Miki S, Ksander B, Shimizu T, Streilein JW. *Reg Immunol* (in press).
4 Miller SD, Man-Sun S, Claman HN. *J Immunol* 1978: 121: 265-273.
5 Miller SD, Man-Sun S, Claman HN. *J Immunol* 1978: 121: 274-280.

Advances in Ocular Immunology
R.B. Nussenblatt, S.M. Whitcup, R.R. Caspi and I. Gery, eds.

187

Immune privilege and induction of tumor-specific effector T cells using IL-2 or IL-4 cDNA transfected tumor cells

B. R. Ksander[a] , S. Miki[b], J. W. Streilein[a] , and E. Podack[b]

[a] Schepens Eye Research Institute and Department of Ophthalmology Harvard Medical School, 20 Staniford Street, Boston, MA, 02114.

[b]Department of Microbiology and Immunology, University of Miami School of Medicine, Miami, FL.

INTRODUCTION

We hypothesize that immunogenic tumors escape immune-mediated elimination by establishing a local microenvironment that conveys immune privilege to the developing tumor site. An immune privileged site is defined as an anatomical site in which immunogenic tissue survives for an extended period of time in an immunocompetent host (1). Since recent evidence from a variety of laboratories indicates that at least some spontaneous human tumors are immunogenic, the site of tumor growth is by definition a privileged site.

Our previous results using a murine model to examine the growth of immunogenic P815 tumor cells within the anterior chamber (AC) of the eye indicate that immune privilege in the AC is maintained by regulation of cellular immunity. P815 tumor cells grow progressively in the AC of BALB/c mice, but inoculation of a similar numbers of tumor cells into non-privileged sites such as the subconjunctiva or subcutaneous tissues of the skin results in rapid tumor. It should be noted, however, that inoculation of large numbers of tumor cells into these same sites results in progressive tumor growth, suggesting that these tumor cells can establish a form of immune privilege at these sites. The failure to eliminate P815 cells from the AC coincides with the failure of T cells to mediate DH and cytolytic killing of tumor cells in vivo. The failure to generate these effector cells results from an inability of precursor cytotoxic T cells (pTc) to terminally differentiate into cytolytic T cells. The experiments of Bando et al (2) indicate that the failure of pTc to differentiate and the failure to generate Tdh cells results from an inability of precursor Th cells to differentiate to Tho cells that secrete IL-2 and IL-4. Thus, the defect in developing tumor-specific effector T cells within the AC appears to be a direct result of the defective differentiation of specific T helper cells.

The purpose of the present series of experiments is to determine if IL-2 or IL-4 cDNA transfected lymphokine-secreting tumor cells can bypass the requirement for Th cells and induce a successful tumor-specific immune response within an immune privileged site. We examined the growth of transfected tumor cells inoculated into two different sites (i) within the AC, a site where immune privilege is already established, and (ii) the subcutaneous tissues in the skin (SQ), a site where tumors must establish privilege. Thus tumor cells were inoculated into the AC to determine if lymphokine-secreting tumor cells could break privilege in the eye; tumor cells were inoculated into the SQ to determine if lymphokine-secreting tumor cells could prevent tumors from establishing immune privilege at this site.

RESULTS AND DISCUSSION

Standard electroporation techniques were used to transfect P815 tumor cells with the pBMGNeo vector that contained either (i) IL-2 cDNA, (ii) IL-4 cDNA, or (iii) no cDNA insert (empty vector). The pBMGNeo vector is an episomal vector that allows the stable expression of inserted cDNA, allowing transfected tumor cells to secrete large amounts of the selected lymphokine. P815 cells transfected with IL-2 cDNA (P815-IL2) secreted 11,000 units/ml (0.5×10^6 cells cultured in 1ml for 48 hr). P815 cells transfected with IL-4 cDNA (P815-IL4) secreted 83,000 units/ml using the same culture conditions. In the first series of experiments we examined the growth of transfected and untransfected P815 cells inoculated in the AC of syngeneic DBA/2 mice. Groups of five mice each received AC inoculations of 2×10^5 tumor cells and the subsequent tumor growth was determined quantitatively by slit lamp examination. The data displayed in Figure 1 indicates the percentage of the AC that contains tumor cells on the designated days post inoculation. All mice that received inoculations of either (i) untransfected P815 cells, (ii) P815-IL2 cells, or (iii) P815-IL4 cells developed ocular tumors that filled 100% of the AC by day 7 pi. Untransfected P815 cells continued to grow progressively into the posterior of the eye after day 7 pi. By contrast, between day 7 and 17 pi P815-IL2 cells were eliminated completely from the AC. Tumor rejection was accompanied by an intense inflammatory response that also resulted in complete destruction of the eye (phthisis). Rejection of P815-IL2 cells was due to the secretion of IL-2 and not due to the pBMGNeo expression vector as demonstrated by progressive growth of P815 tumor cells transfected with the empty vector (data not shown). IL-4 secreting P815 cells were not rejected from the AC and continued to grow progressively. We conclude from these results that within the AC, an established immune privilege site, IL-2 but not IL-4 is effective in preventing tumor growth.

The next series of experiments were performed to determine if IL-2 or IL-4 secreting tumor cells can prevent tumor growth when injected into a non-privileged site such as the SQ. In other words we wished to determine if lymphokine-secreting tumor cells can prevent tumors from establishing their own immune privilege at the developing tumor site. Groups of DBA/2 mice received SQ inoculations of 2×10^6 P815 cells and tumor growth was determined quantitatively. The data displayed in Figure 2 indicate that mice that received inoculations of either (i) untransfected P815 cells, (ii) P815-IL2 cells, or (iii) P815-IL4 cells all formed tumors averaging approximately 5 mm in size by day 10 pi. Untransfected tumor cells continued to grow progressively after day 10 pi, eventually reaching an average size of 23 mm by day 21 pi. By contrast, both P815-IL2 and P815-IL4 transfected tumor cells were eliminated completely between days 10 and 21 pi. We conclude from these experiments that secretion of either IL-2, or IL-4 is sufficient to prevent tumors from establishing immune privilege.

Since secretion of IL-4 by P815 cells was sufficient to prevent tumors from establishing immune privilege within the SQ, but was unable to break immune privilege within the AC, we next wished to determine if lymphokine secretion by P815-IL2, and P815-IL4 cells stimulated different populations of specific T cells. The first series of experiments examined the induction of tumor-specific cytotoxic T cells during rejection of lymphokine-secreting tumor cells from the SQ. Groups of DBA/2 mice received SQ inoculations of either P815, P815-IL2, or P815-IL4 cells as in the previous experiments. Spleen cells were recovered on day 20 pi and restimulated in vitro for 5 days with x-irradiated P815 cells. At completion of the incubation period, the cytotoxic activity was determined using a standard 4 hr chromium release assay against either P815 or third-party EL-4 target cells. The results are displayed in Figure 3. Spleen cells recovered from either normal DBA/2 mice, or mice that received SQ inoculations of untransfected tumor cells did not contain cytotoxic T cells that lysed P815 cells. By contrast, spleen cells recovered from mice that rejected P815-IL2 tumor cells contained cytotoxic T cells that lysed P815 cells (figure 3), but failed to lyse third-party EL-4 target cells (data not shown). Spleen cells from mice that rejected P815-IL4 cells displayed killing of P815 cells that was only slightly above the background level of the negative controls. Thus these data demonstrate that P815-IL2, but not P815-IL4 tumor cells induce specific cytotoxic T cells in the spleen during tumor rejection.

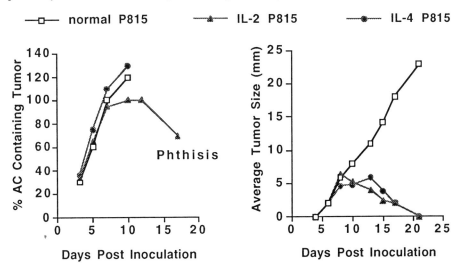

Figure 1. Growth of cDNA transfected
tumor cells within the immunologically privilege AC.

Figure 2. Growth of cDNA
tumor cells within the non-privileged subcutaneous tissue.

In the final series of experiments we examined if rejection of P815-IL2 or P815-IL4 cells from the SQ was accompanied by the induction of DH. Groups of DBA/2 mice received SQ inoculations of tumor cells as in the previous experiments and on day 20 pi mice received injections of 0.5 x 10^6 x-irradiated P815 cells in 10 μl in the right ear pinnae. Ear swelling was measured 48 hrs later as a measure of DH. The results are displayed in Figure 4 and demonstrate that the induction of DH is associated with the rejection of either P815-IL2, or P815-IL4 tumor cells from the SQ.

Our results indicate that secretion of either IL-2, or IL-4 by P815 tumor cells is sufficient to prevent tumors from establishing immune privilege in the subcutaneous tissues of the skin. However, in sites where privilege already exists, IL-2 but not IL-4 is effective in breaking immune privilege. Since both IL-2 and IL-4 secreting tumor cells induced DH, but only IL-2 secreting tumor cells induced specific cytotoxic T cells, the failure of IL-4 to prevent tumor growth within the privileged AC corresponds with the failure to activate specific cytotoxic T cells. Therefore the induction of DH alone is insufficient to initiate tumor rejection in an immune privileged site such as the eye.

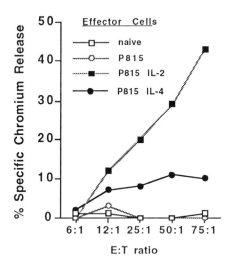

Figure 3. Cytotoxic T cell lysis of P815 target cells.

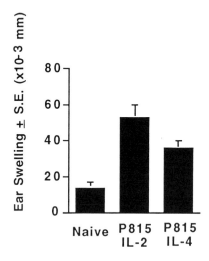

Figure 4. Induction of DH in mice inoculated with cDNA transfected tumor cells.

REFERENCES

1. Ksander BR, Streilein JW. Regulation of the Immune Response within Privilege Sites - in "Mechanisms of Regulation of Immunity", ed. R. Granstein. *Chemical Immunology* Basel, Karger. 1994; vol. 58, 117-145.

2. Bando Y, Ksander BR, Streilein JW. Characterization of T Helper Cell Activity in Mice Bearing Alloantigenic Tumors in the Anterior Chamber of the Eye. *Eur. J. Immunol.* 1991: 21:1923-1931.

© 1994 Elsevier Science B.V. All rights reserved.
Advances in Ocular Immunology
R.B. Nussenblatt, S.M. Whitcup, R.R. Caspi and I. Gery, eds.

Inhibition of cell induced interferon-α production; a novel immunosuppressive activity in human, porcine and rabbit vitreous

M.P. Langford, T.E. Kruger, L. Wood, and J.P. Ganley

Department of Ophthalmology, Louisiana State University Medical Center, Shreveport, LA, 71130 USA

Introduction

We have reported the detection of a factor in human vitreous that inhibits the production of interferon-α (IFN-α) by human peripheral blood lymphocytes (HPBL) co-cultured with cells of tumor origin [1]. The inhibitor is hyaluronidase resistant and is not reactive with antibodies to transformation growth factor β or melanocyte stimulating hormone as reported for these immunosuppressive factors in aqueous [2-4]. In this report, we identify similar levels of an inhibitor of IFN-α production in vitreous of different animal species and low levels of an IFN-α inhibitor in porcine and human aqueous but not in rabbit aqueous or human cerebral spinal fluid (CSF). Also, we show that the factor inhibits an early event in the HPBL-tumor cell interaction that results in the production of IFN-α.

Materials and Methods

Vitreous, aqueous and human CSF. Human liquid vitreous was removed from 12 frozen cadaveric eyes (Northwest Louisiana Lions Eye Bank, Shreveport, LA) as previously described [1]. Aqueous and/or vitreous were aspirated from two human cadaveric (4 days post enucleation), four porcine and eight rabbit eyes. Two infectious agent negative human CSF were obtained from the Neurology Department, LSU Medical Center, Shreveport, LA.

Assay for inhibition of cell induced IFN-α production by vitreous, aqueous, and CSF. HPBL were obtained from the venous blood of volunteer donors using the separation procedures previously described [5]. Vitreous, aqueous and CSF were diluted in culture media and 100 µl added to microtiter plate cultures (Corning, Corning, NY) of HEp-2 cells (human epidermoid carcinoma, American Type Culture Collection, Rockville, MD). 5×10^5 HPBL (50µl) were added to each culture and incubated for 16 to 24 hrs at 37°C and frozen as previously described [6]. The culture fluids were assayed for antiviral activity using a standard virus microplaque reduction assay [7].

Figure 1. Effect of different concentrations of human, porcine and rabbit vitreous humor (VH) on IFN-α production.

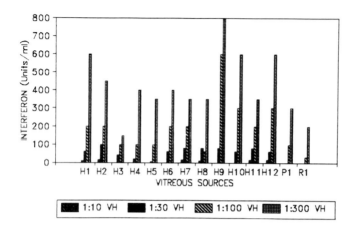

Results

   Inhibition of IFN-α by different concentrations of human, porcine and rabbit vitreous. IFN production by HPBL co-cultured with HEp-2 cells was inhibited equally by vitreous from 12 human eyes, a porcine eye and a rabbit eye in a dose dependent manner (Figure 1). For example, culture media harvested after 16 hrs incubation from co-cultures treated with 10% vitreous (1:10 v/v) contained <10 to 20 units of IFN/ml (>90% reduction), with 1% vitreous (1:100 v/v) contained 20 to 600 units (0->90% reduction) or with 0.3% vitreous (1:300 v/v) contained from 150 to 800 units of IFN/ml (0-50% reduction) (control co-cultures produced 600 to 2,000 units of IFN/ml, not shown).

   Effect of vitreous, aqueous and CSF on IFN-α production. Vitreous was more effective at inhibiting IFN-α than aqueous, and CSF did not inhibit IFN-α production (Table 1). Interestingly, human and porcine aqueous inhibited IFN production by 5-10 fold (≥80%), but rabbit aqueous did not affect IFN production (≤3-fold reduction is not statistically significant).

   Kinetics of the inhibition of IFN-α production by vitreous. IFN-α was detected at 2 hrs post incubation, increased to near maximal levels by 4 hrs and remained at a steady-state level through 16 hrs in media harvested from control co-cultures (Figure 2). Vitreous (10% v/v) added to co-cultures at 0 hr inhibited IFN-α production. Vitreous added at 0.5 and 1.0 hr post incubation suppressed IFN-α production by ≥90%, and vitreous added after 1.0 hr of incubation had no effect on the IFN-α produced through 16 hrs of incubation.

Table 1
Effect of rabbit, porcine and human aqueous and vitreous and CSF on IFN-α production by HPBL co-cultured with HEp-2 cells.

Sample		Units/ml IFN-α produced by:								
		HPBL Donor #1					HPBL Donor #2			
		Aqu[a]	Ctl	Vit	Ctl	CSF	Aqu	Ctl	Vit	Ctl
Rabbit	#243	2,000	<10	100	<10		300	20	30	10
	#244	2,000	<10	100	<10		300	10	100	20
	#245	2,000	<10	600	<10		200	20	60	10
Porcine	#5/94	600	<10	30	<10		100	20	60	10
Human	#40/94	300	<10	30	<10		60	10	<3	30
	#41/94	300	<10	60	<10		100	10	10	10
Human	#6				<10	1,000				
	#10				<10	1,000				
HPBL Ctl					<10					20
HPBL-HEp-2 Ctl				3,000						600

[a]Aqueous (Aqu), vitreous (Vit) and human CSF were added to the medium (10% v/v) of HEp-2 cell cultures prior to the addition of HPBL. Controls (Ctl) consisted of 10% aqueous, vitreous or CSF and HPBL, HPBL alone or HPBL plus HEp-2.

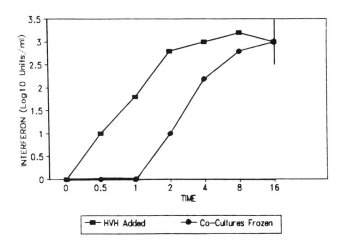

Figure 2. Inhibition of the cell-induced IFN-α production. The kinetics of IFN production in HPBL-HEp-2 co-cultures (-o-) and the IFN levels in co-cultures treated with human vitreous humor (HVH) at different times and incubated for 16 hrs (-x-) are shown. (Vertical bar is the standard error of the IFN assay).

Discussion

IFN-α can be produced by virus-infected lymphocytes/monocytes and by non-sensitized lymphocytes that come in contact with viral or tumor antigens on cells [8]. We have detected a factor in human vitreous that inhibits IFN-α production by HPBL co-cultured with tumor cells [1]. The inhibitor appears to effect an early interaction between the HPBL and tumor cells, since the addition of vitreous to co-cultures after 1.0 hr of incubation does not inhibit IFN-α production. In addition to its rapid effect, the factor appears to be a potent inhibitor, in that concentrations of ≤1% (v/v) of some vitreous inhibit IFN-α production by ≥90%. Also, we have detected a titratable factor in rabbit and porcine vitreous that inhibits IFN-α production as well as human vitreous. This suggests that other animal species produce a vitreal factor that can inhibit the production of cell induced IFN-α. Interestingly, human and porcine aqueous but not rabbit aqueous can inhibit IFN-α production, but the level of inhibition was less than that for vitreous. This suggests that the inhibitor may diffuse into the aqueous, but does not rule out the production of the (an) inhibitor of IFN-α in the anterior chamber of some animals.

The results of these studies extend our previous studies [1] to include vitreous and aqueous of different animal species and suggest that the vitreal factor is a potent inhibitor of a very early "induction signal" that initiates IFN-α production by lymphocytes that "recognize" antigen(s) on tumor cells. Also, we suggest that the inhibitor could suppress the immediate type, IFN-α mediated immune responses to tumor (and possibly viral and embryonic) antigens on cells within the eye.

References

1   Langford MP, Ganley JP, Kruger TE. Reg Immunol 1994;6:(in press).
2   Forrester JV, Balazs EA. J Cell Sci 1980;48:315-331.
3   Cousins SW, McCabe MM, Danielpour D, Streilein JW. Invest Ophthalmol Vis Sci 1991;32:2201-2211.
4   Taylor AW, Streilein JW, Cousins SW. Curr Eye Res 1992; 1:1199-1206.
5   Langford MP, Stanton GJ, Johnson HM. Infect Immun 1978; 22:68-78.
6   Blalock JE, Langford MP, Georgiades JA, Stanton GJ. Cell Immunol 1979;43:197-201.
7   Langford MP, Weigent DA, Georgiades JA, Johnson HM, et al. Methods Enzymol 1981;78:339-346.
8   DeMaeyer E, DeMaeyer-Guignard J. Induction of IFN-α and IFN-β. In: Interferons and Other Regulatory Cytokines. New York: John Wiley & Sons, 1988; 39-66.

Advances in Ocular Immunology
R.B. Nussenblatt, S.M. Whitcup, R.R. Caspi and I. Gery, eds.

ACAID as a potential therapy for established experimental autoimmune uveitis.

S. Okamoto[a], M.M.Kosiewicz[a], R.R. Caspi[b], and J.W.Streilein[b].

[a] The Schepens Eye Research Institute Boston, MA 02114,
[b] Laboratory of Immunology, NEI, NIH, Bethesda, MD 20892

INTRODUCTION

Retina-specific proteins, such as rhodopsin, retinal S antigen and IRBP (Interphotoreceptor Retinoid Binding Protein) have been used as pathogens to induce autoimmune uveitis in experimental animals, including monkey, mice and rats [1]. Anterior chamber associated immune deviation (ACAID) has been induced by these retina-specific proteins, and specific ACAID has been used to prevent experimental autoimmune uveitis (EAU) in mice and rats. Mizuno et al reported that pretreatement of rats with intracameral injection of S-Ag prevented the onset of EAU [2]. Hara et al showed that intracameral injection of IRBP prevented IRBP-specific delayed hyper-sensitivity (DH) and suppressed autoimmune uveitis. In addition, Hara et al. reported that spleen cells from mice that received IRBP via anterior chamber (AC) suppressed uveitis when adoptively transferred into recipients in which EAU had been established [3]. These findings suggest that ACAID-dependent suppressor T cells generated by the intracameral injection of IRBP possess the capacity to suppress ongoing EAU.

Recently Kosiewicz et al have found that ACAID can be induced by AC injection of antigen even in specifically presensitized animals [4]. These results suggest that ACAID may be inducible after the onset of an auto-immune disease. To test this possibility, we determined whether IRBP-specific ACAID could be induced in IRBP-primed mice, and whether ACAID induction *after* the onset of EAU could suppress further clinical progression. Our results indicate that ACAID can be induced in IRBP-immune mice by either AC injection of IRBP, or intravenous (IV) injection of IRBP-pulsed, TGFß-treated peritoneal exudate cells (PEC). Moreover, EAU subsided within 48-78 hr after the injection of IRBP-pulsed, TGFß-treated PEC.

MATERIALS AND METHODS

Animals. BALB/c mice and B10.A mice (6 to 12 wk) were obtained from our domestic mouse breeding facility, or were purchased from Taconic Farm (NY). All animals were treated according to the Association for Research in Vision and Ophthalmology resolution on the use of animals in research. All procedures were performed under ketamine and xylazine mixtures as anesthetics. *Antigens (Ag).* IRBP was isolated from bovine retinas as described previously [5]. Ag was dissolved in PBS and injected directly, or mixed with complete Freund's adjuvant (CFA; Difco Lab., Detroit, MI), containing killed mycobacterial organisms at 2 mg/ml. *Induction of DH* was accomplished as previously described [6]. Mice received an immunizing dose of IRBP (50 µg) emulsified in CFA in a total volume of 100 µl injected S.C. into the nape of the neck. For the assessment of DH, mice received intra-dermal inoculations of

IRBP (5 µg/20 µl) into the right ear pinna. The ear swelling response was then assessed 24 h later using a micrometer (Mitsutoyo 227-101, MTI Corporation, Paramus, NJ). *Induction of uveitis.* As described elsewhere [6], IRBP, 50 µg, was mixed with CFA, and injected into the nape of the neck. Bordetella PTX (Sigma) was injected 500 ng i.p. at the same time as the adjuvant was injected. *Intraocular injections.* AC and subconjunctival (SCon) injections were carried out as described previously [3]. Briefly, anesthetized mice received AC injections with blunted 30 gauge needle attached via plastic tubing to a disposable syringe. For AC inoculations, an oblique transcorneal paracentesis tunnel was formed with a sharp 30-gauge needle, carefully avoiding iris or lens injury. The blunt needle was inserted through this track, followed by inoculation of 3 µl of Ag and a few bubbles of air, sealing the injection tract. For SCon injection, the blunt needle was inserted via the inferior bulbar conjunctiva and a small bleb of fluid and air was raised. The AC or SCon of the right eye of each mouse received 50 µg/3 µl of IRBP. *In vitro ACAID-inducing protocol.* PEC were harvested from naive syngeneic mice that were injected 3 ml of 3% thioglycolate 3 days before, were washed twice. $2x10^5$ cells were cultured in 100µl of complete culture medium containing 1% normal mouse serum in 96 well round bottom plates as previously described [7]. IRBP (50 µg/well) was added as antigen. TGFß (0.1 ng/well) dissolved in PBS was added to the cultures and incubated overnight in CO_2 incubator. After harvesting and 2 washings, the cells were resuspended and infused intravenously (IV) ($2x10^3$ cells/100 µl) into naive syngeneic recipients. *Assessment of uveitis.* Fundus examination of the eye was performed daily after immunization. According to the ocular findings, an arbitrary 4-point score was devised in order to provide a semi-quantitative evaluation as described previously [3]. One point each was awarded for retinal vascular dilation, retinal vasculitis, retinal exudates, and choroidal infiltration, and swelling of the optic disc. A score of 2+ or greater by fundoscopy was taken as clinical evidence of uveitis, and most severe examples of uveitis received a score of 4+. *Statistic evaluations.* Analysis of ear swelling responses was accomplished using a two-tailed Student's t-test. Ocular fundus scores were analyzed with Mann-Whitney test. All probability values less than 0.05 were deemed significant.

RESULTS

Induction of unresponsiveness in IRBP-immune mice by AC injection of IRBP.

Panels of naive BALB/c mice received subcutaneously, IRBP (50µg), mixed with CFA. Seven days prior to sensitization, one panel of mice received 50 µg IRBP injected into the anterior chamber (AC) of right eye, i.e., this panel received a typical ACAID inducing protocol and these mice served as the ACAID control. The other two panels of mice received IRBP injection into the AC or into the SCon space seven days *after* the recipient mice had received conventional sensitization with IRBP. Seven days later DH responses were assessed by ear challenge. The results are displayed in Figure 1. As anticipated, mice that were pre-treated with an AC injection of IRBP prior to sensitization with Ag in CFA failed to develop DH responses. Similarly, pre-immunized mice that received an AC injection of IRBP also failed to show DH responses. These results indicate that the capacity of pre-sensitized animal to express DH can be impaired by exposing the recipient to the same antigen by the intraocular route.

Induction of unresponsiveness in IRBP-primed mice by IV injection of PEC cultured with TGFß and IRBP.

Wilbanks reported that F4/80 positive PEC treated with Iris/ciliary body supernatant or TGFß induce ACAID when injected intravenously [7]. Based on this observation, we determined whether PEC cultured with IRBP in the presence of TGFß could function as a so-called ACAID-inducing signal in IRBP pre-sensitized mice. Two panels of BALB/c mice were sensitized with IRBP mixed with CFA. PEC harvested from naive BALB/c mice were treated with IRBP and TGFß overnight and were injected intravenously into IRBP pre-sensitized BALB/c mice. One week later, DH responses were assessed by ear challenge. The results are displayed in Figure 1. Pre-sensitized mice that received an IV injection of TGFß treated PEC also failed to show DH responses. These results indicate that the capacity of an animal to develop and express DH can be impaired by injecting so-called ACAID inducing signal IV even if the recipients have already been sensitized with the antigen.

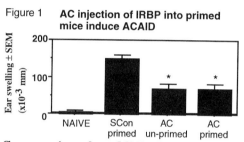

Figure 1 **AC injection of IRBP into primed mice induce ACAID**

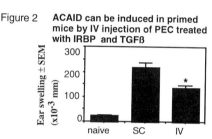

Figure 2 **ACAID can be induced in primed mice by IV injection of PEC treated with IRBP and TGFß**

Suppression of established uveitis by ACAID induction with TGFß treated PEC

To study the effect of ACAID induction on EAU, panels of B10.A mice received a uveitogenic induction regimen of 50 µg IRBP in CFA along with 500 ng PTX. Retinal changes, as revealed by fundoscopy, were graded on an arbitrary 4 point system as described in Material and Methods. When eyes of these mice were estimated to have a score of 2+ to 3+ by fundoscopy, PEC treated with or without TGFß in the presence of IRBP were injected IV in randomized fashion. A summary of a typical experiment is shown in figure 3. As early as day 2, the clinical scores of eyes of the control group had progressed to 3+ or 4+, whereas the eyes of most of the ACAID group retained scores 2+ or 3+. At day 4 , although the eyes of mice in which ACAID was induced displayed scores 2+, or 3+, and some even regressed to 1+, the control group eyes revealed scores 3+ and 4+. After day 7, although the uveitogenic inflammation began to disappear in both groups, eyes of the control group still displayed scores 4+. The retina and retinal vessels showed irreversible changes, even though the inflammation subsided. By statistical analysis, the differences in clinical scores between the ACAID group and the control group were significant at day 2 (p<0.05), day 4 (p<0.01), and day 7 (p<0.01).

Figure 3 ACAID induction after the onset of EAU prevent the progression.

Score	Day 0 ACAID	Control	Day 2 ACAID	Control	Day 4 ACAID	Control	Day 7 ACAID	Control
4	0 %	0 %	19%	65%	0 %	73%	0 %	72%
3	27	9	36	35	64	27	46	18
2	73	91	45	0	18	0	27	9
0-1	0	0	0	0	18	0	27	0

DISCUSSION

Various studies using different protocols have been used to induce antigen-specific T-cell tolerance, such as IV injection, oral inoculation, or AC injection of Ag. There is hope that immuno-therapy of this type might be useful in the clinical setting. The most critical factor isto know whether a therapy can be used to treat an ongoing autoimmune response, or whether it is effective only for prevention. In clinical medicine, an autoimmune disease is usually diagnosed at a time when significant tissue damage has already occurred. At this point, immuno-therapy is needed to prevent further tissue damage and to eliminate or suppress autoreactive T cells. Gaur et al reported that intra-peritoneal injection of myelin basic protein (MBP) prevented the onset of experimental autoimmune encephalo-myelitis (EAE) in mice, and furthermore this procedure reduced the severity of ongoing EAE [8]. In EAU, although the oral administration or AC injection of S-Ag or IRBP can prevent the onset of EAU, specific immunotherapy has not been reported to block ongoing EAU.

The evidence in this communication indicates that ACAID can be induced after prior sensitization and that suppressor cells can be generated even after the onset of an experimentally induced systemic autoimmune disease. More important, in this study we demonstrate that an IRBP-specific ACAID-inducing signal created *in vitro* by exposure of PEC to IRBP in the presence of TGFß can evoke ACAID in mice previously sensitized to IRBP, and that intravenous administration of an ACAID-inducing signal to mice experiencing ongoing EAU results in the failure of progression of the ocular inflammation, and even promotes resolution of the disease.

In the last experiment, promotion of ACAID and suppression of EAU was achieved without recourse to injection of antigen into the eye. Merely an IV injection of cells bearing an ACAID-inducing signal was sufficient to achieve the effect. This outcome suggests that this approach to immunotherapy of ocular autoimmune disease may have clinical merit.

REFERENCES

1 Nussenblatt, R.B. Invest. Ophthalmol. Vis. Sci. 1991; 32: 3131-3141, 1991.

2 Mizuno, K., Altman, N.F., Clark, A.F. et al. Curr. Eye Res. 1989;8:113-121.

3 Hara, Y. Caspi, R.R., Wiggert, B., et al. J. Immunol. 1992; 148: 1685-1692.

4 Kosiewicz, M., Okamoto, S., Miki, S., et al. J. Immunol (in press).

5 Redomond, T.M., Wiggert, B., Robey, F.A., et al. Biochemistry 1985; 24: 787

6 Caspi, R.R., Chan, C.C., Leake, W.C. J. Autoimmun. 1990; 3: 237

7 Wilbanks, G.A., Mammolenti, M., Streilein, J.W. Eur. J. Immunol. 1992; 22: 165-173.

8 Gaur, A., Wiers, B., Liu, A., et al. Science. 258; 1491-1494, 1992.

Advances in Ocular Immunology
R.B. Nussenblatt, S.M. Whitcup, R.R. Caspi and I. Gery, eds.

199

In vitro-ACAID induction by culturing blood monocytes with transforming growth factor-beta

Yoshiko Okano[1], Yoshiyuki Hara[2], Yu-Feng Yao[3], and Yasuo Tano[3]

[1]Department of Ophthalmology, Tane Memorial Eye Hospital, 1-1-39, Sakaigawa, Nishi-ku, Osaka, 550 Japan

[2]Department of Ophthalmology, Sumitomo Hospital, 5-2-2, Nakanoshima, Kita-ku, Osaka, 530 Japan

[3]Department of Ophthalmology, Osaka University Medical School, 2-2, Yamada-oka, Suita-city, 565 Japan

INTRODUCTION

An impaired delayed hypersensitivity following anterior chamber (AC) injection of soluble antigen is one of the most characteristic phenomenon of the systemic immune reaction termed Anterior chamber-associated immune deviation (ACAID)(1). The mechanism of the induction of ACAID is thought that the aqueous humor is supposed to possess some properties that can endow antigen presenting cells (APC) with ACAID-inducing signal(s). Now one of the signals is identified transforming growth factor-beta (TGF-ß) (2,3). We wished to determine whether TGF-ß can endow extraocular APC; especially APC from peripheral blood, with an ACAID-inducing signal when cultured together in the presence of an soluble antigen.

MATERIALS AND METHODS

Animals.

Six to 12-week-old male or female BALB/c were obtained from Nippon Clea Co. Ltd (Tokyo, Japan). All animals were treated according to the Association for Research in Vision and Ophthalmology resolution on the use of animals in research; all procedures were carried out under sodium pentobarbital anesthesia or ketamine and xylazine mixtures as anesthetics.

Transforming growth factor-beta.

Transforming growth factor (TGF)-ß2 from porcine (R&D Systems, Minneapolis, MN, U.S.A.) was used for culturing peritoneal exudate cells. Briefly, TGF-ß2 was diluted with Bovine serum albumin and 4mM HCL into 20ng/20ml, and stocked under -40°c. When peritoneal exudate cells were cultured, TGF-ß2 were added either 0.1ng/ culture well or appropriate amount.

Preparation of APC.

Peritoneal exudate cells (PEC) were obtained from naive mice receiving 3 ml of a 3% thioglycolate solution intraperitoneally 4 days earlier. Peripheral blood cells were obtained by cardiac puncture with 18 gage needle and heparin coated syringe.

Methods of APC Injections.
The method of APC injections has been described previously (4).

In vitro incubations of APC.
APC from naive mice were washed and resuspended into single cell suspensions with culture media (RPMI-1640; Nikken Bio Medical Laboratory, Kyoto, Japan). TGF-ß2 was then added 1.0ng/well. PBS was added instead of TGF-ß2 as controls. After overnight culture, the microwells contained the cells were kept 30 minutes in the refrigerator. The cells were then harvested and washed in iced RPMI, pipetting vigorously to dislodge adherent cells.

DH assay.
Delayed hypersensitivity (DH) was assessed by ear swelling responses as described previously (5).

Statistical analysis.
Analysis of ear swelling responses was accomplished using a two-tailed Student's t-test. All probability less than 0.05 were deemed significant.

RESULTS

In vitro-ACAID induction by TGF-ß2.
Peritoneal exudate cells (PEC) were incubated in vitro with 0.1ng of TGF-ß2 in each culture well, and incubated overnight at 37°c. Twenty-four hours later, cells were suspended into 2×10^3/100ml, and injected i.v. into naive syngeneic mice. DH assay by ear injection were performed seven days after immunization with BSA with CFA. As Figure 1 shows, the group of mice that had received PEC pulsed with BSA plus TGF-ß2 indicated an impaired DH response, whereas the group of mice that had received PEC with BSA plus PBS indicated vigorous DH.

In vitro-ACAID induction by adoptive transfer of ACAID splenocytes
Single cell suspensions were prepared from spleens of mice that had received TGF-ß2 treated PEC. Naive syngeneic mice received 50×10^6 splenocytes in each. One week later, immunization with BSA was performed, and then DH responses were measured 7 days after immunization. The group of mice which received in vitro-ACAID-splenocytes generated ACAID (data not shown).

Dose dependency of TGF-ß2 in in vitro-ACAID induction.
Groups of mice received PEC pulsed with either 10.0ng, 1.0ng, 0.01ng of TGF-ß2 or zero in one culture well. The only the group that had received 1.0ng-treated-PEC impaired DH (data not shown). Neither higher amount of TGF-ß2 nor lower amount of that were sustained. Since Figure 1 indicates that 0.1ng of TGF-ß2 treated PEC also impair DH, taken these together, the range of 0.1ng to 1.0ng of TGF-ß2 is the most adequate amount to induce in vitro-ACAID.

In vitro-ACAID induction by peripheral blood monocytes.

The conception of the usage of blood monocytes comes from the fact that the monocytes in peripheral blood may also act as macrophages and APC as well as PEC. Whole blood cells were separated into red cells and mononuclear cells. Each cells treated *in vitro* with antigen and TGF-ß2 were incubated overnight, and injected i.v. into naive syngeneic mice one week before immunization with BSA plus CFA subcutaneously. As Figure 2 shows, the group of mice that received TGF-ß2 treated monocytes displayed lower DH response rather than "red blood cells" group.

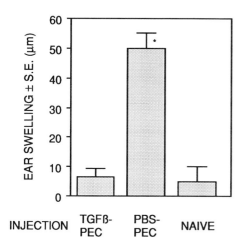

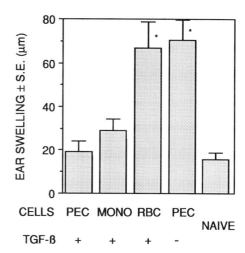

FIGURE 1. ACAID is induced by culturing PEC in vitro with bovine serum albumin (BSA) in the presence of TGF-ß2. Data presented as mean ear swelling responses (± standard error of mean). Asterisk indicates statistically higher than others (* P < 0.01).

FIGURE 2. ACAID is generated by peripheral blood monocytes. Whole blood cells harvested by cardiac puncture are separated into red blood cells(RBC) and blood monocytes. DH assay by ear injection were performed seven days after immunization (* P < 0.01).

DISCUSSION

We have already reported that peritoneal exudate cells (PEC) can play a significant role as antigen presenting cells (APC) when cultured with eye-derived fluids (6). It is important that ACAID could be induced *in vitro* by culturing not only PEC but also peripheral blood monocytes with an antigen in the presence of TGF-ß. The results we have shown here indicates that the conventional macrophages may have the potential to carry the signal which generates the systemic immune

(5,7). The APC in the iris and ciliary body process BSA peptide and acquire an ACAID-inducing signal in the AC, they migrate through the trabecular meshwork via blood stream and reach the spleen, where they confer an antigen specific ACAID-inducing signal upon splenic suppressor T cells (8). Taken these together, it is certain that TGF-ß can endow the any kind of APC with an ACAID-inducing signal that can generates antigen specific suppressor T cells.

Successful induction of *in vitro*-ACAID by TGF-ß and blood monocytes lead us to consider the possible application in immunotherapy of autoimmune diseases and graft rejection.

Address for correspondence; Yoshiyuki Hara, M.D. Department of Ophthalmology, Sumitomo Hospital, 5-2-2, Nakanoshima, Kita-ku, Osaka 530 Japan.

REFERENCES

1   Kaplan HJ, Streilein JW. J Immunol 1977; 118: 809-814.
2   Streilein JW, Bradley D. Invest Ophthalmol Vis Sci 1991; 32: 2700-2710.
3   Cousins SW, MaCabe MM, Danielpour D, Streilein JW. Invest Ophthalmol Vis Sci 1991; 32: 2201-2211.
4   Wilbanks GA, Mammolenti M, Streilein JW. Eur J Imm 1992; 22: 165-173.
5   Williamson JP, Streilein JW. Reg. Immunol 1988; 1: 15-23.
6   Hara Y, Dorf ME, Streilein JW. J Immunol 1993; 151: 5162-5171.
7   Wilbanks GA, Streilein JW. J Immunol 1991; 146: 2610-2617.
8   Wilbanks GA, Mammolenti M, Streilein JW. J Immunol 1991; 146: 3018-3024.

Advances in Ocular Immunology
R.B. Nussenblatt, S.M. Whitcup, R.R. Caspi and I. Gery, eds.

PHENOTYPE OF SUPPRESSOR CELLS INDUCED BY ORCHIDIC INJECTION OF S-ANTIGEN (S-Ag)

Jianming Ren and Hitoshi Shichi

Kresge Eye Institute, Department of Ophthalmology, Wayne State University School of Medicine, Detroit, MI 48201, USA

INTRODUCTION

Experimental autoimmune uveoretinitis (EAU) induced in animals by immunization with a retina soluble antigen (S-Ag) has been studied extensively as a model for human autoimmune ocular diseases (1, 2). The onset of S-Ag-induced EAU in Lewis rats is prevented by intracameral injection (3, 4) or feeding of S-Ag (5).

We have previously shown that the EAU is also inhibited by an injection of S-Ag in the testis (6, 7). Induction of immunological tolerance by this treatment (designated orchidic tolerance) has the following characteristics: (i) Induction of orchidic tolerance is initiated promptly, i.e. within 24 hours, after intraorchidic antigen injection (6). (ii) In orchidically tolerized rats, delayed-type hypersensitivity is inhibited but serum anti-S-Ag antibody levels are not affected (6). (iii) Systemic immunotolerance induced is antigen-specific (7). (iv) Tolerance can be transferred by injection of splenocytes of tolerized rats to naive recipients (7). (v) Splenocytes of tolerized rats suppress in vitro lymphoproliferation. These characteristics indicate that orchidic tolerance results from the generation of "suppressor cells" rather than anergy of T lymphocytes.

In this work, therefore, we have attempted to analyze the phenotype of the suppressor cells generated in orchidic tolerance.

MATERIALS AND METHODS

Intraorchidic injection of S-Ag, footpad immunization and preparation of splenic lymphocytes (uveitogenic cells and suppressor cells) were performed as described previously (6, 7). To determine suppressor activity, suppressor cells and S-Ag were added to uveitogenic cells. After incubation for 48 hours, [^{3}H]-thymidine was added and the mixed lymphocytes were incubated for additional 12 hours. All procedures used in this study conformed to the ARVO Resolution in the Use of Animals in Research. Suppressor cells were prepared from the spleens of rats orchidically treated 7 days before sacrifice.

CD4+-depleted or CD8+-depleted suppressor cells were prepared by the panning technique (4) using microculture plates coated with mouse anti-rat CD4 and CD8 monoclonal antibodies (Harlan Bioproducts for Science, Inc.). The cells bound to anti-CD4 or anti-CD8 antibodies were separated from the culture plates by shaking and used as CD4+- or CD8+-enriched cells. Analysis of CD4+-depleted or CD8+-depleted cells by FITC fluorescence flow cytometry indicated that %CD8+ cells (or %CD4+ cells) in the CD4+-depleted cell population (or CD8+-depleted cell population) did not increase by more than two consecutive pannings.

RESULTS

Effect of CD4- or CD8-enriched suppressor cells on in vitro lymphoproliferation

Uveitogenic splenocytes (2.5 x 10^5 cells) were mixed with T suppressor cells in

204

various ratios and [³H]-thymidine uptake by the mixed population of cells following S-Ag stimulation was determined. As shown in Fig. 1, a 60% decrease in [³H]-thymidine incorporation was observed when uveitogenic cells were incubated with an equal number of suppressor cells, compared with culture of uveitogenic cells alone. This decrease was paralleled by a lower cell count (data not shown). [³H]-Thymidine uptake by 1:6 mixtures of uveitogenic cells and suppressor cells was not significant indicating that suppressor cells themselves did not proliferate under the conditions. It is worthy of note that both CD4-enriched and CD8-enriched suppressor cells inhibited [³H]-thymidine uptake by uveitogenic T cells.

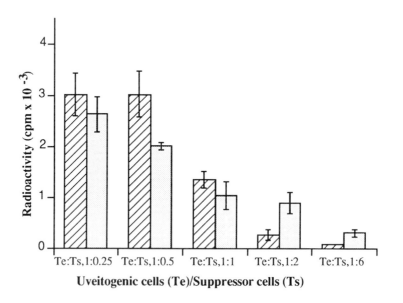

Figure 1.   Suppression of uveitogenic lymphocyte proliferation by CD8⁺-enriched (grated columns) and CD4⁺-enriched (dotted columns) suppressor cells. To a constant population of uveitogenic cells (2.5×10^5), increasing numbers of CD4⁺-enriched or CD8⁺-enriched suppressor cells were added. Bars are S.D. (n=5).

Effect of CD4- or CD8-depleted suppressor cells on the onset of S-Ag-induced EAU

To investigate the capability of suppressor cells to block the onset of EAU, splenocytes from tolerized rats were treated either with anti-CD4 or anti-CD8 antibodies and CD4-depleted or CD8-depleted suppressor cells thus prepared were injected intraperitoneally into recipients which were subsequently immunized with S-Ag. Compared with control animals, 50% of rats that received CD4-depleted cells were protected against EAU (Table 1). In contrast CD8-depleted cells provided only moderate protection and delayed the onset of EAU.

Table 1

Suppressor Cell Phenotypes And Prevention of EAU

Cells transferred*	Days after immunization (EAU rats/total of rats)						
	10	12	13	14	16	18	23
CD4 depleted	0/14	2/14	4/14	5/14	7/14	7/14	7/14
CD8 depleted	4/9	6/9	7/9	8/9	8/9	9/9	9/9
PBS	9/10	10/10	10/10	10/10	10/10	10/10	10/10

*5×10^8-1×10^9 cells transferred per recipient.

Protocol for this experiment

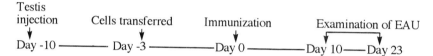

DISCUSSION

The present results indicate that the suppressor cells generated in orchidic tolerance are of both CD4+ and CD8+ phenotypes. The suppressor cells induced following S-Ag challenge in the anterior chamber were reported to be OX8+ (i.e. CD8+) and OX8⁻ cells, both of which suppressed the proliferation of the uveitogenic helper cell line (4). OX8⁻ cells were positive for the W3/25 (i.e. CD4+) surface marker (4). Inhibition of S-Ag-primed lymphoproliferation by the suppressor cells produced by feeding of S-Ag to rats was alleviated by anti-CD8+ antibody, suggesting that the suppressive activity depended upon CD8+ cells (5).

Several suppressor phenotypes (i.e. CD4+, CD8+ and CD4⁻ CD8⁻) have been reported in the experimental autoimmune encephalomyelitis system (8). It is likely that the predominant suppressor phenotype induced depends on the method of antigen administration and that both CD4+ and CD8+ suppressor subsets are required for suppression. For example, in vaccination-induced suppression of murine autoimmune thyroiditis, CD4+ and CD8+ cells appear to act cooperatively (9). It has been suggested that CD4+, MHC class II-restricted inducer/suppressor cells function in the early stage of immune response, while CD8+ cells regulate ongoing immune responses (10). It is interesting to note that suppressor cells generated in orchidic tolerance not only blocked the early stage of immune response, i.e. generation of uveitogenic cells, but also showed mild inhibition (or delaying of the onset) of EAU induced by adoptive transfer of uveitogenic cells (7). Although most of CD8+ suppressor clones so far described are not cytotoxic cells (8), it is not known whether CD8+ cells generated in orchidic tolerance act as cytotoxic T cells. It is also unknown at present whether the suppressor cells exert their effects by secreting soluble factors (e.g. cytokines).

ACKNOWLEDGEMENTS

We thank Debra A. Jones for typing the manuscript. This work was supported by NIH grant EY03807 and a departmental grant from Research to Prevent Blindness, Inc.

CORRESPONDENCE

Hitoshi Shichi, Ph.D., Kresge Eye Institute, Department of Ophthalmology, Wayne State University School of Medicine, 4717 St. Antoine, Detroit, MI 48201, USA.

REFERENCES

1.   Wacker W. Invest Ophthalmol Vis Sci 1991; 32: 3119-3128.
2.   Nussenblatt RB. Invest Ophthalmol Vis Sci 1991; 32: 3131-3141.
3.   Mizuno K, Clark AF, Streilein JW. Invest Ophthalmol Vis Sci 1989; 30: 772-774.
4.   Caspi RR, Kuwabara T, Nussenblatt RB. J Immunol 1990; 140: 2579-2584.
5.   Nussenblatt RB, Caspi RR, Mahdi R, Chan CC, Roberge F, Lider O, Weiner HL. J Immunol 1990; 144: 1689-1695.
6.   Peng B, Yoshitoshi T, Shichi H. Autoimmunity 1992; 14: 149-153.
7.   Ren J, Shichi H. Regional Immunol 1994; 6: in press.
8.   Arnon R, Teitelbaum D. Int Arch Allergy Immunol 1993; 100: 2-7.
9.   Flynn J, Kong Y. Clin Immunol Immunopathol 1991; 60: 484-494.
10.   Dorf ME, Kuchroo VK, Collins M. Immunol Today 1992; 13: 241-243.

Advances in Ocular Immunology
R.B. Nussenblatt, S.M. Whitcup, R.R. Caspi and I. Gery, eds.

Effects of corneal surgical wounds on ocular immune privilege

Y. Sano and J.W. Streilein

Schepens Eye Research Institute, and Department of Ophthalmology, Harvard Medical School, Boston, MA., USA

INTRODUCTION

Cells comprising each of the layers of the normal mouse cornea have been demonstrated to secrete factors that contribute to the immunosuppressive microenvironment of the tissues that surround the anterior chamber of the eye (1). Moreover, the absence of blood vessels in the normal stroma, and the lack of significant numbers of Langerhans cells in the central epithelium of the normal cornea have each been found to be important in conferring immune privilege upon the anterior chamber (2, 3). Induction of ACAID by injection of antigenic material into the anterior chamber (AC) of normal eyes is an important expression of immune privilege, and induction of ACAID to graft alloantigens has been implicated in the extraordinary success of orthotopic corneal allografts (4). In both laboratory animals and in man, orthotopic corneal allografts are often accepted for indefinite intervals of time, and these grafts appear as normal, functional corneal tissue. We have recently attempted to induce ACAID in eyes bearing orthotopic corneal grafts. Injection of bovine serum albumin (BSA) into the AC of eyes bearing healthy syngeneic (or even allogeneic) grafts failed to prevent these animals from developing intense BSA-specific delayed hypersensitivity (DH). This was surprising because (a) the grafts were devoid of neovascularization at the time of ACAID testing, and (b) the graft epithelium contained few if any Langerhans cells (5). In an effort to explain the failure of ACAID induction under the conditions of grafting, we designed experiments to determine whether the trauma of corneal surgery - in the absence of actual grafting - is sufficient to rob the AC of its capacity to support ACAID induction.

MATERIALS AND METHODS

Animals: BALB/c mice of 6 to 8 weeks of age, obtained from our domestic mouse breeding facility were used in these experiments. All animals were treated according to the Association for Research in Vision and Ophthalmology resolution on the use of animals in research.

Corneal incision: In one group of mice, a circumferential incision was made with a micro surgical knife, adjacent to the limbus but within the cornea. In another set of mice, a crossed incision was made such that the corneal surface displayed an X with the cross at the center of the cornea, and incisions extended to the limbus. The depth of the incisions was sufficient to penetrate through the epithelium and the upper 2/3 of the stroma. The experiments were performed after 7 days when the corneal surface was completely epithelialized and appeared normal.

Enumeration of Langerhans cells in corneal epithelium: Corneal epithelial sheets were prepared by removing corneas from incised eyes 1 week later, and soaking cornea in EDTA-PBS buffer (6). Langerhans cells were quantified using anti I-A^d antibody in an immunofluorescence assay.

Mixed Lymphocyte Reaction: Cornea and I/CB from eyes that received corneal incisions were placed, one piece of tissue per well, in 100 µl mitogen-free medium in a round bottomed 96-well plate and incubated at 37 °C for 3 days prior to addition of the MLR cells. Responder (BALB/c) spleen cells (1×10^5 cells/well) were added to irradiated stimulator (C57BL/6) spleen cells (1×10^5 cells/well) in the 96 well plate. 4 days later, the cultures were pulsed with tritiated thymidine at a concentration of 0.5 µCi/well. The cells were harvested on day 5 and the thymidine incorporation was measured.

Antigen inoculation: Animals received 50 µg of bovine serum albumin (BSA) into the anterior chamber (AC) of incised eyes. Subconjunctival inoculation of eyes of non-treated animals served as positive control, and AC inoculations of eyes of non-treated animals served as the ACAID control. Seven days later, all animals received an immunizing dose of BSA (50 µg) emulsified 1:1 in complete Freund's adjuvant (CFA) in a total volume of 100 µl injected subcutaneously (s.c.) into the nape of the neck.

Assessment of DH: Seven days after s.c. immunization with BSA in CFA, mice received intradermal inoculation of BSA (400 µg/20 µl) into the right ear pinna. The ear swelling response was then assessed 24 and 48 hr later by using a micrometer.

Detection of nerve fibers in corneal stroma: Corneal tissues were removed 1 week after incisions, and stained with an antibody NAP 4, directed against a neurofilament protein NF-H, (a gift from Dr. Gerry Shaw, Univ. of Florida) (7). Tissues were then analyzed in immunofluorescence assay.

RESULTS

Density of Ia$^+$ cells in epithelium of eyes with corneal incisions. The density of Ia$^+$ cells of corneal epithelial sheets from 5 mice that received either corneal circumferential or crossed incision was examined by counting Ia$^+$ cells. No significant increase in number of Ia$^+$ cells was found in the center of the cornea that received either circumferential or crossed incision (data not shown).

Effects of cultured corneal and I/CB cells from incised eyes on Mixed Lymphocyte Reaction. Cornea and I/CB were removed from 5 mice that received either circumferential or crossed incision. After 3 days culture, responder and stimulator cell reactants of an MLR were added to these wells. Whereas corneas from normal eyes inhibited MLRs significantly, corneas that had sustained either circumferential or crossed incision failed to inhibit T cell activation (p < 0.0005). By contrast, I/CB tissues obtained from eyes with either circumferential or crossed corneal incisions retained their ability to secrete immunosuppressive factors in a MLR (Fig. 1).

Induction of ACAID by intraocular injection of soluble antigen. 5 mice with circumferential corneal incision and 5 mice with crossed corneal incision received AC inoculation of BSA followed by s.c. immunization of BSA in CFA at 7 days. At 14 days their ears were challenged with BSA and the swelling response was assessed 24 and 48 hr later. The group of mice with crossed corneal incision acquired ACAID, however, the group of mice with circumferential corneal incision failed: they developed DTH significantly greater than ACAID control ($p < 0.05$) (Fig. 2).

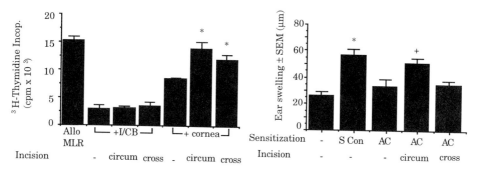

Figure 1. MLR with cultured corneas or I/CB tissues from incised eyes.

Figure 2. DTH response to BSA of animals which received corneal incisions.

Staining neurofilaments in incised cornea. Corneal tissues were removed 1 week after incisions, and stained with anti-NAP 4 antibody. In the corneal stroma which received crossed incision, neurofilaments were found to extend from the limbus to the central cornea. In the corneal stroma which received circumferential incision, neurofilaments were also found in the limbus. However, they extended only to the site of the incision, not beyond to the central cornea (Fig. 3).

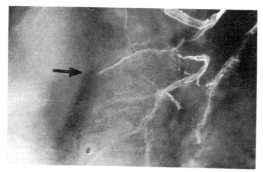

Figure. 3 Neurofilaments in the stroma of incised cornea (an arrow indicates the incision site).

DISCUSSION

Several local features of the cornea have been found to contribute to ocular immune privilege (1-3). Our results reveal that corneal incisions, either circumferential or crossed, rob corneas of their ability to secrete immuno-suppressive factors, whereas I/CB from incised eyes retain this ability. Moreover, ACAID failed **only** in eyes which received circumferential corneal incisions, even though neither Langerhans cells nor neovessels were detected in the incised corneas. This effect of circumferential corneal incision seems to be related to the denervation of the central cornea, since corneas with crossed incisions, which do not interrupt corneal innervation, retain this ability. Because corneal nerves are interconnected with the nerves that supply the I/CB, and because I/CB cells secrete factors which are necessary to induce ACAID (such as transforming growth factor beta) (8), it is possible that disruption of these neuronal interconnections interferes with *in vivo* secretion of immunosuppressive factors. Since aqueous humor contains neuropeptides which possess ACAID-inducing properties (such as alpha-melanocyte stimulating hormone, vasoactive intestinal peptide) (9), it is also possible that denervation of the cornea depletes these neuropeptides from aqueous humor and results in a failure to support ACAID induction.

From the results of this series of experiments, we suspect that the inability of eyes with healed, clear orthotopic corneal grafts to support ACAID induction may result from the unavoidable denervation of the central cornea that occurs during the grafting procedure.

REFERENCES

1. Streilein J.W, Bradley D, Sano Y. ARVO abstracts. Invest Ophthalmol Vis Sci 1994: 35 (suppl): 1737.
2. Sano Y, Streilein J.W. Regional Immunol Proceedings for the Third International Symposium on Recent Developments in the Immunopathology of Intraocular Inflammation. (in press).
3. Williamson J.SP, DiMarco S, Streilein J.W. Invest Ophthalmol Vis Sci 1987: 28: 1527-1532.
4. Sonoda Y, Streilein J.W. J Immunol 1993: 150: 1727-1734.
5. Sano Y, Streilein J.W. ARVO abstracts. Invest Ophthalmol Vis Sci 1994: 35 (suppl): 1686.
6. Gillette TH, Chandler JW. Curr Eye Res 1981: 1: 249-253
7. Harris J, Ayyub C, Shaw G. J. Neurosci. Res. 1991: 30: 47-62
8. Wilbanks G.A, Mammolenti M, Streilein J.W. Eur. J. Immunol 1992: 22: 165-173.
9. Okamoto S, Streilein J.W. Regional Immunol Proceedings for the Third International Symposium on Recent Developments in the Immunopathology of Intraocular Inflammation (in press).

1. Ocular Immunology and Inflammation
c. Therapeutic approaches

© 1994 Elsevier Science B.V. All rights reserved.
Advances in Ocular Immunology
R.B. Nussenblatt, S.M. Whitcup, R.R. Caspi and I. Gery, eds.

Induction of oral tolerance in CD8 cell deficient mice.

N.P. Chanaud III[1,2], N.J. Felix[1,2], P.B. Silver[1], L.V. Rizzo[1], R.R. Caspi[1],
R.B. Nussenblatt[1], I. Gery[1]

[1]Laboratory of Immunology, National Eye Institute, Bethesda, MD,
[2]Autoimmune Inc., Boston, MA

Introduction

Oral tolerance has been identified in recent years as an effective procedure for prevention or treatment of animal diseases such as experimental autoimmune encephalomyelitis (EAE) [1] or uveoretinitis (EAU) [2]. Moreover, oral tolerance was reported to be a beneficial treatment in multiple sclerosis [3] or rheumatoid arthritis [4] and is currently being tested in uveitis.

Accumulating data indicate that at least two mechanisms are involved in the induction of oral tolerance: (i) clonal anergy, mainly when high doses of the antigen are used [5,6], and (ii) active suppression, mediated by suppressor cells, mainly CD8, when low antigen doses are administered [1,6,7]. It is of interest that the latter mechanism of oral tolerance resembles the one that mediates another immunosuppressive process, anterior chamber associated immune deviation (ACAID) [8]; in both systems the suppressor cells were shown to produce their effect by releasing a cytokine, TGF-ß [8,9].

The present study examined the necessity for CD8 T-cells in the induction of oral tolerance. The approach we used was to test the induction of oral tolerance in mice deficient in CD8 lymphocytes due to genetic manipulation, i.e., "knock-out" of the ß2m molecule. These mice do not express MHC class I molecules on their cell surface and they lack mature CD8 lymphocytes [10,11]

Materials and Methods

ß2m(-/-) and 129J mice, 6-10 weeks old, provided by the NCI animal facility and Jackson Lab, respectively, were maintained in a pathogen free environment. Groups of mice were gavage fed every other day with 1 mg ovalbumin (OVA) or control antigen (either bovine serum albumin (BSA) or myosin, as indicated). Three days after the last feeding all mice were immunized with 20µg OVA emulsified in complete Freund's adjuvant (CFA). Cellular immune responses against OVA were determined 11 or 14 days post-

214

immunization, by collecting draining lymph node cells and performing a standard lymphocyte proliferation assay. The results are expressed as mean stimulation indices (S.I.).

Results

Groups of ß2m(-/-) and their normal 129J controls were fed with either OVA or an unrelated antigen and the development of oral tolerance was assessed by comparing the two groups for their lymphocyte responses to OVA, following a challenge with OVA, emulsified in CFA. A state of tolerance is indicated when the lymphocyte response in mice fed with OVA is lower than that in mice fed with the control antigen. Fig. 1 summarizes a typical experiment in which the groups of mice were fed 5 times. The pattern of response of the ß2m(-/-) mice closely resembled that of their 129J controls: in both groups the response to OVA was much lower in mice fed with OVA than in those fed with BSA.

In order to obtain a state of oral tolerance of lower magnitude, additional groups of ß2m(-/-) and 129J mice were fed 3 times with OVA or a control antigen, myosin. As shown in Fig. 2, the state of tolerance induced by three feedings was only slightly less effective than that induced by the five feedings and, again, the level of tolerance in the ß2m(-/-) mice resembled that in the 129J controls.

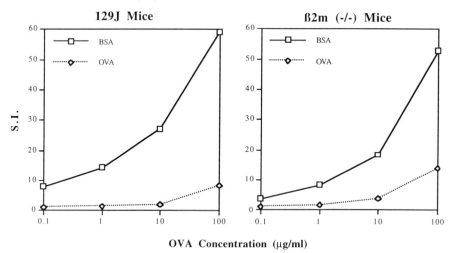

Fig. 1.   Lymphocyte proliferation response of ß2m(-/-) mice and their 129J controls after five feedings with either 1 mg OVA or a control antigen (BSA) and a challenge with OVA in CFA. Oral tolerance is similarly induced in ß2m(-/-) mice and their 129J controls.

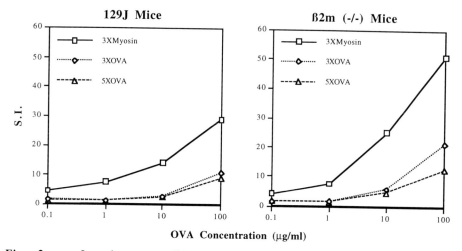

Fig. 2. Lymphocyte proliferation response of ß2m(-/-) mice and their 129J controls after three feedings with either 1 mg OVA or a control antigen (myosin), or five feedings with OVA.

Discussion

The data recorded here show that oral tolerance can be induced in ß2m(-/-) mice, which are CD8 cell deficient [10,11]: feeding with OVA inhibited in these mice the response to a subsequent challenge with this antigen and the level of inhibition was very similar to that seen in the normal 129J controls (Figs. 1 and 2). The schedule of feeding with OVA used in this study was defined by Melamed and Friedman [5] to be a "low dose" schedule, in which active suppression should play a major role in the process of tolerance induction [1,6]. Our finding could be explained by the assumption that the tolerance in the mice used in the present study was mediated by anergy rather than by active suppression. Alternatively, it is conceivable that the active suppression was mainly carried out by CD4 T-lymphocytes of the Th2 subset; these cells secrete cytokines such as IL-4 and IL-10, that may inhibit the generation of effector cells [1,12]. More studies are needed to further examine these hypothetical explanations.

It is of note that in a recent study, Hara et al have shown that ß2m(-/-) mice are incapable of developing ACAID [8]. Our finding, that oral tolerance was readily induced in these animals, thus shows that the mechanism that mediated oral tolerance in the system used here is different from the one that brings about the immunosuppression in ACAID.

The role of CD8 T-cells in oral tolerance is currently being tested in another system in which CD8 cells are eliminated by treating rats with monoclonal antibody against these cells (antibody OX-8). Preliminary data indicate that treated rats, in which almost all CD8 cells were eliminated, developed oral tolerance similarly to their normal controls.

Summary

ß2m(-/-) mice, deficient in CD8 T-cells, resembled their 129J control mice in developing oral tolerance. This result thus indicates that CD8 cells do not play a major role in the induction of oral tolerance in the experimental system used in the present study, a system in which a relatively small dose of antigen was used for feeding.

References

1   Weiner H, Friedman A, Miller A, et al.   Annu. Rev. Immunol. 1994; 12: 809-837
2   Nussenblatt R, Caspi R, Mahdi R, et al.   J. Immunol. 1990; 144: 1689-1695
3   Weiner H, Mackin G, Matsui M, et al.   Science 1993; 259: 1321-1324
4   Trentham D, Dynesius-Trentham R, Orav E, et al.   Science 1993; 261: 1727-1730
5   Melamed D, Friedman A.   Eur. J. Immunol. 1993; 23: 935-942
6   Gregerson D, Obritsch W, Donoso L.   J. Immunol. 1993; 151: 5751-5761
7   Miller A, Lider O, Weiner H.   J. Exp. Med. 1991; 174: 791-798
8   Hara Y, Okamoto S, Rouse B, Streilein J.   J. Immunol. 1993; 151: 5162-5171
9   Miller A, Al-Sabbagh A, Santos L, et al.   J. Immunol. 1993; 151: 7307-7315
10   Zijlstra M, Bix M, Simister N, et al.   Nature 1990; 344: 742-746
11   Koller B, Marrack P, Kappler J, Smithies O.   Science 1990; 248: 1227-1230
12   O'Garra A, Murphy K.   Current Opinion in Immunology 1993; 5: 880-886

Advances in Ocular Immunology
R.B. Nussenblatt, S.M. Whitcup, R.R. Caspi and I. Gery, eds.

ENHANCEMENT OF ORAL TOLERANCE BY BACTERIAL PRODUCTS.

Alexander T. Kozhich , Robert B. Nussenblatt, Igal Gery

Laboratory of Immunology, National Eye Institute, Bethesda, MD, USA

INTRODUCTION

Pathogenic autoimmune processes can be inhibited or even treated by several procedures in which specific unresponsiveness toward the pathogenic antigen(s) is induced. One of these procedures is the administration of the antigen through the enteric route that produces a state of unresponsiveness termed "oral tolerance". Oral tolerance was reported to effectively inhibit several immune mediated diseases in animals, such as experimental autoimmune encephalomyelitis (EAE) [1], or uveoretinitis (EAU) [2], as well as arthritis [3,4] and diabetes in non-obese mice [5]. Furthermore, oral tolerance has been recently reported to be effective in multiple sclerosis [6] and rheumatoid arthritis [7] and is currently being tested in patients with uveitis.

Since amelioration of disease by feeding is usually incomplete, procedures to enhance oral tolerance are sought for. It was reported recently that bacterial lipopolysaccharide (LPS) when given orally in conjunction with myelin basic protein (MBP) enhances the protective effects of MBP feeding in EAE [8].

The present study was aimed at testing the capacity of LPS and other bacterial immunomodulators to enhance the induction of oral tolerance in a system in which feeding with a uveitogenic antigen inhibits the induction of EAU and immune response in rats immunized with the same antigen in adjuvant. The uveitogen used here was peptide 1179-1191 of bovine interphotoreceptor retinoid-binding protein (IRBP) [9]. The bacterial products included LPS, N-acetyl-D-glucosaminyl-ß(1-4)-N-acetyl-L-muramyl-L-alanyl-D-isoglutamine (GMDP), its des-(N-acetyl-D-glucosaminyl) analog (MDP) and Salmonella typhimurium Mitogen (STM). These materials exert multiple effects on cells of the immune system, in particular they activate macrophages, enhance expression of MHC molecules and monokines such as interleukin-1 (IL-1) or tumor necrosis factor (TNF) and stimulate proliferation of B-cells [10,11].

MATERIALS AND METHODS

8-11 week old male Lewis rats were fed by gavage 0.3 µmol IRBP1179-1191 dissolved in PBS on days -7, -2 prior to immunization with 1nmol of the peptide IRBP1181-1191 in complete Freund's adjuvant. Control rats were similarly fed with PBS. LPS from *Escherichia coli* strain 0127:B8 (Sigma Chemical Co., St.Louis, Mo), GMDP (a generous gift of Prof. V.T. Ivanov, Shemyakin and Ovchinnikov Institute of Bioorganic Chemistry, Moscow, Russia), MDP (Sigma) and STM (Ribi Immunochem. Research, Inc., Hamilton, MT), dissolved in PBS, were fed either in combination with antigen or alone at indicated doses. Immunized rats were examined daily for clinical ocular changes and occurrence and severity of the disease were verified by histology. Draining lymph node cells (LNC) were obtained 14-19 days after immunization and their proliferative responses were measured as described in detail elsewhere[12]. Clinical and histological data were compared using Snedecor and Cochran 's test of nonparametric data [13]. The probability values of ≤ 0.05 were considered significant.

RESULTS AND DISCUSSION

Table 1 summarizes repeated experiments which examined the effects of feeding with bacterial products on the development of EAU, induced by the challenge with IRBP1181-1191. Feeding rats with GMDP or LPS alone moderately exacerbated the disease. In contrast, feeding these two agents together with IRBP1179-1191 augmented the immunosuppression effect, as shown by protecting larger portions of the rats, further delaying the disease onset and reducing the severity, as compared to the group of rats fed with the IRBP peptide alone. Two other bacterial products, MDP and STM, on the other hand, had no detectable effect when fed together with the IRBP peptide.

Table 1
Effect of bacterial products on prevention of EAU by oral tolerance.

Feeding agents[a]	Incidence	Onset day (mean)	Severity (mean)
PBS	18/18	11.7	1.5
GMDP	3/3	11.0	2.0
LPS	3/3	11.0	1.7
IRBP1179-1191	15/18	12.5	0.6[b]
IRBP1179-1191+GMDP	7/18	13.4	0.3[c]
IRBP1179-1191+LPS	11/18	12.9	0.5
IRBP1179-1191+MDP	3/3	12.6	0.8
IRBP1179-1191+STM	3/3	12.3	0.8

[a]Doses of the bacterial products used per feeding were: GMDP, 0.5mg; LPS, 1mg; MDP, 0.5mg; STM, 0.5mg. Data represent several combined experiments.
[b]$P< 0.02$ vs PBS.
[c]$P<0.02$ vs IRBP1179-1191.

Fig 1 summarizes experiments that tested the effects of GMDP and LPS on the cellular immunity of the experimental rats, measured by the lymphocyte proliferation assay. In line with its effect on EAU development feeding GMDP alone enhanced the immune response (Fig 1A), while feeding it together with IRBP1179-1191 remarkably suppressed the lymphocyte response, as compared to the response after feeding with IRBP1179-1191 alone (Fig 1B). LPS, however, only minimally affected the cellular immune response, when given alone (Fig 1A) or mixed with IRBP1179-1191 (Fig 1B). Feeding with the two other bacterial products, MDP and STM, had essentially no effect on the lymphocyte response (data not shown).

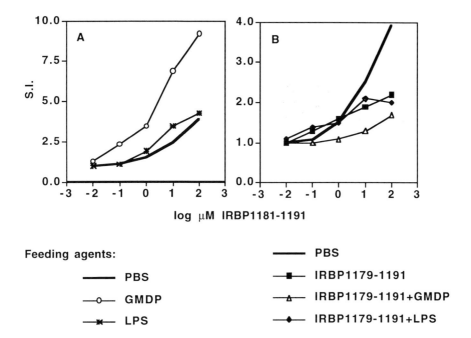

Fig 1. Effect of feeding on proliferative responses of LNC form fed rats.

The effects of LPS in the system described here are generally in accord with those recorded by Khoury et al [8] in the EAE system. Of particular interest are our data with GMDP: this agent was found superior to LPS in its effects, both as an immunostimulant when fed alone, and when tested for augmentation of the oral tolerance induced by the peptide. Two other immunostimulatory bacterial products tested here, MDP and STM, had no detectable effect in our systems.

The lack of effect of MDP is noteworthy, since this molecule, that differs from GMDP by a single carbohydrate residue, has been shown to resemble GMDP in numerous other biological systems [14]. The difference noted here may be due to the superior ability of GMDP to stimulate the expression of IL-1 and MHC class II, two molecules that were suggested to play important roles in the induction of oral tolerance [8].

CONCLUSIONS

These data thus show that the immunosuppressive processes that are triggered by feeding with an antigen can be enhanced by adding bacterial immunostimulants to the fed antigen.

REFERENCES

1. Higgins PJ, Weiner HL. J Immunol 1987; 140: 440-445.
2. Nussenblatt RB, Caspi RR, Mahdi R, Chan CC, et al. J Immunol 1990; 144: 1689-1695.
3. Thompson HS, Staines NA. Clin Exp Immunol 1986; 64: 581-586.
4. Zhang ZJ, Lee C, Lider O, Weiner HL. FASEB J 1990; 4: A2258.
5. Zhang ZJ, Davidson L, Eisenbarth G, Weiner HL. Proc Natl Acad Sci USA 1991; 88: 10252-10256.
6. Weiner HL, Mackin GA, Matsui M, Orav EJ, et al. Science 1993; 259: 1321-1324.
7. Trentham DE, Dynesius-Trentham RA, Orav EJ, Combtchi D et al. Science 1993; 261: 1727-1730.
8. Khoury SJ, Lider O, Al-Sabagh A, Weiner HL. Cell Immunol 1990; 131: 302-310.
9. Sanui H, Redmond TM, Kotake S, Wiggert B, et al. J Exp Med 1989; 169: 1947-1960.
10. Georgiev VS. Medicinal Res Rev 1991; 11: 81-119.
11. Audibert FM, Lise LD. Immunology Today 1993; 14: 281-284.
12. Hu L-H, Redmond TM, Kuwabara T, Crawford MA, et al. Cell Immunol 1989; 122: 251-261.
13. Snedecor GW, Cochran WG. Statistical Methods (6th Edition). Ames, IO: Iowa State Univ Press, 1967; 246-248.
14. Andronova T, Ivanov V. Sov medical Rev D Immunol 1991; 4: 1-63.

© 1994 Elsevier Science B.V. All rights reserved.
Advances in Ocular Immunology
R.B. Nussenblatt, S.M. Whitcup, R.R. Caspi and I. Gery, eds.

EFFECT OF INTERLEUKIN-2 ON THE INDUCTION OF ORAL TOLERANCE IN EXPERIMENTAL AUTOIMMUNE UVEORETINITIS.

Luiz V. Rizzo, Nancy E. Miller-Rivero, Chi-Chao Chan, *Barbara Wiggert, Robert B. Nussenblatt and Rachel R. Caspi. From the: Laboratory of Immunology and * Laboratory of Cell and Molecular Biology, National Eye Institute, Bethesda, MD 20892, USA.

Inflammatory eye diseases of suspected autoimmune ethnology are responsible for 70,000 new cases of uveitis every year in the united states and account for 10% of all cases of legal blindness. Experimental autoimmune uveoretinitis (EAU) is an animal model for these diseases and it can be induced in rodents and primates. In susceptible mouse strains, EAU can be induced by a single dose immunization with the interphotoreceptor retinoid-binding protein (IRBP) or by the adoptive transfer of uveitogenic T cell lines and clones. Recently, immunotherapeutic approaches have become an attractive alternative to the drugs conventionally used in the treatment of autoimmune diseases in general and uveitis in particular. In the National Eye Institute we have an ongoing clinical trial on the use of antigen feeding for the treatment of uveitis of putative autoimmune nature. The purpose of this study was to test the feasibility of potentiating the induction of oral tolerance to retinal proteins by immunomanipulation. We show that a single dose of recombinant IL-2 at the time of immunization was sufficient to convert a non-protective feeding regimen into a protective one. Furthermore, we have also shown that feeding can be used to treat already established disease.

MATERIALS AND METHODS

Animals. Female B10.A mice, 5 to 12 weeks old were obtained from the National Cancer Institute breeding facility in Frederick, Maryland, and were kept under specific pathogen-free conditions.

Induction of oral tolerance and treatment with IL-2. Mice were fed 0.2 mg of bovine IRBP (1) either three or five times by gavage. Animals receiving three feedings were gavaged on days -7, -5 and -3 before immunization. Animals receiving five feedings were gavaged on days -11, -9, -7, -5 and -3 before immunization. Some groups of mice were treated with recombinant human IL-2 (Cetus, Emeryville, CA) injected intraperitoneally at the times and doses indicated. Some animals were fed by gavage every other day after immunization for 35 days, others were fed the same dose of IRBP every other day starting 7 or 14 days after immunization.

Induction and scoring of EAU. Mice were immunized with 50 µg of IRBP emulsified in complete Freund's adjuvant given subcutaneously in the thighs and base of tail, and received 0.5 µg pertussis toxin intraperitoneally. Eyes were collected for histopathology 21 to 42 days after immunization. Serial sections (hematoxylin and eosin) were graded in a masked fashion by one of us, who is an ophthalmic pathologist (C.C.C.). EAU severity was scored on a scale of 0 to 4 in half-point increments using a semiquantitative grading system based on the number, size and type of lesions present (2). Statistical analysis was by Snedcor and Cochran's test for linear trend in proportions (nonparametric, frequency based)

(3). Each mouse, not each eye, was treated as a statistical event. Probability values of ≤ 0.05 were considered significant.

Measurement of cytokine production. Peyer's Patches (PP) of each animal were removed 21 days after immunization. The cells were cultured in 96-well plates (5×10^5 cells in each 0.2 ml well) with 20 μg/ml IRBP or with 2.5 μg/ml ConA in supplemented (4) DMEM (GIBCO) containing 0.5% fresh-frozen mouse serum. Supernatants were collected for cytokine assays after 24-36 h. TGF-β was assayed by inhibition of the mink lung carcinoma (CCL-64) cell line proliferation using ^{3}H-thymidine uptake. Total TGF-β was detected after heat activation of the supernatants at 80°C for 5 min. and the active moiety was detected without pretreating the supernatants. IL-2 and IL-4 were assayed on HT2 cells (as ^{3}H-thymidine uptake) using the monoclonal antibodies S4B6 (anti-IL-2) and 11B11 (anti-IL-4) to neutralize the reciprocal cytokine. IFN-γ and IL-10 were measured by ELISA using the antibody pairs obtained from PharMingen (La Jolla, CA). Biological activity in units or concentration in pg/ml was calculated from a standard curve established with the respective recombinant cytokine.

Results

B10.A mice were fed 0.2 μg of IRBP three times or five times prior to immunization with a uveitogenic dose of IRBP. Histopathological examination of the eyes was performed in a masked fashion 21 days after immunization. The results indicated that animals fed IRBP 5 times were protected against the development of uveitis after a uveitogenic challenge with IRBP (Table 1). The data also indicated that animals fed three times were not protected. Interestingly, if a single dose of 1,000 U of recombinant human IL-2 was given intraperitoneally to the 3 times fed animals at the time of the antigenic challenge, it was sufficient to induce protection against the development of EAU (Table 1).

Table 1. Interleukin-2 Converts a Non-Protective Feeding Regimen Into a Protective Regimen

Groups	EAU Score	INCIDENCE
Control	2.1 ± 1.0†	10/10
3x	2.4 ± 1.2	6/7
3x + IL-2	0.5 ± 0.5	7/10
5x	0.6 ± 1.1	3/5
5x + IL-2	1.0 ± 1.0	4/5

†· Standard deviation

To understand the mechanism(s) involved in the development of protection by the combination of antigen feeding and IL-2 treatment, we looked at the lymphokine profile of cells from the Peyer's Patches and mesenteric lymph nodes of fed animals. Table 2 shows that cells from mice fed IRBP three times or five times (not treated with IL-2) did not secrete significant levels of IL-4, IL-10 or TGF-β following *in vitro* stimulation with antigen. Furthermore, whereas cells from animals fed three times and injected with IL-2 produced high levels of IL-4, IL-10 and TGF-β after antigenic challenge *in vitro*, cells from 5 times fed IL-2 injected animals failed to secrete any of these cytokines in appreciable amounts (Table 2).

Table 2. Lymphokine Production by the Mesenteric Lymph nodes and Peyer's Patches from IRBP-Fed B10.A Mice.

Groups	TGF-β in pg/ml	IL-4 in U/ml	IL-10 in U/ml
Control	197 ± 30†	497 ± 210	< 10
3x	346 ± 190	314 ± 125	N.D.
3x + IL-2	4,130 ± 490	6,506 ± 571	66 ± 10§
5x	129 ± 50	195 ± 176	N.D.
5x + IL-2	117 ± 60	209 ± 104	N.D.

†Standard Deviation. N.D. Not done. § Measured in a separate experiment.

Since one of the final goals of medical research in animal models of disease is to develop novel therapeutic approaches, we used antigen feeding to treat B10.A mice <u>after</u> immunization with a uveitogenic dose of IRBP. Animals were fed IRBP every other day. Animals that were fed from day 7 after immunization were divided into 2 groups, one received recombinant IL-2 i.p. at every feeding and the other did not. Mice fed from day 14 after immunization were also dived in similar groups. Table 3 shows that mice fed from day 7 were protected against the development of EAU. Interestingly if these animals were also treated with recombinant IL-2 every feeding they became less protected, in contrast to what was seen if the animals were fed before the antigenic challenge with IRBP. Furthermore, animals that had already developed EAU and were fed from day 14, had a better outcome than control, unfed animals. Interestingly, here IL-2 treatment at every feeding does not seem to affect the result of feeding and IL-2 treated or non-treated animals had similar histopathological scores 45 days after antigenic challenge with IRBP. However, the incidence of disease was lower on the IL-2 treated animals (Table 3).

Table 3. Prolonged IL-2 Treatment is not Efficient to Potentiate Oral Tolerance

Groups	EAU Score	Incidence
Control	3.8 ± 0.3†	3/3
3x + IL-2	1.4 ± 0.5	4/5
Feeding from day 7	0.7 ± 0.1	1/5
Feeding from day 7 + IL-2 from day 7	1.9 ± 1.1	4/5
Feeding from day 14	2.7 ± 0.9	5/5
Feeding from day 14 + IL-2 from day 14	2.6 ± 1.2	3/5

†Standard Deviation.

Conclusions

Our data suggest that antigen feeding can be used as a therapeutic strategy for the treatment of uveitis since animals fed after disease had developed had a better outcome than unfed animals. We have shown that IL-2 can convert a non-protective 3x feeding regimen into a protective regimen. We propose that IL-2 treatment enhances protection from EAU at least in part by stimulating regulatory cells able to secrete anti-inflammatory cytokines. Moreover, the respective lymphokine production patterns suggest that protection induced by the 3x + IL-2 regimen may involve a different mechanism than the one induced by the 5x regimen. Whereas in the former case protection could involve anti-inflammatory cytokines, anergy or deletion of uveitogenic T cells might play a role in the latter. We have also shown that the effectiveness of the IL-2 treatment is time dependent. The importance of the timing for the effectiveness of the IL-2 treatment probably involves the mechanism by which IL-2 potentiates tolerance, i.e., by inducing regulatory T cells that secrete anti-inflammatory cytokines. If IL-2 treatment is given prior to immunization with a uveitogenic dose of IRBP but after induction of regulatory cells by feeding, the most likely targets of expansion by IL-2 will be these regulatory cells. Whereas, if IL-2 is given after immunization, especially after disease is established, uveitogenic cells elicited by antigenic stimulation will have matured and will probably compete with the regulatory cells for this extra stimulus.

References

1   Redmond, T. M., B. Wiggert, F. A. Robey, N. Y. Nguyen, M. S. Lewis, L. Lee, and G. J. Chader. 1985. Isolation and characterization of monkey interphotoreceptor retinoid-binding protein, a unique extracellular matrix component of the retina. *Biochemistry* 24:787-793.

2   Caspi, R. R., F. G. Roberge, C. C. Chan, B. Wiggert, G. J. Chader, L. A. Rozenszajn, Z. Lando, and R. B. Nussenblatt. 1988. A new model of autoimmune disease. Experimental autoimmune uveoretinitis induced in mice with two different retinal antigens. *J. Immunol.* 140:1490-1495.

3   Snedcor, G. W., and W. G. Cochran. 1967. Statistical Methods (6th Edition). Iowa State Univ. Press, Ames, IO. P. 248-248 pp.

4   Caspi, R. R., F. G. Roberge, C. G. McAllister, M. el Saied, T. Kuwabara, I. Gery, E. Hanna, and R. B. Nussenblatt. 1986. T cell lines mediating experimental autoimmune uveoretinitis (EAU) in the rat. *J. Immunol.* 136:928-933.

Advances in Ocular Immunology
R.B. Nussenblatt, S.M. Whitcup, R.R. Caspi and I. Gery, eds.

INHIBITION OF ENDOTOXIN-INDUCED UVEITIS BY NITRIC OXIDE (NO) SYNTHASE INHIBITOR; EFFECT ON INTRAOCULAR TNF AND NO SYNTHESIS.

J. Bellot[a], O. Goureau[b], B. Thillaye[a], L. Chatenoud[c] and Y. de Kozak[a].

[a]INSERM U86, 15 rue de l'Ecole de Médecine, 75270 Paris 06, France.
[b]INSERM U118, 29 rue Wilhem, 75016 Paris, France.
[c]INSERM U25, 161 rue de Sèvres, 75015 Paris, France.

ABSTRACT

Nitric oxide (NO) and tumor necrosis factor (TNF) have been implicated in the pathogenesis of several human inflammatory processes. In this study, we show that NO is involved in endotoxin-induced uveitis in Lewis rats. Indeed, two intraperitoneal injections of NO synthase inhibitor, N^G-nitro-L-arginine-methyl ester (L-NAME) inhibits clinical inflammation induced by foot pad injection of lipopolysaccharide from *Salmonella typhimurium* and decreases NO and TNF release in aqueous humor of treated rats compared to controls. Therefore down regulating of NO and TNF represents a potential means of modulating human uveitis.

INTRODUCTION

Nitric oxide (NO) is a free radical gas synthesized from L-arginine by NO synthase (NOS). It has been identified as a potent and pleiotropic mediator in some physiologic and pathologic processes such as vascular relaxation and inflammation (reviewed in 1). The inducible NO-synthase (NOS) is activated by endotoxin and cytokines in different cell types, such as macrophages. High levels of NO are then released and responsible for cellular toxic effects in immune-mediated phenomena and in some pathological conditions (1).

Footpad injection of bacterial endotoxins (LPS) in rats induces an acute and self-limited uveitis characterized by an infiltration of inflammatory cells principally in the anterior segment of the eye (2), but also into the posterior segment (3). Local synthesis of TNF occurs in the eye of Lewis rats developing EIU (4, 5). Retinal Müller glial cells activated in vitro secrete TNF (5) and NO (6) into the culture medium. These facts suggest that both factors could be implicated in the pathogenesis of EIU. In the present study, we have investigated the effects on EIU of N^G-nitro-L-arginine-methyl ester (L-NAME), a well-characterized NOS inhibitor.

MATERIAL AND METHODS

Male Lewis rats weighing 200 to 250 g were injected in one hind footpad with 150 µg of lipopolysaccharide (LPS) from *Salmonella typhimurium* (Sigma, St. Louis, Mo). Experimental groups were treated with two intraperitoneal injections of L-NAME (Sigma, St. Louis, Mo) diluted in sterile saline solution. A first dose of 75 mg/kg of L-NAME was administered 30 minutes before LPS injection; the second, of

50 mg/kg, was injected two hours after. Control rats received sterile saline injections. Clinical signs of uveitis were graded at slit lamp examination from 0 to 4 as described (3). Rats were sacrificed with chloroform, 2 and 16 hours after LPS injection. Aqueous humor (AH) was collected for TNF and NO determination. TNF levels were measured by a bioassay using murine L 929 cells (7). NO release was evaluated as the accumulation of the stable end-product nitrite by Griess reaction (8). Statistical analysis of results was made by Student t test for normally distributed data or Mann-Whitney U test as non-parametric test.

RESULTS

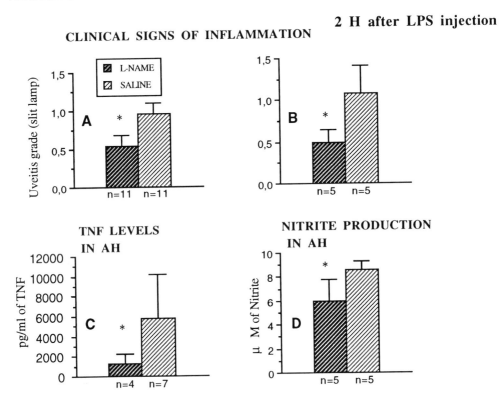

Figure 1. A, B. Clinical signs of inflammation at slit lamp observation 2 h after LPS injection in L-NAME treated rats in two different experiments. C, D. TNF and NO release in AH from both groups of rats. * p<0.005.

Nitrite level, which reflects NO production, is increased in HA at 2 h after LPS injection compared to HA of uninjected animal (< 3 μM) (Figure 1D). At 16 h, a marked increase of nitrite is detected in AH (Figure 2D). In AH from L-NAME treated rats, nitrite amounts are significantly decreased compared to LPS injected control rats. This L-NAME treatment inhibited clinical inflammation in two distinct experiments at 2 h (Figure 1A, B) and 16 h (Figure 2A, B) after LPS injection. Counting of inflammatory cells on paraffin sections of ciliary body showed a significant inhibition of cell infiltration in L-NAME treated rats at 16 h compared to controls (data not skown) Concerning TNF, a large release of cytokine in AH is detected during EIU at 2 and 16 h, compared to uninjected animals (800 pg/ml in ref. 5) (Figure 1C, 2C). TNF levels in AH are largely lower in L-NAME treated groups than in control groups at both times (Figures 1C and 2C).

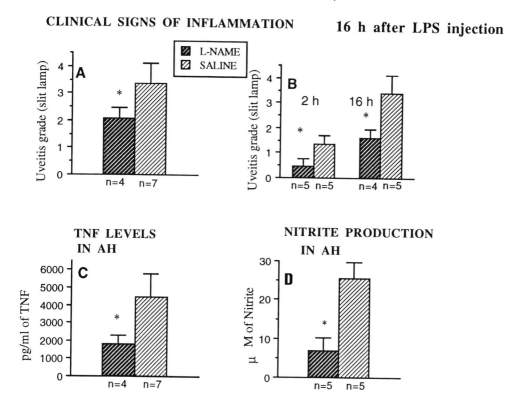

Figure 2. A 16 h after LPS injection, effect of 2 injections of L-NAME on clinical inflammation. B. In this experiment, rats were observed at slit lamp 2 h and 16 h after LPS injection. C, D. Detection of TNF and NO in AH at 16 h. * p<0.05.

DISCUSSION

EIU is a widely used model of intraocular acute inflammation for human ocular diseases such as the Reiter's syndrome. Different mediators, such as cytokines, have been implicated in the pathogenesis of this experimental disease and, based on these results, new therapeutical approaches have been investigated to improve the treatment of immunogenic uveitis in man. Recently, NO has been implicated as a potent mediator in the pathogenesis of several inflammatory processes (1) and in this study, we demonstrate that NO is involved in experimental uveitis.

We have found that EIU is correlated with an increase of nitrite level in AH. This increase is due to an NOS activity, since treatment with the NOS inhibitor (L-NAME) decreases nitrite amounts in AH. Furthermore, this treatment inhibits clinical inflammation and local TNF release, demonstrating that NOS activity is involved in the development of EIU. This protection of uveitis by L-NAME is in agreement with recent experiments from Parks et al. (9). NO is secreted by inflammatory cells such as polymorphonuclear leukocytes and macrophages activated by cytokines (1). In the eye, we recently demonstrated that retinal Müller glial (RMG) and pigmented epithelial (RPE) cells are able to produce TNF and NO in an inducible manner, after stimulation by endotoxin and cytokines (5, 6, 8). Indeed, TNF and NO were detected in the vitreous of EIU rats (data not shown). From these results, NO and TNF produced during EIU could originate from either resident cells (RMG and RPE cells) or inflammatory cells. We have also observed that inhibition of NO synthesis by L-NAME leads to a decrease in TNF in AH. This fact could be explained by a reciprocal regulation of both factors, since TNF is an NO inducer (1) and NO is described as a modulator of TNF production (10).

Further investigations are needed for better understanding of the role of NO in uveitis, particularly the kinetics of NO release during EIU and the cell types responsible for NO production. Treatments based on the inhibition of NO synthesis would improve the management of human uveitis.

REFERENCES

1   Nussler AK, Billiar TR. J Leukoc Biol 1993; 54:171-178.
2   Rosenbaum JT, McDevitt HO, Guss RB, Egbert PR. Nature (London) 1980; 266:611-615.
3   Ruiz-Moreno JM, Thillaye B, de Kozak Y. Ophthalmic Res 1992; 24:162-168.
4   De Vos AF, Van Haren MAC, Verhagen C, Hoekzema R, et al. Invest Ophthalmol Vis Sci 1994; 35:1100-1106.
5   De Kozak Y, Hicks D, Chatenoud L, Bellot J, et al. Reg. Immunol. 1994. In press.
6   Goureau O, Lepoivre M, Becquet F, Courtois Y. Proc Natl Acad Sci USA 1993; 90:4276-4280.
7   Ferran C, Sheenan K, Dy M, Schreiber R, et al. Eur J Immunol 1990; 20:509-515.
8   Goureau O, Hicks D, Courtois Y, de Kozak Y. J Neurochem 1994; 69: In press.
9   Parks DJ, Cheung MK, Chan CC, Roberge FG. Arch Ophthalmol 1994; 112:544-546.
10 Van Dervort AL, Yan L, Madara PJ, Cobb JP, et al. J Immunol 1994;152:4102-4109.

Advances in Ocular Immunology
R.B. Nussenblatt, S.M. Whitcup, R.R. Caspi and I. Gery, eds.

Effect of acetazolamide on the pharmacokinetics of cyclosporine in rabbits

Y. M. El-Sayed,[a] K. F. Tabbara,[b] and M. W. Gouda[a]

[a]Department of Pharmaceutics, College of Pharmacy, King Saud University, P.O. Box 2457, Riyadh 11451, Saudi Arabia

[b]Department of Ophthalmology, College of Medicine, King Saud University and King Khaled Eye Specialist Hospital, Riyadh, Saudi Arabia

INTRODUCTION

Cyclosporine, a neutral lipophilic cyclic polypeptide with unique immunosuppressive properties, has been extensively used in transplant patients. [1,2] More recently, cyclosporine has been evaluated for use in a variety of other immune-mediated disorders. [3-7] Following intravenous administration, cyclosporine is rapidly (within about 10 minutes) distributed between blood cells (60 to 70%) and plasma. Most of the cyclosporine in blood cells is taken up by erythrocytes (41% to 58%), whereas most of the drug in plasma is bound to lipoproteins (34%). [8,9] Subsequently, the majority of the cyclosporine dose is distributed outside the blood with a large apparent volume of distribution. [10] Cyclosporine is extensively (99%) metabolized in the liver, exhibits linear elimination kinetics, and is considered a drug of low-to-intermediate clearance. [10]

Acetazolamide, a heterocyclic sulfonamide, acts as a noncompetitive inhibitor of the enzyme carbonic anhydrase. Its action on the renal tubule results in a bicarbonate diuresis and a mild self-limiting metabolic acidosis. [11] The presence of carbonic anhydrase in a number of intraocular structures, including the ciliary processes, and the high concentrations of bicarbonate in the aqueous humor were the factors that called attention to the role that the enzyme and its inhibitor might play in the production of aqueous humor. Acetazolamide reduces the rate of aqueous humor formation, leading to a decrease in intraocular pressure in patients with glaucoma. [11]

Acetazolamide is 70% to 90% protein-bound and is widely distributed throughout body tissues, especially those with high carbonic anhydrase concentrations (renal cortex and red blood cells). [12] The drug is not metabolized in the body and is mainly eliminated unchanged in urine. [12]

When administered in conjunction with cyclosporine, acetazolamide has been shown to cause a five-fold increase in cyclosporine trough serum levels as well as pronounced nephrotoxicity and neurotoxicity. [13]

Cyclosporine has been used widely in the treatment of many forms of uveitis. Since intraocular pressure can increase in patients with uveitis and cause secondary glaucoma, it is sometimes necessary to use cyclosporine concomitantly with acetazolamide to control the glaucoma. One of the authors of the present study noted an increase in the serum level of cyclosporine following the coadministration of acetazolamide in a patient with uveitis. We therefore decided to study the effect of concomitant intravenous administration of acetazolamide and cyclosporine on cyclosporine's pharmacokinetic parameters in rabbits.

MATERIALS AND METHODS

Cyclosporine (Sandimmun®, 250 mg/5 ml) was obtained from Sandoz Ltd. (Basel, Switzerland). Acetazolamide in vials (Diamox®, 500 mg/10 ml) was obtained from Lederle Laboratories (American Cyanamid Company, NY, USA).

The study design was parallel; the acetazolamide-treated group and the control group each comprised six rabbits. All procedures involving animals were conducted in accordance with the ARVO Statement for the Use of Animals in Ophthalmic and Vision Research.

New Zealand white male rabbits, weighing from 3.0 kg to 4.3 kg, were used. The animals were fasted for 12 hours before the experiment began as well as during the experiment, although water was allowed *ad libitum*. The animals were immobilized in a restraining box when drugs were administered and when blood samples were taken.

The dose of cyclosporine (15 mg/kg) was mixed with normal saline (0.9%) (50:50% v/v) and administered as an IV bolus over a period of 3 to 4 minutes in the marginal ear vein. Immediately following cyclosporine administration, six rabbits received an intravenous dose (10 mg/kg) of acetazolamide in the marginal vein of the opposite ear. The marginal vein of one ear was cannulated with a polyethylene tube (Terumo 22 G) for blood sampling. Multiple blood samples (1.5 ml) were collected in evacuated glass tubes containing ethylene diamine tetraacetic acid (EDTA) anticoagulant at 0, 0.5, 1.0, 1.5, 2.0, 3.0, 4.0, 6.0, 8.0, 10.0, 12.0 and 24.0 hours following administration of the drugs. All samples were then refrigerated (4°C) until analysis, which was performed within 1 week.

Whole blood cyclosporine was measured by a specific and selective monoclonal antibody-based radioimmunoassay (RIA) (Sandimmun-Kit®, Sandoz Ltd, Basel, Switzerland) which has been shown to be specific for cyclosporine with negligible metabolite cross-reactivity. [14,15] The maximum interassay coefficient of variation was 11.4%. Significant correlation was found between whole-blood RIA cyclosporine and a whole-blood HPLC assay that had been developed and validated in our laboratory. The ratio of RIA and HPLC measurements in whole blood was not significantly different from unity.

A non-linear regression program known as PCNONLIN (Version 4.2; Statistical Consultants, Inc., Lexington, KY, USA) was used to fit individual blood cyclosporine concentrations to a first order, two-compartment open model. Selection of the most appropriate model was based upon the application of Akaike's criterion. [16] Initial estimates of coefficients and exponentials required by PCNONLIN were obtained from exponential curves by the use of the stripping technique. [17] Other pharmacokinetic parameters were calculated from the fitted parameters, including the terminal elimination rate constant (ß), the terminal elimination half-life (t½ß), and the area under the blood concentration-time curve (AUC).

Model-independent parameters were also computed. These included the total body clearance of cyclosporine (Cl), the steady-state volume of distribution (Vdss), [18] the area under the first moment curve (AUMC), the mean residence time of the drug in the body (MRTB), [19] the mean residence time of the drug in the general circulation (MRTC), the mean residence time of the drug in the peripheral tissues (MRTP) and the intrinsic mean residence time in peripheral tissue (IMRTP), [20,21] using the following equations:

$$Cl = Dose/AUC$$

$$Vdss = Dose \cdot AUMC/(AUC)^2$$

$$MRTB = AUMC/AUC$$

$$MRTC = AUC/C(O)$$

$$MRTP = MRTB - MRTC$$

$$IMRTP = \frac{MRTP}{1 + \dfrac{C(O)^2}{C^1(O).AUC}}$$

where,

$$AUMC = \int_0^\infty tC(t)\,dt$$

$$AUC = \int_0^\infty C(t)\,dt$$

$$C(O) = A+B$$

and, as defined by Veng-Pedersen [20,21]

$$C^1(O) = -(A\alpha + B\beta)$$

where A, α, B and ß are hybrid constants of the two-compartment model.

The data are presented as mean ± SD. Evaluation was performed in a statistics program (SAS, Statistical Analysis System) using analysis of variance and Student's t test for unpaired data. Differences between two related parmacokinetic parameters were considered significant for p values less than or equal to 0.05.

RESULTS

The administration of cyclosporine (15 mg/kg) to the rabbits in the control group and the rabbits in the acetazolamide-treated group produced blood concentration-time profiles that were adequately described by the two-compartment model with linear pharmacokinetics. Figure 1 depicts the time course of the blood cyclosporine level with and without acetazolamide. The calculated compartmental and non-compartmental pharmacokinetic parameters are shown in Table 1. There was no significant difference in the weights of the rabbits used in the control group (3.82 ± 0.49 kg) and the acetazolamide-treated group (4.07 ± 0.22 kg). The terminal elimination half-life ($t\frac{1}{2}\beta$) of cyclosporine in the acetazolamide-treated group was significantly longer than it was in the control group. Compared with the control group, the total body clearance (Cl) of cyclosporine was significantly lower in the acetazolamide-treated rabbits resulting in higher plasma concentrations and a larger area under the blood concentration vs time curve (AUC) in this group. The steady-state volume of distribution of cyclosporine was significantly higher in the acetazolamide-treated rabbits than in the control group. Cyclosporine's mean residence time in the general circulation (MRTC), mean residence time in the body (MRTB), mean residence time in the peripheral tissue (MRTP) and its intrinsic mean residence time in the peripheral tissue (IMRTP) all dramatically increased when administered in conjunction with acetazolamide (Table 1).

Table 1. Pharmacokinetic parameters of cyclosporine after administraton of a single IV dose (15 mg/kg) of cyclosporine with and without coadministration of a single IV dose (10 mg/kg) of acetazolamide to rabbits.

Parameter	Cyclosporine alone*	Cyclosporine with acetazolamide*	p-value**
AUC (ug.min/ml)	970 ± 108.2	1441.3 ± 320.2	0.007
Cl (ml/min/kg)	15.62 ± 3.78	11.0 ± 43.44	0.016
Vdss(L/kg)	4.69 ± 0.95	7.57 ± 2.38	0.021
MRTB(h)	5.2 ± 1.4	11.7 ± 2.9	0.001
MRTC(h)	1.40 ± 0.2	3.6 ± 1.9	0.019
MRTP(h)	3.8 ± 1.3	8.1 ± 2.6	0.004
IMRTP(h)	7.4 ± 1.3	12.6 ± 3.2	0.004
B (h^{-1})	0.125 ± 0.02	0.069 ± 0.02	0.001
t½ß (h)	5.7 ± 0.9	10.5 ± 2.2	0.001

* each value represents mean ± SD of six rabbits
** p-value of the analysis of variance

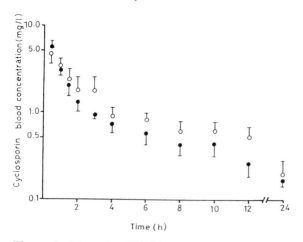

Figure 1. Mean (± SD) blood concentration of cyclosporine with (o) and without (●) acetazolamide coadministration.

DISCUSSION

Concomitant administration of cyclosporine and acetazolamide was reported to result in increased cyclosporine levels and toxicity (renal impairment and neurotoxicity) in a 50-year-old cardiac transplant patient. [13] Symptoms of toxicity subsided following withdrawal of acetazolamide and reduction of the cyclosporine dose.

The results of our investigation demonstrate that coadministration of acetazolamide affected the disposition kinetics of cyclosporine significantly. Acetazolamide administration resulted in a significant decrease in the elimination rate constant (55%) and the total body clearance (29.3%), and a significant increase in the steady-state volume of distribution (61.4%). The reduction in the clearance is confirmed by the significant increase both in the area under the blood concentration-time curve (48.6%), and in the terminal elimination half-life (84%).

Cyclosporine and acetazolamide are known to bind avidly to erythrocyte. [8,10,22] The increase in the steady-state volume of distribution of cyclosporine can be explained, at least in part, by acetazolamide's inhibition of carbonic anhydrase in the red blood cells which may change the way cyclosporine is incorporated into the red blood cells. Another possibility is that acetazolamide displaces cyclosporine from its binding sites. According to Gibaldi and McNamara, [23] the apparent volume of distribution (Vdss) can be related to the free fraction of a drug in blood as follows:

$$Vdss = V_B + V_T f_B/f_T$$

where,

V_B = Blood volume

V_T = Volume of tissue

f_B = Free fraction in blood

f_T = Free fraction in tissue

The above equation indicates that the apparent volume of distribution at steady-state increases when tissue-binding increases and blood-binding decreases. Perturbation in f_B would therefore alter Vdss.

The decrease in total body clearance of cyclosporine is difficult to explain. Cyclosporine is mainly eliminated metabolically, [10] whereas acetazolamide is mainly eliminated unchanged in urine. [12] Furthermore, cyclosporine is a low-to-intermediate extraction-ratio drug, [10] and therefore, its total body clearance will depend on its free fraction in blood as well as on its free intrinsic blood clearance according to the following equation:

$$Cl = f_B.Cl_{int\ (blood)}$$

where,

$Cl_{int\ (blood)}$ = Intrinsic clearance of unbound drug.

Total body clearance can be expected to increase if the free fraction of cyclosporine in blood increases as a result of altered binding. In contrast, the total body clearance of cyclosporine decreases following acetazolamide administration, suggesting that metabolism inhibition may be responsible. It is possible that acetazolamide coadministration induces metabolic acidosis which results in the reduced hepatic metabolism of cyclosporine, although this warrants further investigation.

The increase in the terminal elimination half-life ($t\frac{1}{2}\beta$) and mean residence time in the body (MRTB) can be explained as follows:

$$t\frac{1}{2}\beta = 0.693 \; Vdss/Cl$$

$$MRTB = Vdss/Cl$$

An increase in Vdss and a decrease in Cl will result in a significant increase in the $t\frac{1}{2}\beta$ and MRTB.

The calculated mean time parameters which reflect the tissue distribution of cyclosporine are of considerable importance from a toxicokinetic point of view. The mean residence time in the peripheral tissue (MRTP) and the intrinsic mean residence time in the peripheral tissue (IMRTP) both increased dramatically (213% and 70% for MRTP and IMRTP, respectively) with coadministration of acetazolamide. The MRTP is the mean total time the drug molecules spend in the peripheral tissue, while, the IMRTP is the average total time which drug molecules spend in the peripheral tissue before being eliminated (centrally or peripherally) from the body. [20,21] It is possible, therefore, to explain the observed toxicity (nephrotoxicity and neurotoxicity) of cyclosporine following acetazolamide administration[13] as being the result of increased distribution into, as well as prolongation of the transit time in, the target organs.

In conclusion, this study demonstrates a possible interaction between acetazolamide and cyclosporine. The most plausible explanation for this is an alteration in the disposition kinetics (distribution and elimination) of cyclosporine. Further studies are needed, however, to identify the exact mechanism of such an interaction.

Cyclosporine and acetazolamide are often given concomitantly in patients with uveitis and secondary glaucoma. This study has shown that the toxicity of cyclosporine may be enhanced by the coadministration of acetazolamide. Consquently, when concomitant use of these drugs is indicated for the treatment of patients with uveitis, a reduction in the dose of cyclosporine and/or acetazolamide may be required to prevent blood cyclosporine levels rising to unacceptable levels.

ACKNOWLEDGEMENTS

This study was supported by the Research Center, College of Medicine, King Saud University (Grant no. CMRC 89-263), and the Abdul-Rahman Al Rashed Fund for Research in Ophthalmology (Grant no. 4-7-92).

The authors wish to acknowledge with thanks the technical assistance of Mr. M. M. Al-Dardiri and Mr. A. A. Abdulraziq.

REFERENCES

1 Freeman DJ. Pharmacology and pharmacokinetics of cyclosporin. Clin Biochem 1991;24:9-14.
2 Faulds D, Goa KL, Benfield P. Cyclosporine: A review of its pharmacodynamic and pharmacokinetic properties, and therapeutic use in immunoregulatory disorders. Drugs 1993;45:953-1040.
3 Chavis PS, Antonios SR, Tabbara KF. Cyclosporine effects on optic nerve and retinal vasculitis in Behcet's disease. Doc Ophthalmol 1992;80:133-142.
4 Christophers E, Mrowietz U, Henneicke H-H, Farber L, Welzel D. Cyclosporine in psoriasis: A multicenter dose-finding study in severe plaque psoriasis. J Am Acad Dermatol 1992;26:86-90.
5 Schrezenmeier H, Schlander M, Raghavachar A. Cyclosporine A in aplastic anemia: Report of a workshop. Ann Hematol 1992;65:33-36.
6 Sherman KE, Pinto PC. Cyclosporine treatment of type 1 autoimmune chronic active hepatitis. Hepatology 1992;16:194A. Abstract 597.
7 Moolman JA, Bardin PG, Rossoaw DJ, Joubert JR. Cyclosporine as a treatment for interstitial lung disease of unknown aetiology. Thorax 1991;46(suppl):S92-S95.
8 Gupta SK, Benet LZ. High-fat meals increase the clearance of cyclosporine. Pharm Res 1990;7:46-48.
9 Kahan BD. Cyclosporine. N Engl J Med 1989;321:1725-1738.
10 Fahr A. Pharmacokinetics, metabolism and biological activity of cyclosporine (Sandimmun®). Clin Pharmacokinet 1993;24:472-495.
11 Gilman AG, Goodman LS, Gilman A, eds. The pharmacological basis of therapeutics. 7th ed. New York, NY: Macmillan Publishing Co, 1985.
12 Bennett WM, Aronoff GR, Golper TA. Drug prescribing in renal failure. Philadelphia, PA: American College of Medicines, 1987.
13 Keogh A, Esmore D, Spratt P, Savdie E, McCluskey P. Acetazolamide and cyclosporine. Transplantation 1988;46:478-479.
14 Ball PE, Munzer H, Keller HP, et al. Specific ^{3}H radioimmunoassay with a monoclonal antibody for monitoring cyclosporin in blood. Clin Chem 1988;34:257-260.
15 Holt DW, Johnston A, Vernillet L, et al. Monoclonal antibodies for radioimmunoassay of cyclosporine: A multicenter comparison of their performance with the Sandoz polyclonal radioimmunoassay kit. Clin Chem 1988;34:1091-1096.
16 Akaike, H. An information criterion (A.I.C.). Math Sci 1976;14:5-9.
17 Gibaldi M, Perrier D. Pharmacokinetics. New York: Marcel Dekker Inc; 1982.
18 Benet LZ, Galeazzi R. Noncompartmental determination of the steady-state volume of distribution. J Pharm Sci 1979;68:1071-1074.
19 Yamaoka K, Nakagawa T, Uno T. Statistical moments in pharmacokinetics. J Pharmacokinet Biopharm 1978;6:547-558.
20 Veng-Pedersen P. Mean time parameters in pharmacokinetics: Definition, computation and clinical implications (part I). Clin Pharmacokinet 1989;17:345-366.
21 Veng-Pedersen P. Mean time parameters in pharmacokinetics: Definition, computation and clinical implications (part II). Clin Pharmacokinet 1989;17:424-440.
22 Wallace SM, Riegelman S. Uptake of acetazolamide by human erythrocyte in-vitro. J Pharm Sci 1877;52:729-731.

23 Gibaldi M, McNamara PJ. Apparent volumes of distribution and drug binding to plasma
proteins and tissues. Eur J Clin Pharmacol 1978;13:373-380.

© 1994 Elsevier Science B.V. All rights reserved.
Advances in Ocular Immunology
R.B. Nussenblatt, S.M. Whitcup, R.R. Caspi and I. Gery, eds.

Thalidomide and Supidimide downregulate the inflammation in endotoxin-induced uveitis.

Yan Guex-Crosier[1], Nancy Pittet[2] and Carl P. Herbort[2].

[1] National Institutes of Health, National Eye Institute, Bldg. 10 , Room 10 N 112, 9000 Rockville Pike, Bethesda, MD, 20892, USA

[2] Hôpital Jules Gonin, Department of Ophthalmology, University of Lausanne, 15 av. de France, 1004 Lausanne, Switzerland

1. Introduction :

Thalidomide, N-alpha-phthalimidoglutarimide was synthesized in 1963. This drug was widely used as a sedative untill 1961. In 1961 the tragedy of phocomelia marked the end of the clinical use of thalidomide [1, 2]. New interest in thalidomide was based on the discovery of its immunomodulating properties in 1965 : Sheskin observed in 6 patients disappearance of erythema nodosum leprosum lesions within 12 hours after administration of thalidomide as a sedative [3].

Thereafter, this drug was used in the therapy of immunologic diseases : erythema nodosum leprosum [4], actinic prurigo [5], discoid lupus erythematosus [6], Behçet's syndrome [7], orogenital ulceration [8], rheumatoid arthritis [9]. Recently Vogelsang reported the benefit of thalidomide in the treatment of graft-versus-host disease after bone marrow transplantation [10-12].

In ophthalmic literature, the use of thalidomide was reported in sporadic cases of Behçet's disease. Thalidomide used as a monotherapy, was not sufficient to reduce ocular inflammation and had some beneficial effect on orogenital lesions [7]. Low doses of thalidomide (50 mg three nights weekly) were used in the prophylaxis of recurrence in Behçet's disease [13]. But its effect on uveitis is still controversial and thalidomide has not yet been tested in the animals models of ocular inflammation. In this study, we tested the effect of thalidomide and supidimide (a thalidomide derivative characterized by a much lower rate of teratogeny in the experimental tests [14,15]) in endotoxin-induced uveitis in Lewis rats.

2. Materials and Methods :

Uveitis was induced in male inbred Lewis rats (6 weeks old) with subcutaneous injection of lipopolysaccharide (LPS) (100µg/rat). The animals were treated with intraperitoneal injections of thalidomide in 0.5 %

methylcellulose suspension. Thalidomide was kindly provided by Grünenthal®
(Strolberg, Germany). The powder was 99.9% pure.

The treatment schedule of thalidomide is represented in table 1. The animals
were sacrificed 20 hours after LPS injection. The inflammation was evaluated
by measuring protein concentration and leukocyte number in the aqueous
humor. Aqueous humor was collected using tuberculine siringue with a 30
gauge needles. Protein determination was performed by the Bio-rad® protein
assay on samples of 2 µl of aqueous humor. To determine AC cell count, 1µl of
aqueous humor was dropped on a slide using a Hamilton precision syringue
(Hamilton®, Co, Reno, Ne). After air drying the slides were stained with the
Wright's stain and cells were counted.

The Sudent's t test was used for protein comparison and the Mann Whittney
for the cells count comparison of the diffenrent groups.

Table 1 :
Thalidomide injection 400 mg/kg/day (Time 0 = LPS injection)

Hours / LPS injection :	24 h. before	4 h. before	4 hours after
THAL-1	X	X	X
THAL-2		X	X
Late THAL			X

3. Results :

The antiinflammatory effect of thalidomide was clearly seen with doses over
300 mg/kg/day. Both protein exudation and anterior chamber (AC) cells
infiltration were decreased in the rats treated by high doses of thalidomide. That
was clearly seen in the THAL-1 group, treated with thalidomide 24 hours, 4
hours before and 4 hours after LPS injection (table 2; exp. 1). Two injections of
thalidomide (400mg/kg/day ; THAL-2), given 4 hours before and 4 hours after
LPS injection, also decreased both protein exudation and cell infiltration into the
AC (table 2; exp. 2). In the group, Late THAL, treated with only one injection of
thalidomide (400 mg/kg/day) given 4 hours after LPS injection, a significant
reduction inflammation was also seen.

In a third set of experiment, lower dosages of thalidomide were tested
(300 and 150 mg/kg/day). Thalidomide given at a dose of 150 mg/kg/day was
not sufficient to reduce inflammation (table 2; exp. 3).

In another set of experiments Supidimide, a thalidomide derivative, was
tested. Supidimide (400 mg/kg/day) was injected 4 hours before and 4 hours
after LPS injection. But inflammation was reduced in a lesser degree (table 2;
exp. 4).

Table 2 :
AC inflammation 20 hours post LPS injection :

Exp. 1	n	p	prot ± SEM g/l	p	Cells ± SEM c/µl
THAL-1	13	<0.001	2.69 ± 0.61	<0.001	469 ± 240
Late Thal	3	<0.001	0.85 ± 0.35	<0.001	16 ± 14
Controls	14		7.63 ± 0.65		1665 ± 389
Exp. 2	**n**	**p**	**prot ± SEM g/l**	**p**	**Cells ± SEM c/µl**
THAL-2	11	<0.001	2.19 ± 0.61	≤0.012	66 ± 29
Controls	10		6.31 ± 0.59		242 ± 76
Exp. 3	**n**	**p**	**prot ± SEM g/l**	**p**	**Cells ± SEM c/µl**
Thal high	6	≤0.023	17.42 ± 1.29	<0.06	1304 ± 389
Thal low	6	≤0.125	19.78 ± 0.91	>0.06	2246 ± 625
Controls	5		22.15 ± 0.58		3025 ± 408
Exp. 4	**n**	**p**	**prot ± SEM g/l**	**p**	**Cells ± SEM c/µl**
Supidim.	8	≤0.053	3.44 ± 0.98	<0.06	153 ± 119
Controls	5		5.69 ± 0.58		443 ± 219

4. Discussion :

Thalidomide was shown to reduce inflammation in endotoxin-induced uveitis in Lewis rats (EIU) at doses over 300 mg/kg/day. Since thalidomide has been widely used for more than 10 years the kinetic and the adverse side effects are well known. More than 44 % patients complain of sleepiness and drowsiness, 8% have some difficulty in accommodation, and rare patients complain of abdominal pain and mouth and ocular dryness. Care must be taken to monitor for the development of possible peripheral neuropathy [16].

The mechanism of action of thalidomide is still unknown. It has no effect on arachidonic acid metabolism [17]. However thalidomide seems to act both on migratory pattern of inflammatory cells and cytokine release. In two other experiments (data not shown) oral thalidomide, dissolved in olive oil, was tested in posterior uveitis models : lens induced uveitis and experimental autoimmune uveitis. In these two models thalidomide was not sufficient to reduce the severity of histologic scoring of uveitis, but cell infiltration was somewhat lower in the thalidomide treated groups. The inhibition of inflammatory cells migration into the tissues could be one of the mechanism of action of thalidomide.

Another effect of thalidomide is specific reduction of TNF alpha production in response to various stimuli in particular LPS, BCG, or products of mycobacterium leprae [18-20]. But the precise role of TNF alpha in EIU has still to be further investigated.

These two drugs with their well known toxicity profile have shown their efficacy in reducing inflammation in EIU. Clinical use is limited by the possible development neurotoxic distal neuropathy. But others more potent thalidomide derivatives have still to be tested.

This work was supported by a grant from "Fonds National Suisse de Recherche Scientifique", from the "Fischer Foundation" and from the "Fonds du 450ème anniversaire de l'Université de Lausanne".

References :

1. McBride WG. Lancet 1961; ii:1358.
2. Lenz W. Lancet 1962; ii:45-46.
3. Sheskin J. Clin Pharmacol Ther 1965; 6:303-306.
4. Hastings RC, Trautman JR, Enna CD , Jacobson RR. Clin Pharmacol Ther 1970; 11:482-487.
5. Calnan CD, Meara RH. Clin Exp Dermatol. 1977; 2:365-372.
6. Knop J, Bonsmann G, Happle R, Ludolph A, Matz DR, Mifsud EJ, Macher E. Br J Dermatol 1983; 108:461-466.
7. Saylan T, Saltik I. Arch Dermatol 1982; 118:536.
8. Jenkins JS, Allen BR, Maurice PDL, Powell RJ, Littlewood SM, Smith NJ . Lancet 1984; 22:1424-1426.
9. Guttierrez-Rodriguez O. Arth Rheumatism 1984; 27:1118-1121.
10. Vogelsang GB, Hess AD, Friedman KJ, Santos GW. Blood 1989; 74:507-511.
11. Vogelsang GB, Farmer ER, Hess AD, Altamonte V, Beschorner WE, Jabs DA, Corio RL, Levin LS, Colvin OM, Wingard JR, Santos GW. N Engl J Med 1992; 326:1055-1058.
12. Lopez J, Ulibarrena C, Garcia-Larana J, Odriozola J, Perez de Oteyza J, Sastre JL, Navarro JL. Bone Marrow transplant 1993; 11:251-252.
13. Denman AM, Graham E, Howe L, Lightman S. La Revue de Medecine Interne 1993; 14 (Suppl.1):49s.
14. Helm FC, Frankus E, Friderichs E, Graudums I, Flohé L. Arzneimmittelforschung 1981; 31:941-949.
15. Neubert R, Nogueira AC, Neubert D. Arch Toxicol 1993; 67:1-17.
16. Hess CW, Hunziker T, Kupfer A, Lüdin HP. J Neurol 1986; 233: 83-89.
17. Maurice PDL, Barkley ASJ, Allen BR. Br J Dermatol; 1986; 115:677-680.
18. Sampaio EP, Sarno EN, Galilly R, Cohn ZA, Kaplan G. J Exp Med 1991; 173:699-703.
19. Fazals N, Lammas DA, Raykundalia C, Bartlett R, Kumararatne DS FEMS Microbiol Immunol 1992; 105:337-346.
20. Moreira AL, Sampaio EP, Zmuidzinas A, Frindt P, Smith KA, Kaplan G J Exp Med 1993; 177:1675-1680.

Advances in Ocular Immunology
R.B. Nussenblatt, S.M. Whitcup, R.R. Caspi and I. Gery, eds.

241

ANTI-INFLAMMATORY PROPERTIES OF XANTHINE OXIDASE INHIBITORS.

George E. Marak Jr.[1], Hagen Schmal[2], Kimberly E. Foreman[2], Hans
P. Friedl[3], Peter A. Ward[2], Gerd O. Till[2].
[1]Center for Sight, Georgetown University, Washington, D.C.;
[2]Department of Pathology, University of Michigan, Ann Arbor,
MI; [3]Universitätsspital Zurich, Switzerland

It is well known that agents that inhibit xanthine
oxidase (XO) activity reduce tissue damage in acute ocular
inflammation[1] and ocular reperfusion injury[2] as well as in a
variety of other tissues and organs[3-6].

The classical Arthus reaction form of experimental
phacoanaphylactic endophthalmitis (EPE) is produced by lens
injury to Lewis rats that have been sensitized by a series of
alternate weekly injections of 10 mg rabbit lens protein in
0.5 ml complete Freunds's adjuvant for the first and
incomplete Freund's adjuvant for the subsequent three
sensitizing injections[7]. Experimental animals received 3 iv
injections of 50 mg/kg oxypurinol at 0,4 and 8 hours after
lens injury. Control animals received iv saline injections at
these intervals. Oxypurinol treatment produced a significant
reduction in a morphometric index of inflammation[8] and almost
completely eliminated the extensive hemorrhage and vasculitis
observed in positive controls.

Reperfusion injury was produced in Lewis rats by
occluding the retinal circulation with a modified
ophthalmopneumoplethysmograph. The ophthalmoscopically
verified occlusion was maintained for 30 minutes and various
parameters evaluated after intervals of reperfusion. Injury
was assessed by vascular leakage of radiolabelled albumin[8].
Allopurinol treatment markedly ameliorated the reperfusion
injury.

Interrelated pathologic processes occur in both acute
inflammation and reperfusion injury that involve free radials
or toxic oxygen metabolites (TOM)[9]. Neutrophil generated TOM
are of major importance in both reperfusion injury and acute
inflammation. XO activity is important in neutrophil
accumulation at the pathologic site[3,10].

The mechanisms involved in XO inhibitor-mediated
suppression of acute inflammatory responses are not
understood. There are a number of potential antiphlogistic
mechanisms of action of XO inhibitors including effects on
complement, histamine, iron chelation, hydroxyl radical
scavenging, superoxide generation, neutrophil chemotaxis,
adhesion molecule effects, and cytokine activity that may

involve protective effects.

Serum complement levels as determined by total hemolytic complement activity and the crossed immunoelectrophoresis method of Chapman and Ward were not altered by treatment with lodoxamide or oxypurinol[11].

As an estimate of iron chelation, iron binding was assessed by the bleomycine-dependent degradation of DNA described by Gutteridge et al[12]. Iron binding was unaffected by XO inhibitor treatment. Histamine levels were measured by radio-immune assay. XO inhibitors had no effect on serum histamine levels.

Hydroxyl radical scavenging by XO inhibitors occurs in vitro but little or no additional scavenging occurs in biological fluids (serum) with treatment by XO inhibitors at the dose levels employed in our experiments[12,13].

Superoxide generation by neutrophils as measured by the superoxide dismutase inhibitable reduction of ferricytochrome c demonstrated that XO inhibitors had no effects on FMLP induced superoxide generation by neutrophils[14].

The treatment of TNF-stimulated human umbilical vein endothelial cell (HUVEC) cultures with XO inhibitors had only a minimal effect on neutrophil adhesion although very high concentration of lodoxamide did significantly inhibit neutrophil adhesion. The principle adhesive mechanisms in this system involve E-selectin and ICAM-I[15]. The effects of XO inhibitors on the ß2 integrin adhesive molecules are being evaluated by different methods.

It has been speculated that XO generated TOM up-regulate endothelial cell adhesion molecules by interfering with the production of nitric oxide which down-regulates adhesion molecules[16]. Technical essay problems prevent any reliable description at this time of the effects of XO inhibitors on NO production.

A major antiphlogistic effect of XO inhibitors is a dose dependent interference with stimulated neutrophil chemotaxis. Each of the XO inhibitors tested lodoxamid, allopurinol, and oxypurinol markedly interfere with neutrophil chemotaxis at therapeutic levels.

In addition to some inhibition of neutrophil adhesion, inhibiting the chemotaxis of neutrophils appears to be an important mechanism by which XO inhibitors protect against tissue damage in acute inflammation and reperfusion injury. Whether this effect is on ligand signal transduction pathways, cytoskelatel organization, expression or activity of adhesion molecules, or responses to various cytokines or chemokines (as well as other potential mechanisms) is now being evaluated. XO inhibitors appear to have a direct effect on neutrophils. The specific relationship of this chemotactic inhibitory effect to neutrophil XO metabolism is not yet clear.

REFERENCES

1. Marak GE Jr, Till GO and Ward PA. 1990. *Int Ophthalmol* 14:345-347.

2. Marak GE Jr, Till GO, Paul JP, Friedl HP, et al. 1990. *Invest Ophthalmol Vis Sci* 31:568.

3. Grisham MB, Hernandez LA and Granger DN. 1986. *Am J Physiol* 251:G567-574.

4. Freidl HP, Till GO, Trentz O. and Ward PA. 1989. *Am J of Pathol* 135:203-217.

5. Till GO, Guilds LS, Mahrougui M, Friedl HP, et al. 1989. *Am J Pathol* 135:195-202.

6. Till GO, Friedl HP and Ward PA. 1991. *Free Radic Biol* 10:379-386.

7. Till GO, Lee S, Mulligan M, Walter JR, et al. 1992. *Invest Ophthalmol Vis Sci* 33:3417-3422.

8. Howes EL and Cruse VR. 1978. *Arch Ophthalmol* 96:1668-1676.

9. McCord JM 1986. *Adv in Free Rad Biol Med* 2:325-345.

10. Granger DN 1988. *Am J Pysiol* 255:H1269-H1275.

11. Chapman WE and Ward PA. 1976. *J Immunol* 117:935-938.

12. Gutteridge JMC, Rowley DA and Ilalliwell B. 1981. *Biochem J* 199:263-265.

13. Joh J, Kline A, Rangan I and Bulkley G. 1994. *FASEB J* 8:A678.

14. Zimmerman BJ, Parks DA, Grisham MB and Granger DN. 1988. *Am J Physiol* 255:H202-H206

15. Babior BM, Kipnes RS and Curnutte JT. 1973. *J Clin Invest* 52:741-753.

16. Kubes P and Granger DN. 1992. *Am J Physiol Circ Physiol* 262:H611-H615.

Advances in Ocular Immunology
R.B. Nussenblatt, S.M. Whitcup, R.R. Caspi and I. Gery, eds.

Loteprednol etabonate: A novel ocular steroid with improved safety profile

Ron Neumann[a] and John F. Howes[b]

[a]Pharmos Ltd., Kiryat Weizmann, Rehovot 76326, Israel

[b]Pharmos Corp., 2 Innovation Drive, Alachua, FL 32615, USA

INTRODUCTION

Corticosteroids are the mainstay of therapy for ocular inflammation and though effective, IOP elevation, cataract progression and potentiation of fungal and herpetic diseases are major drawbacks to their chronic use in the eye. Among these complications IOP elevation is the most common accounting for approximately 30% of steroid users (1). Loteprednol etabonate (LE) is a "site active" drug having a specific esterase sensitive site leading to a predictable one step deactivation to an inactive metabolite (PJ-91) (2). Thus, it can be hypothesized that ocular esterases may reduce active drug level at the trabecular meshwork leading to lower propensity to elevate IOP. Over the last years LE had been studied extensively in animals and in clinical studies. The results suggest a unique ocular steroid that is highly efficacious, yet with reduced potential to elevate IOP.

RECEPTOR AFFINITY

Using the rat lung cytosol preparation LE displaced tritiated triamcinolone acetonide with a potency 1.5 times that of dexamethasone (unpublished data). The Hill coefficient for the LE data was 1.32 - 1.51 indicating more than one binding site for this steroid. In the presence of cortienic acid (10^{-5}M) which saturates transcortin binding sites, LE demonstrated a potency 4.3 times that of dexamethasone and a Hill coefficient of close to 1.0. These data indicate that LE binds competitively to transcortin, in common with other non-fluorinated corticosteroids. The putative metabolite of LE (PJ-91) did not displace tritiated triamcinolone acetonide from the glucocorticoid receptor, indicating that this molecule lacks significant glucocorticoid activity.

OCULAR PHARMACOKINETICS

The penetration of LE into rabbit eyes was studied using ^{14}C-labelled LE (3). Highest level of LE was found in the conjunctiva with negligible metabolism (Table 1). Penetration to the cornea was substantial with considerable metabolism resulting in significant accumulation of the PJ-91. Of greatest interest was the very low level of the active drug with the relatively high level of inactive metabolites in the aqueous humor as it suggests lower level of the active drug bathing the trabecular meshwork. Moreover, persistent higher level of the drug at the iris-ciliary body may suggest high efficacy in iridocyclitis.

TABLE 1: Mean level of LE and its metabolites (ngr/gr tissue) in discrete ocular tissues at various time points after drug application.

Time (Hours)		0.5	1.0	2.0	4.0	6.0	8.0
Conjunctiva	(L)	305 ± 119	215 ± 62.1	*163 ± 95.8	115 ± 33	25 ± 5.3	53 ± 26.6
	(M)	*35 ± 11	18 ± 2.8	*12 ± 4.6	*8 ± 2.9	4 ± .25	10 ± 4.1
Cornea	(L)	38 ± 2.7	21 ± 1.1	*13 ± 3.4	9 ± 1.1	6 ± 1.1	11 ± 3.7
	(M)	49 ± 3.4	41 ± 2.9	*32 ± 4.3	22 ± 2.1	18 ± 2.5	22 ± 1.5
Iris	(L)	19 ± 5.0	*11 ± 1.6	*7 ± 1.5	*7 ± 1.6	2 ± 0.7	9 ± 3.1
	(M)	4 ± 0.9	3 ± 0.6	*2 ± 0.3	3 ± 0.5	1 ± 0.1	2 ± 0.5
Aqueous	(L)	0.27 ± .02	0.16 ± .02	*.07 ± .006	.03 ± .005	.02 ± .004	.02 ± .008
	(M)	0.17 ± .01	0.23 ± .02	*0.25 ± .01	0.11 ± .015	.07 ± .003	.06 ± .001

N = 4 unless otherwise noted   (L) Loteprednol   (M) Metabolite   *N = 3

OCULAR ANTI-INFLAMMATORY ACTIVITY

Three groups of rabbits (N = 8 per group) were given 200 ng endotoxin intravitreally in both eyes. The left eyes of each rabbit were treated with LE suspension (1%), Prednisolone (1%), or vehicle placebo. Animals were dosed at -4 hrs and -2 hrs prior to endotoxin administration, and then at time 0, 3, 6, 9 and 19 hrs post endotoxin injection. At 20 hours post injection there were no differences in clinical signs between the groups, yet leukocytes were significantly reduced in the prednisolone (3295 ± 804 cell/mm^2) and LE (4440 ± 620) treated groups as compared to placebo (8880 ± 2450). Similarly, myeloperoxidase activity was reduced to 0.13 ± .08 units/mg tissue and 0.23 ± .05 in the prednisolone and LE groups respectively compared to 0.38 ± .08 in the placebo control. LE did not suppress protein transudation in this study as opposed to prednisolone acetate.

In another study, four groups of rabbits were given 300 ng endotoxin in both eyes (4) and were treated with LE (0.5%; n = 6 animals), FML (0.1%; n = 6) Dexamethasone (0.1%; n = 3), or vehicle placebo (n = 3). Animals were dosed four times daily, starting at the time of the intraocular endotoxin injection for three consecutive days. Aqueous leukocytes were reduced in all treatment groups to the same degree compared to placebo treated animals; aqueous protein was also reduced in LE treated animals compared to placebo, but not to the other groups. LE was superior to placebo in alleviating all clinical signs but dexamethasone and FML were superior in reducing conjunctival redness and fibrin formation.

Studying the effect of LE in a model of chronic ocular inflammation, 10 μl of complete Freund adjuvant were injected intravitreally to groups of 3-6 rabbits (Table 2). LE, FML and dexamethasone were given q.i.d. in a masked fashion starting at the time of the intraocular injection for nine consecutive days. On the tenth day, the rabbits were sacrificed and aqueous protein and leukocyte contents were measured showing reduced cellular response in the LE treated animals compared to all other groups. Aqueous protein in LE treated animals was also reduced compared to placebo group, but not to the other groups. Clinical inflammation was reduced to the same degree by LE and dexamethasone though FML was superior to both in reducing conjunctival injection (Table 2).

TABLE 2: Comparative evaluation of anti-inflammatory effects of 0.1% FML, 0.1% Dexamethasone, 1% LE, and placebo in chronic intraocular inflammation in rabbits ± standard error of the mean.

Clinical Scoring	FML N = 6	Dexa N = 3	LE N = 6	Placebo N = 3
Conjunctival Injection	*#0.5 ± .05	*1.1 ± 0.2	*1.4 ± 0.1	2.1 ± 0.2
Corneal Edema	*0.2 ± .05	*0.4 ± .08	*0.3 ± .06	2.1 ± 0.2
Corneal Neovascularization	*0.22 ± .07	*5.0 ± 2.6	*0.9 ± .04	25.5 ± 9.9
Aqueous Cells	*0.8 ± .07	1.4 ± .2	*1.1 ± 0.1	1.5 ± .15
Aqueous Flare	*0.5 ± .09	*0.6 ± .08	*0.5 ± .06	1.1 ± .15
Iris Hyperemia	*0.22 ± .07	*5.0 ± 2.6	*0.9 ± .04	25.5 ± 9.9
Aqueous Cells (x 10^4/ml)	*16.1 ± 2.3	*15.1 ± 6.4	*9.3 ± 3.1	48.4 ± 15.1
Protein (μg/ml)	*1077 ± 159	*925 ± 159	*1386 ± 168	1956 ± 162

*$p < 0.05$ for placebo vs. treatment group; #$p < 0.05$ for Loteprednol vs. FML.
(Duncan's post-hoc studies following significant ANOVA with repeated measure)

CLINICAL STUDIES
Efficacy:

The anti-inflammatory effect of LE was studied in contact lens induced giant papillary conjunctivitis (GPC) and in seasonal allergic conjunctivitis. A phase II GPC study (5) in 110 patients treated with either LE or placebo in a double masked fashion for 28 days, resulted in a statistically significant improvement of the papillae redness and size in the LE treated group compared to the placebo treated group. Similarly, investigator's clinical judgement composed of papillae severity, itching, and bulbar conjunctival injection favored LE treatment (p = .017).

In a phase III study in 223 patients treated with either LE or placebo the lenses were not removed throughout the study to increase data resolution. Patients treated with LE showed improvement throughout the study in all parameters as early as 2 days after initiation of therapy. Papillae size and redness were reduced by approximately two fold in the LE compared to the placebo treated group; similarly, itching and lens tolerance (ability to continue lens wearing) were highly significantly improved (An intent to treat analysis showed p < 0.002 for all parameters). (Final data analysis will be presented by our "Ocular Allergy Study Group"). A similar study in additional 220 patients is now being analysed.

LE or placebo drops were given to 293 patients with a documented history of ocular seasonal allergy, starting approximately two weeks prior to the peak pollen and/or cedar season for 42 days. An intent to treat analysis showed a highly significant improvement for itching and conjunctival redness (p < 0.001) in the LE treated patients compared to placebo.

Safety (IOP elevation)

TABLE 3: IOP elevation in 257 LE treated patients compared to other steroids based on our studies and reviewed literature

	Dexamethasone Betamethasone	FML	LE
IOP elevation in the general population			
☞Percentage[#]	30%[1]		3.0%*
☞Mean rise of IOP (mmHg)	4.6^1-9.08^2	4.82^2	0.93
IOP elevation in steroid responders			
☞Percentage[#]	100%	60.5%[3]	33%[6]
☞Mean rise of IOP (mmHg)	23.7^4	6.9^4-8.1^5	4.1^6

* 36 patients who had an incidental IOP elevation of 6 mmHg or more that did not recur despite continuation of therapy were not considered responders.
#Percentage of subjects elevating IOP on therapy for 6 mmHg or more
Steroids were given q.i.d. for three to 11 weeks in the various studies cited.
1. Becker *et al.*   Arch. Ophth. 1963;   70:500-507
2. J. S. Mindel *et al.*   Am J. Ophth.1980;   96:1577-1578
3. R. Stewart *et al*   Arch. Ophth. 1979;   97:2139-2140
4. Y. Kitazawa   Am. J. Ophth 1976;   82:492-495
5. M. Kass *et al.*   Am. J. Ophth 1986;   102:159-163
6. J. Bartlett *et al.*   J. Ocular Phar 1993; 9:157-165

IOP elevation of the general population was derived from the 257 patients receiving LE for 42 days in the GPC and seasonal allergic conjunctivitis studies described in the previous section. These data combined with previous data on steroid responders (5) suggest that LE has the lower propensity to elevate IOP compared to other steroids including FML.

CONCLUSIONS

LE is a novel ocular steroid with high affinity to the glucocorticoid receptor and a unique ocular pharmacokinetic profile due to its esterase sensitive structure. LE is effective in models of ocular inflammation in animals and it has been *highly effective* in human ocular allergic diseases. Moreover, LE exhibits the lowest propensity to elevate IOP among the currently used ocular steroids. Thus, LE is a unique ocular steroid combining high efficacy with low tendency to elevate IOP.

REFERENCES

1. Armaly MF. Invest Ophthalmol 1965; 4: 187-197.
2. Bodor N. J Ocular Pharm   1994; 10: 3-15
3. Druzgala P, Whei-Mei WU, Bodor N. Curr Eye Res 1991; 10: 933-937.
4. Howes JF, Baru H, Vered M, Neumann R. J Ocular Phar 1994; 10: 289-293.
5. Bartlett JD, Howes JF, Ghormley NR, Amos JF, Laibovitz R, Horwitz B. Curr Eye Res 1993; 12: 313-321.

© 1994 Elsevier Science B.V. All rights reserved.
Advances in Ocular Immunology
R.B. Nussenblatt, S.M. Whitcup, R.R. Caspi and I. Gery, eds.

249

Treatment of Allergic Conjunctivitis in Murine Model

Bo Peng, Qian Li, Deborah Luyo, Scott M. Whitcup, Francois G. Roberge, and Chi-Chao Chan

Laboratory of Immunology, National Eye Institute, NIH, Bethesda, MD.

Introduction

Allergic conjunctivitis (AC) is a common external ocular disease with sight-threatening complications.[1] An experimental model of AC has been developed in the C57BL/6 mouse following the topical application of compound 48/80 (C48/80).[2] C48/80 induces mast cell degranulation, leading to the subsequent release of histamine and other inflammatory mediators.[3,4] Therefore, the current model of AC is a passive anaphylactic response in the conjunctiva of mice. The histopathological changes of AC are characterized by infiltration of neutrophils, monocytes and eosinophils into the conjunctiva, peaking at 24 hours.

Prednisolone, a corticosteroid with non-specific anti-inflammatory effect,[1] and nedocromil, a newly developed mast cell stabilizer,[5,6] have been widely used for anti-allergy therapy to achieve dramatic improvements on the outcome of AC. But the safety and efficacy of long term treatment in some cases remain to be a challenge for clinicians. Rapamycin is a macrolide antibiotic with potential inhibitory effect on type I hypersensitivity. Rapamycin has been studied primarily for its cellular mediated immunosuppressive properties,[7,8] however, its topical anti-allergic effect has not been previously investigated.

We conducted a series of experiments to test the effects of topical nedocromil, rapamycin, and prednisolone on allergic conjunctivitis, specifically assessing the efficacy of these drugs on inhibiting leukocyte and monocyte infiltration associated with an IgE reaction.

Materials and Methods

Animals
Female 6-8 week old C57BL/6 mice were obtained from Charles River Raleigh, Raleigh NC. The mice were kept under standard pathogen-free conditions, and this research adhered to the ARVO statement for the Use of Animals in Research.

Reagents
C48/80 was purchased from Sigma Chemical Company, MO, and was prepared by dissolving 40 mg in 100 μl PBS and adjusting to pH 7.4 with 5M NaOH.

Rapamycin was kindly provided by Wyeth-Ayerst Research, Princeton, NJ, and was prepared in a concentration of 2 mg/ml in olive oil.

Nedocromil sodium was kindly provided by Fisons pharmaceuticals, UK, and was freshly prepared in a concentration of 5% in PBS.

Predforte, 1% prednisolone acetate, was purchased from Allergan Pharmaceuticals, Irvine, CA.

Induction of AC

Mice were anesthetized by Metofane (Methoxyflurane, Pitman-Moore Inc. Mundelein, IL) inhalation. Initially 2 mg of C48/80 in 5 μl PBS was instilled onto the conjunctival lower cul de sac of each eye.

Treatment

The treatment consisted of three groups which received rapamycin, 5% nedocromil, Predforte respectively. Two control groups received PBS or olive oil. One drop (5 μl) of solution was applied to each group 15 minutes after application of the C48/80, and treatment was continued thereafter at 6 hours intervals.

Histology

Eyes and lower lid conjunctiva were collected at 6, 24 and 48 hours after C48/80 challenge. One lower lid bulbar and tarsal conjunctiva attached the globe of each animal was immediately fixed in 4% glutaraldehyde for 30 minutes, then transferred to 10% Formalin for at least 24 hours before processing. The tissue was embedded in methacrylate. Sections were stained with H&E for neutrophils, toluidine blue for mast cells, and PAS for Goblet cells.

Immunohistochemistry

The other eye and lower lid of each animal were embedded in O.C.T. compound (Miles Inc., Elkhart, IN), snap frozen and stored at -70⁰ C until sectioning. Immunohistochemical staining to detect CD4, CD8, CD11c/CD18 and CD19 cells was performed on cryostat sections using the Avidin-biotin-peroxidase complex (ABC) (Vector Lab., Burlingame, CA) method.[2] The slides were read and recorded by independent masked observers.

Results

Clinical examination demonstrated mice treated with rapamycin, nedocromil and prednisolone have less edema, erythema and discharge in comparison to control animals treated with either PBS or olive oil.

The analysis of histopathology illustrated that neutrophil infiltration decreased significantly 6, 24, and 48 hours after treatment in all treated-groups (Fig. 1). Macrophage infiltration decreased significantly 24 hours after treatment with rapamycin, nedocromil and prednisolone, but no marked changes at 6 and 48 hours after treatment. The number of mast cells, Goblet cells, T cell subsets and B lymphocytes did not differ significantly between the treated-groups and the controls using analysis of variance (Tables 1 and 2). However, persistent loss of

Goblet cells were observed in the groups treated with rapamycin, prednisolone, and olive oil.

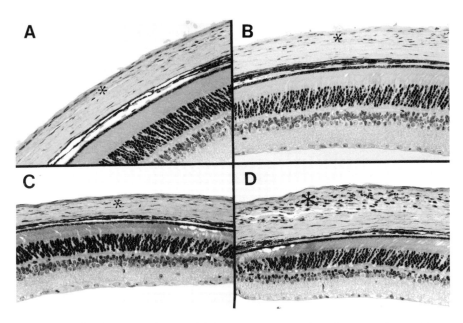

Figure 1. Conjunctiva (asterisk) from rats treated with rapamycin (A), nedocromil (B), prednisolone (C) and olive oil (D) at 24 hours. Inflammatory cellular infiltration was significantly reduced in treated groups. (Hematoxylin and eosin, x200)

Table 1
Numbers of neutrophils (mean± S.E.M) infiltrating the conjunctiva

Treatment	6hr.	24hr.	48hr.
Rapamycin	15.2±12.5(9)**	13.4±12.3(12)**	7.1 ± 4.8 (9)**
Nedocromil	19.4± 8.3 (7)**	14.1± 5.1 (8) **	9.0 ± 7.8 (7)*
Prednisolone	25.0±16.7(6)*	14.0±10.3 (6) **	8.7 ± 8.0 (7)*
PBS	54.0±18.2(5)	61.0±28.2 (7)	18.2 ± 4.4 (6)
Oil	50.7±20.3(6)	95.2±70.3 (4)	23.0±10.7(5)

(n) = number of animals,   * P<0.03,   ** P<0.01

Table 2
Number of macrophages (mean ± S.E.M) infiltrating the conjunctiva

Treatment	6hr.	24hr.	48hr.
Rapamycin	43.6±48.9 (5)	14.6±10.6 (5)**	9.6 ± 3.0 (5)
Nedocromil	44.5± 46.8(4)	33.0±10.6 (4)**	9.5 ±11.0 (4)
Prednisolone	37.7±37.6 (5)	22.7± 15.6(5)**	9.5 ± 7.8 (5)
PBS	56.1±30.1 (6)	63.3±10.9 (6)	15.3 ± 14.5 (6)
Oil	63.4±66.7 (5)	44.0±21.6 (5)	10.0± 10.9 (5)

(n) = number of animals,   ** P<0.01

Discussion

Topical rapamycin, nedocromil and prednisolone significantly decreased subacute cellular inflammation in this animal model of allergic conjunctivitis. This is the first study demonstrating a topical anti-allergic effect of rapamycin. The mechanism of this anti-allergic effect may involve its inhibition of IgE receptor-mediated exocytosis from mast cells and of other cytokine-mediated activities.   The predominant result of treatment with rapamycin, nedocromil and prednisolone was a decrease in infiltrating neutrophils. The mast cell has been shown to induce the recruitment of leukocytes,[9] and the decrease of neutrophils appeared to be a direct result of therapy. Macrophage infiltration was only decreased 24 hours after C48/80 in the animals receiving rapamycin, nedocromil or prednisolone, suggesting that early influx of macrophages was less inhibited. It is also noteworthy that rapamycin more strongly inhibited macrophage infiltration than either nedocromil and prednisolone. However, only nedocromil showed rapid recovery of Goblet cells in the conjunctiva.

C48/80-induced conjunctivitis in murine model appears useful for evaluating therapy for allergic conjunctivitis. This study demonstrated that topical rapamycin, nedocromil and prednisolone were effective in reducing C48/80-induced conjunctival inflammation in mice, and suggests that these medications may be effective in treating allergic conjunctivitis in humans.

References

1. M. H. Friedlaender. Annals of Allergy, 1991; 67: 5-14.
2. Q. Li, N. Hikita et al: IOVS, 1993; 34: 857.
3. I. J. Udell, M. B. Abelson. Am. J. Ophthalomal., 1981; 91: 226-230.
4. M. R. Allensmith et al: Acta Opthalmologica., 1989; 67:145-153.
5. M. Blumenthal, T. Casale et al: Am. J. Ophthalmol., 1990; 113: 56-63.
6. I. G. Knottnerus et al: Ocul. Immunol. Inflam., 1992; 1: 27-30.
7. T. Hultsch, R. Martin et al: Am. Society for Cell Biolog, 1992; 3: 981-987.
8. F. G. Roberge et al: Ocul. Immunol. Inflam., 1993; 1: 269--273.
9. B. K. Wershil, Z-S. Wang et al: J. Clin. Invest., 1991; 87: 446-453.

© 1994 Elsevier Science B.V. All rights reserved.
Advances in Ocular Immunology
R.B. Nussenblatt, S.M. Whitcup, R.R. Caspi and I. Gery, eds.

The Efficacy of Leflunomide in Experimental Models of Ocular Disease

Stella M. Robertson*, Laura S. Lang*, and Jerry Y. Niederkorn^

* Alcon Laboratories, Inc., 6201 South Freeway, Fort Worth, TX, 76134-2099 (USA)

^ Univ. of Texas Southwestern Medical Center, 5323 Harry Hines Blvd., Dallas, TX, 75235-9057(USA)

INTRODUCTION

Autoimmune responses in the eye can have severe clinical consequences. Autoimmune uveitis, one form of uveitis, is an inflammation of the uveal tract and retina. Severe posterior uveitis is particularly devastating because it can end in blindness. In addition, immunological rejection of corneal tissue after transplantation is currently the leading cause of corneal graft failure.

Topical or systemic administration of corticosteroids, often as long-term therapy, has been the standard treatment regimen for many types of uveitis and as part of therapy post transplantation. The lengthy administration of steroids with their known risk of inducing secondary glaucoma renders them less than optimal. For several years, cyclosporin A (CSA) has been an experimental alternative treatment in the more difficult cases of uveitis and corneal transplantation. Leflunomide (LEF) is a new immunomodulator with an immunopharmacological profile similar to, yet distinct from CSA [1]. We demonstrate here the efficacy of LEF and CSA in two rat *in vivo* models: experimental autoimmune uveitis (EAU) and corneal allograft rejection.

MATERIALS & METHODS

Test Compounds

Leflunomide, an isoxasol derivative, was obtained from Hoechst AG, Wiesbaden, Germany and was evaluated as an aqueous suspension. A77 1726A, a salt of the active metabolite of LEF, was also obtained from Hoechst AG and administered as a solution. A clinical formulation of cyclosporin A (SANDIMMUNE, Sandoz, East Hanover, NJ) was obtained commercially and diluted prior to use. Dexamethasone was obtained from Sigma (St. Louis, MO) and formulated as a suspension.

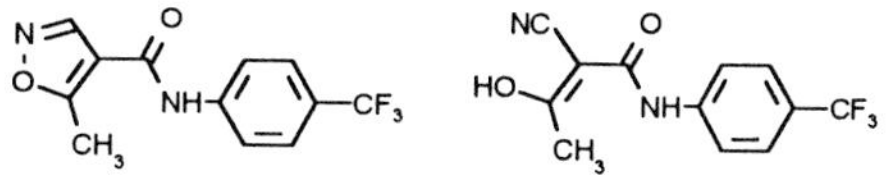

Leflunomide   A77 1726

Fig. 1. Leflunomide and its primary metabolite, A77 1726.

Experimental Autoimmune Uveitis

EAU was induced in male Lewis rats using a modified method of Dorey et al. [2]. Briefly, 0.5 mg/ml of purified bovine S-antigen (S-Ag) was emulsified in complete Freund's adjuvant containing an additional 2.5 mg/ml of M. tuberculosis. One hindpaw of each rat received a single 100 µl injection (50 µg) of the S-Ag emulsion. Animals were dosed with test compounds or vehicle immediately following injection with S-Ag (Day 0) through the day before sacrifice. Compounds were administered topically in a volume of 5 µl to the right eye (OD) QID or orally by gavage once per day. Leflunomide was administered at concentrations ranging from 0.2 to 10 mg/kg/day, CSA at 1 to 10 mg/kg/day and dexamethasone at 0.1 mg/kg/day. Individual eyes were examined daily from disease onset (Day 10 post injection) up until one day before sacrifice by direct ophthalmoscopic examination. Disease signs and symptoms of EAU were assigned numerical scores according to the disease intensity in the anterior and posterior chambers and were totaled for a daily disease score per animal as described elsewhere [3,4].

Corneal Allograft Rejection

Forty eight (48) female Lewis rats were given 3.0 mm full-thickness corneal grafts from Wistar-Furth donor rats as described elsewhere [5]. Prior to transplantation, donor corneas were treated with sterile latex beads to induce centripetal migration of peripheral Langerhans cells in the donor tissue. Daily treatment with oral LEF (10 mg/kg/day), CSA (10 mg/kg/day), A77 1726A (6.5 mg/kg/day), or vehicle was initiated two days prior to transplantation surgery and continued for 30 days post-surgery. One group of animals was grafted but received no treatment. Grafted corneas were examined to determine the mean graft survival time in each group. Corneal graft rejection was assessed based on severity of graft opacity, edema, and neovascularization as described previously (5).

RESULTS

The onset and development of experimental autoimmune uveitis was inhibited with daily oral doses of either LEF or CSA at 10 mg/kg/day (Fig. 2A). Animals treated with daily oral doses of dexamethasone (0.1 mg/kg/day) demonstrated a delayed disease onset with limited improvement in the disease severity. Vehicle treated animals developed severe inflammation in the anterior and posterior chambers with accompanying retinal destruction. The inflammation peaked around Days 11-13 and with time gradually declined (Days 16-21). This decline possibly reflects the depletion of the autoimmune stimulus (S-Ag) due to the retinal destruction in this model.

Continued administration of LEF and CSA is necessary to prevent disease onset and control uveitic disease. As shown in Fig. 2B, upon cessation of treatment with LEF or CSA, disease onset initiates within 4 days. Both LEF and CSA mitigate this breakthrough, however the peak ocular disease score obtained with LEF is less than that seen with CSA treated animals.

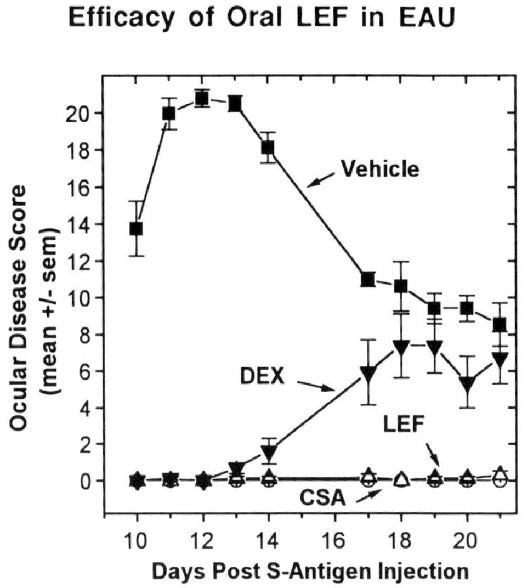

Efficacy of Oral LEF in EAU

Fig. 2A. Kinetics of EAU progression in rats treated with a daily oral dose of LEF or CSA (10 mg/kg/day) or DEX (0.1 mg/kg/day) or vehicle control.

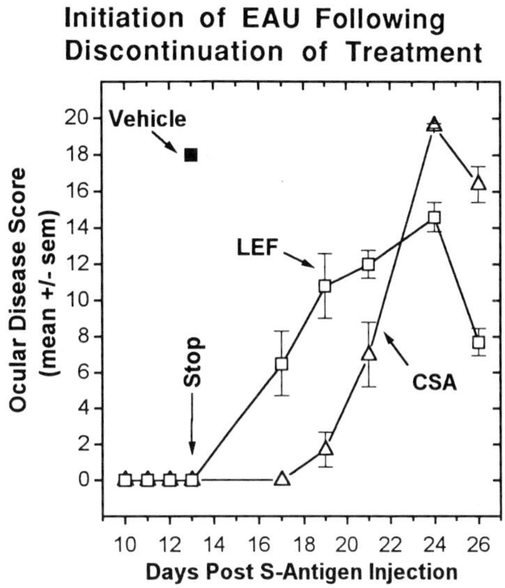

Initiation of EAU Following Discontinuation of Treatment

Fig 2B. Kinetics of disease breakthrough upon discontinuation (D13) of LEF or CSA oral treatment (10 mg/kg/day).

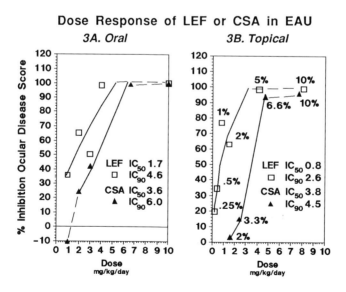

Dose Response of LEF or CSA in EAU

3A. Oral

3B. Topical

Fig. 3A,B. Dose-dependent inhibition (I) of LEF (□) and CSA (▲). The numbers by the symbols refer to the topical concentration (Fig. 3B). The %I ocular disease score was calculated for each group during the peak of the disease (D 10-13). IC values were calculated based on linear regression for log %I vs log dose.

LEF and CSA inhibit the development of EAU in a dose-dependent fashion when administered orally or topically (Fig. 3). Two inhibitory concentration (IC) values were calculated, an IC_{50}, representing the concentration necessary for inhibition of the general inflammatory response, and an IC_{90}, because our previous results indicated that a 90% inhibition of the ocular disease score was necessary to maintain a histologically normal retina [4]. LEF was more effective (lower IC values) than CSA in inhibiting EAU whether administered orally or topically as shown in Fig. 3A,B.

Leflunomide, it's active metabolite (A77 1726A), CSA, and a vehicle control were also evaluated for their effect on mean survival time of corneal allografts in rats after oral administration. The results of this study are shown in Table 1. Neither CSA (10 mg/kg/day) or vehicle control were seen to prolong the graft survival time over that seen in untreated control grafts, with a mean graft survival time of 14.6 and 14.7 days versus 11.0 days, respectively. However, oral dosing with either LEF (10 mg/kg/day) or A77 1726A (6.5 mg/kg/day) resulted in a significant survival time of the corneal allografts. Five of the 10 LEF-treated grafts demonstrated survival nearly 3 times that seen in the untreated control group, and 3 of these 5 corneas survived at least 21 days after drug treatment was discontinued on day 30. Two of the LEF-treated grafts survived until the end of the study (Days 60-61) with no signs of graft rejection [6]. Treatment with Leflunomide's active metabolite resulted in a similarly dramatic prolongation of graft survival (Table 1).

Table 1

Effect of Leflunomide on Corneal Graft Survival

Treatment	N	MST	P	Number of Grafts Surviving	
				>22 Days*	After drug removal
None	11	11.0	-	0	0
CSA	9	14.6	0.06	0	0
Olive Oil	10	14.7	0.18	1	1
Leflunomide	10	29.7	0.002	5	3
A77 1726A†	8	32.4	0.005	5	5

p values were determined using one-way analysis of variance and a Mantel Haenszel survival analysis program.

*Graft survival 22 days or longer represents a doubling of the MST (mean survival time)

†Salt of the active metabolite of leflunomide

CONCLUSIONS

A new immunomodulator, leflunomide (LEF) and its active metabolite, A77 1726, were compared to the immunosuppressant cyclosporin A (CSA) and corticosteroid dexamethasone in two ocular models of autoimmune inflammatory disease: experimental autoimmune uveitis and corneal keratoplasty. LEF and CSA, when administered topically or orally, were both effective at inhibiting the development of EAU in a dose-dependent fashion. However, the inhibitory concentrations needed to reduce the ocular disease score (IC_{50} and IC_{90}) and preserve the retina (IC_{90}) in EAU were lower for LEF than for CSA. Discontinuation of LEF or CSA treatment resulted in uveitic disease onset. Dexamethasone had a limited effect on disease progression in this model of autoimmune uveitis. LEF or A77 1726 administered orally to rats receiving full-thickness corneal allografts significantly prolonged graft survival by nearly three fold when compared to untreated controls. CSA did not enhance graft survival time in this study, which may be the result of the dosage chosen to minimize CSA's oral toxicity or bioavailability of the compound. Our results suggest that leflunomide has therapeutic potential for treating ocular autoimmune disease.

REFERENCES

1   Bartlett RR, Dimitrijevic M, Mattar T, Sielinski T, Germann T, Rude E, Thoenes GH, Kuchle CCA, Schorlemmer HU, Bremer E, Finnegan A and Schleyerbach A Agents and Actions 1991; 32:10-21.
2   Dorey C, Cozette J, Faure JP Ophthalmic Res 1982; 14:249-255.
3   Lang LS, Glaser RL, Weimer LK, and Robertson SM. In: Dernouchamps JP, Verougstraete C, Caspers-Velu L and Tassignon MJ, eds. Third International Symposium on Uveitis. Amsterdam: Kugler Publications, 1993; 529-534.
4   Robertson SM and Lang LS Agents and Actions 1994 in press.
5   Callanan DG, Luckenbach MW, Fischer BJ, Peeler JS, Niederkorn JY Invest Ophthalmol Vis Sci 1989; 30:413-424.
6   Niederkorn JY, Lang LS, Ross J, Mellon J, Robertson SM Invest Ophthalmol Vis Sci 1994; in press.

Advances in Ocular Immunology
R.B. Nussenblatt, S.M. Whitcup, R.R. Caspi and I. Gery, eds.

Gold salts modify the Th1-Th2 balance in Experimental Autoimmune Uveoretinitis (EAU)

R. Sheela[1], A. Saoudi[1], Y. de Kozak[2], K. Huygen[3], P. Druet[1] and B. Bellon[1]

[1]INSERM U28, Hopital Broussais, 96 Rue Didot, 75674 Paris, France.

[2]INSERM U86, Institut des Cordeliers, Paris, France.

[3] Institut Pasteur van Brabant, Brussels, Belgium.

Summary

Gold compounds, used in rheumatoid arthritis (RA) therapy, are known to trigger adverse immune reactions related to T helper (Th) 2 response in certain patients. Since RA is presumed to be a Th1 dependent disease, gold salts may act by skewing the immune response towards Th2 type. In this study we analysed the effect of gold salts in the development of Th1 mediated experimental autoimmune uveoretinitis induced by retinal S antigen (SAg) in (Lewis X Brown Norway)F1 rats. Immunization of F1 rats on day 7 after the first injection with gold salts induced a clearcut Th2 response. Production of IL-4 was increased while that of IL-2, IFN-γ and TNF-α were reduced in *in vitro* cultures of spleen and lymph node cells from gold salt-treated SAg immunized rats (Au-SAg); concomitantly, production of nitric oxide was reduced in these rats. Analysis of the isotypes of anti-SAg antibodies showed that IgG1 levels were significantly elevated in Au-SAg rats, while the levels of IgG2a was significantly elevated in the H2O-SAg rats. No significant clinical protection was observed in gold salts treated rats, as against the complete protection observed after treatment with HgCl2, another Th2 activating chemical. One of the possible reasons for this lack of protection may be that gold salt-induced Th2 response is not strong enough to protect completely against this Th1 mediated disease. But under mild disease conditions this skewing of the immune response from Th1 to Th2 may be sufficient enough to contain the disease.

Introduction

T helper cells comprise of two subsets on the basis of their cytokine profile. Th1 cells which primarily secrete IL-2 and IFN-γ are involved in cellular immune responses and Th2 cells which secrete IL-4, IL-5 and IL-10, in humoral immune responses (1). Experimental autoimmune uveoretinitis (EAU) is an ocular autoimmune disease mediated by T cells recognising retinal S antigen (SAg) and can be induced in Lewis (LEW) rats by immunization with SAg (2,3); EAU can be adoptively transferred by T cell lines which produce IL-2 and IFN-γ, and prevented by treatment with monoclonal antibodies against IL-2 receptor or IFN-γ (4,5). These features characterize EAU as a TH1 mediated disease.

Previous studies have shown that HgCl2 and gold salts induce an auto-immune disease in Brown Norway (BN) rats with increases in autoantibodies and serum IgE levels which are characteristic of a Th2 mediated disease (6,7). Treatment of (LEW X BN)F1 rats with HgCl2 resulted in the development of Th2-like response against the immunizing antigen concomitantly preventing the development of the disease (8). In this study, we analysed the effects of gold salts on the development of EAU since gold salts used in RA therapy (9) are believed to contain the disease by skewing the immune response to Th2-type.

Materials and Methods

Eight to thirteen week old (LEW X BN)F1 female rats were immunized with SAg in Freund's complete adjuvant in the rear footpads simultaneously with intraperitoneal vaccination with killed *Bordetella pertussis*, on day 7 after the first injection of gold salts (Au-SAg) or control solution (H2O-SAg). The eyes were examined daily after SAg injection in order to assess the development of EAU clinically. On day 28 after injection of SAg, the eyes of one set of rats were removed, dissected and fixed in Bouin's solution for histological analysis.

Fourteen days after immunization, spleen and lymph node cells were stimulated with 20μg/ml SAg *in vitro* at a concentration of 2×10^6 cells/ml and supernatants were collected after 24, 48 or 72 hours of incubation. Nitric oxide (NO) synthesis was determined as nitrite release in the 72h supernatants using the spectrophotometric method based on the Griess reaction. IL-2 was measured by CTLL-2 bioassay in 24h supernatants. IFN-γ was measured in 48h supernatants using reduction of cytopathic effect of VSV on normal rat kidney cells. TNF-α levels were determined in a bioassay using L-929 mouse fibroblasts in which the concentration of TNF-α is proportional to fibroblast lysis. IL-4 levels were detected by polymerase chain reaction (PCR) using mRNA extracted from spleen and lymph node cells obtained *ex vivo*.

Titers of anti-SAg antibody isotypes were measured in sera from Au-SAg and H2O-SAg rats on day 14 after SAg immunization. Sera were titered by comparison with a reference curve built with a pool of sera from LEW rats immunized thrice with S-Ag (8).

Results

Table 1
Production of IL-2 and IFN-γ

	Rat #	IL-2 (cpm) None	IL-2 (cpm) SAg	IFN-γ (U/ml) None	IFN-γ (U/ml) SAg
H2O-SAg	1	8,497	136,252	14	161
	2	427	81,584	228	271
	3	531	66,211	136	543
Au-SAg	1	1,177	23,033	3	57
	2	209	332	3	3
	3	761	18,862	3	24

Gold salt-treated rats exhibit a Th2-type response to SAg

As shown in Fig.1, the expression of IL-4 mRNA was increased in the spleen and lymph node cells from Au-SAg rats and not in those from H2O-SAg rats. Concomitantly, low levels of IL-2 and IFN-γ were observed in supernatants derived from Au-SAg rats in contrast to H2O-SAg rats after *in vitro* stimulation of spleen cells with SAg (Table 1). No significant levels of IL-2 or IFN-γ were observed in supernatants derived from naive rats under similar conditions (data not shown).

In addition to IL-2, IFN-γ and IL-4, the expression of TNF-α was observed only in response to antigenic stimulation in H2O-SAg rats and not in Au-SAg rats (Fig.2). The synthesis of NO was also decreased in Au-SAg rats (Fig.3). Similar results were observed with lymph node cells (data not shown).

Analysis of anti-SAg antibody isotypes

On day 14 after immunization, Au-SAg rats showed significantly increased anti-SAg antibodies for IgG1 isotype (p < 0,05) when compared to H2O-SAg rats. On the other hand, the levels of IgG2a were significantly elevated in H2O-SAg rats (p < 0,05; Fig.4). The IgG2b levels were not different between the two groups.

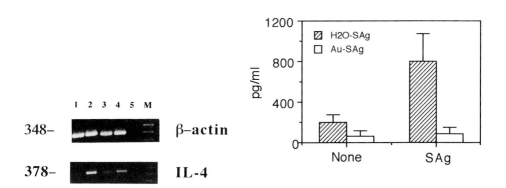

Fig 1 Expression of IL-4 mRNA in spleen (1,2) and lymph node (3,4) cells from H2O-SAg (1,3) and Au-SAg (2,4) rats, negative control (5).

Fig 2. Production of TNF-α

Discussion

Gold salts, which have beneficial effects in RA, have also been shown to induce an increase in serum IgE concentrations and/or autoimmune manifestations in susceptible individuals (9). The effects of gold salts may be mediated by the preferential skewing of the immune response to an antigen towards Th2 type as is evident from this study where we demonstrate that (LEW X BN)F1 rats immunized with the retinal SAg and treated with gold salts develop a

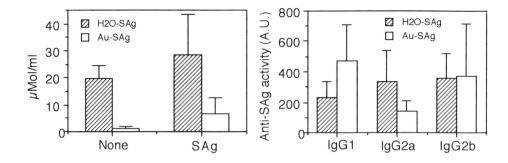

Fig 3. Production of NO   Fig 4. Anti-SAg antibody isotypes

Th2 rather than Th1 dependent response against SAg. The shift in the immune response is not sufficient for inducing protection against Th1 mediated EAU (data not shown) unlike that we have reported with HgCl2, a chemical which also induces a Th2 response (8). One possibility is that the mechanism of induction of Th2 response by HgCl2 and gold salts may be different. A more likely explanation is that the Th2 response induced by gold salts is not as strong as that of HgCl2. The latter view is supported by the observation that autoimmune disorders induced by gold salts in contrast to that induced by HgCl2 are milder (7).

Nonetheless, the observed beneficial effects of gold salts in RA suggests that mild skewing of the immune response towards Th2 type may lead to decreases in the intensity of the disease. Also, in RA, continuous treatment with gold salts is required to contain the disease over a long time (10). The association of the shift towards Th2 and induction of certain autoimmune disorders implies that a balance between suppression of deleterious Th1 response along with minimal Th2 induced side effects is required in the treatment of Th1 mediated autoimmune diseases.

References

1. Mosmann TR and Moore KW. Immunol Today 1991; 12: A49-A53.
2. Wacker WB, Donoso LA, Kalsow CM, Yankeelov JA, Organisciak DT. J Immunol 1977; 119: 1949-1958.
3. de Kozak Y, Sakai J, Thillaye B, Faure P. Curr Eye Res 1981; 1:327-337.
4. Atalla LR, Yoser S, Rao NA. Ocular Immunol. Today, Usui M, Ohno S, Aoki K Eds . Elsevier , 1990; 65.-68.
5. Higuchi M, Diamantstein T, Osawa H, Caspi RR. J. of Autoimmunity 1991; 4: 113-124.
6. Sapin C, Hirsch F, Delaporte JP, Bazin H, Druet P. Immunogenetics 1984, 20: 227-236.
7. Tournade H, Pelletier L, Guéry JC, Pasquier R, et al. Nephrol Dial Transplant 1991; 6: 621-630.
8. Saoudi A, Kuhn J, Huygen K, de Kozak Y, et al. Eur J Immunol 1993; 23: 3096-3103.
9. Bretza J, Wells I, Novey HS. Am J Med 1983; 74: 945-951.
10. Serre H, Sany J, Rosenberg F. Ann Med Interne 1976; 127: 552-560.

Advances in Ocular Immunology
R.B. Nussenblatt, S.M. Whitcup, R.R. Caspi and I. Gery, eds.

263

EFFECT OF ANTI-CD3 ANTIBODIES ON THE DEVELOPMENT OF EAU IN MICE

H. Yokoi, T. Kezuka, M. Takeuchi, J. Sakai and M. Usui.

Department of Ophthalmology, Tokyo Medical College Hospital, Tokyo, Japan.

INTRODUCTION

Experimental autoimmune uveoretinitis (EAU) can be induced in animals by immunization with the retinal self-antigen, interphotorecepter retinoid-binding protein (IRBP). Recent investigations utilizing a novel protocol of immunization have shown that EAU can be induced in susceptible mouse strains, even though mice were previously considered resistent to induction [1]. Subsequently, many reseachers have created murine EAU models by that and other similar protocols.

Depending on various conditions, anti-CD3 monoclonal antibodies (mAb) are known to be both immunosuppressive or mitogenic to T cells *in vitro*, and have recently been studied as a mode of immunomodulation in experimental models and human disease. Various aspects of these mAb have been analyzed *in vivo*, and they have also begun to be used clinically in the field of transplantation immunology [2-6].

In this study, using anti-CD3 mAb, we investigated the immunosuppressive effects of this monoclonal antibody on the induction of EAU.

MATERIALS AND METHODS

Mice
Four-to six-week-old B10.A mice were used in this study.

Antigen
Bovine IRBP was purified using the method described by Redmond [7].

Immunization
To induce EAU, mice were immunized on day zero with 100 µg of IRBP in a 1:1 (v/v) emulsion with complete Freund's adjuvant, containing 2.5 mg/ml of *Mycobacterium tuberculosis* strain H37RA, in a total volume of 0.1 ml injected in the hind footpad. *Bordetella pertussis* bacteria (10^{10}) in a volume of 0.2 ml were injected intraperitoneally at the same time.

Anti-CD3 mAb preparation
Monoclonal antibody was prepared by immunizing 145-2C11 hybridoma cells into SCID mice and collecting the ascites, from which antibody was purified by 50% ammonium sulfate precipitation, followed by gel filtration on a Protein G column.

Treatment schedule
Mice were injected with varying concentrations (10, 30, 100, 300 and 900 µg) of mAb on days -1, 0 and 1. The antibody was suspended in a volume of 200 µl PBS, and injected intraperitoneally. Mice injected with only 200 µl of PBS were prepared as controls.

Histopathological assessment of EAU

All mice were sacrificed 1 month after immunization, with the eyes enucleated and fixed in Bouin's fixative for histopathological study. Samples were embedded in paraffin and 4 to 6 μm sections were stained with hematoxylin and eosin.

Cytokine assay

Splenic lymphocytes from mice were obtained and assessed for cytokine production. Spleens were dissociated into single-cell suspensions, with lysing of erythrocytes using Tris NH4Cl. The cells were cultured in flat-bottomed plates at a density of $5x10^6$ cells/2 ml well in RPMI 1640 medium with HEPES, supplemented with 2 mM L-glutamine, 0.1 mM nonessential amino acids, streptomycin (100 μg/ml), 10% fresh fetal calf serum, and 2-mercaptoethanol at $5x10^{-5}$ M (conditioned medium). The cells were stimulated with 10 ug of IRBP, and cell cultures were incubated at 37 °C in 6% CO_2. The supernatants were removed from each well 48 hours after the initiation of culture, and cytokine (IL-2, IFN-γ, IL-4, IL-10) production was assayed by ELISA.

ELISA protocol was as follows. 1) Dilute purified anti-cytokine capture mAb to 5 μg/ml in coating buffer (0.1 M NaHCO3, pH 8.2). Add 50 μl to well of an enhanced protein binding ELISA plate. 2) Cover plate and incubate overnight at 4 °C. 3) Wash with PBS/Tween and block with Block Ace at 200 μl per well. 4) Incubate at 37 °C for 2 hours and wash. 5) Add standards and samples at 100 μl per well (diluted in PBS/10% serum). 6) Incubate overnight at 4 °C and wash. 7) Dilute biotinylated anti-cytokine detecting mAb to 2 μg/ml in PBS/10% serum. 8) Incubate at room temperature for 1 hour and wash. 9) Dilute avidin, biotinylated-peroxidase to manufacturer's recommendation in PBS/10% serum. Add 100 μl per well. 10) Incubate at room temperature for 30 minutes and wash. 11) Add 10 mg of o-phenylenediamine and 10 μl of H2O2 per 10 ml of citrate-phosphate buffer. Add 100 μl per well and allow to develop at room temperature. Color reaction can be stopped by adding 50 μl of 4N H2SO4. 12) Read plate at OD 490 nm.

RESULTS

Suppression of EAU with anti-CD3 mAb treatment

In control mice, 7 of 13 mice were observed to develop EAU by immunization with IRBP. On the other hand, in anti-CD3 mAb treated mice, full suppression of EAU was clearly observed in the majority of animals at each dose of mAb (Table 1). Moreover, in animals that did exhibit inflammation, the extent was much diminished when compared to control mice with EAU (Figure 1).

Cytokine assay

There were distinct differences in cytokine production between anti-CD3 mAb treated mice and control mice 1 month after IRBP immunization. In control mice, cytokine production of IL-2 and IFN-γ was found, but not IL-10. On the other hand, in anti-CD3 mAb treated mice, cytokine production of IL-10 was found, but not IL-2 at each dose (Table 2).

Table 1
Incidence of EAU in Control and Treated mice

dose (µg)	Anti-CD3 mAb treatment					Control treatment
	10 x 3	30 x 3	100 x 3	300 x 3	900 x 3	(-)
EAU	1/6	0/6	1/5	0/6	0/6	7/13

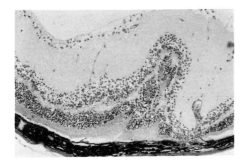 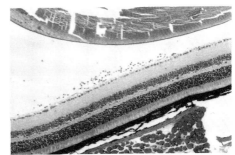

Figure 1. Histopathology of EAU in Control (a) and Treated (b) mice

Table 2
Cytokine Production

Treatment	n	IL-2 (µg/ml)	IFN-γ (U/ml)	IL-4 (µg/ml)	IL-10 (µg/ml)
Control	7 (EAU +)	0.64 ± 0.14	52.0 ± 18.3	< 0.1	< 0.1
	6 (EAU -)	< 0.1	< 1.0	< 0.1	< 0.1
Anti-CD3 mAb					
10 µg x 3	6	< 0.1	> 1000	< 0.1	1.10 ± 0.17
30 µg x 3	6	< 0.1	> 1000	< 0.1	1.03 ± 0.15
100 µg x 3	5	< 0.1	38.0 ± 7.21	< 0.1	0.40 ± 0.11
300 µg x 3	6	< 0.1	80.7 ± 39.3	< 0.1	0.93 ± 0.13
900 µg x 3	6	< 0.1	23.7 ± 8.02	< 0.1	0.58 ± 0.12

DISCUSSION

With regards to immunosuppression using anti-CD3 mAb, many studies have been conducted. It was reported that anti-CD3 mAb prolonged skin graft survival, and thus it is starting to be utilized clinically [2]. On the other hand, Chavin KD et al. demonstrated that the combination of anti-CD3 and anti-CD2 mAb resulted in significant prolongation of allograft survival, greater than with using anti-CD3 mAb alone [6].

In this study, we administered anti-CD3 mAb alone to mice. As a result, the suppression of EAU was clearly observed in mAb treated mice at each dose. Thus, judging from our results, immunosuppression of anti-CD3 mAb is very effective in the murine EAU model. However, our study looked at only relatively short term (1 month) effects, and we need to conduct a more long term study in the future. In skin grafts, anti-CD3 mAb therapy has been found to have only limited short term effects (< 1 month).

We also analyzed cytokine production in the treated and control mice. In T cell-mediated autoimmune disease, various cytokines are thought to be involved in the induction process. In recent years, it has been discovered that T cells are divided into at least two types of clones, TH1 and TH2, according to cytokine production patterns. TH1 cells synthesize IL-2, IFN-γ, whereas these cytokines are not expressed by TH2 cells. Conversely, only TH2 cells synthesize detectable amounts of IL-4, IL-6, and IL-10. TH1 cells are responsible for cell-mediated immune reactions, and TH2 cells for assisting in IgE and IgG1 antibody production [8-11]. In the EAU model of autoimmune disease, it is believed that TH1 cells act in the development of disease, while TH2 cells act in the suppression of disease [12].

In this study, spleen cells from anti-CD3 mAb treated mice at all doses tested produced IL-10, which is considered to be a suppressive cytokine, but not IL-2. Anti-CD3 mAb may be influencing patterns of cytokine production, thereby causing suppression of IRBP-induced EAU in these mice.

REFERENCES

1   Caspi RR, Roberge FG, Chan CC, Wiggert B, et al. J Immunol 1988;140:1490-1495.
2   Hirsch R, Eckhaus M, Auchincloss H Jr, Sachs DH, et al. J Immunol 1988;140:3766-3772.
3   Hirsch R, Gress RE, Plyznik DH, Eckhaus M, et al. J Immunol 1989;142:737-743.
4   Ferran C, Sheehan K, Dy M, Schreiber R, et al. Eur J Immunol 1990;20:509-515.
5   Chatenoud L, Bach JF. Immunol Ser 1993;59:175-191.
6   Chavin KD, Qin L, Lin J, Woodward JE, et al. Ann Surg 1993;218:492-503.
7   Redmond T, Wiggert B, Robey F, Nguyen N, et al. Biochemistry 1985;24:787.
8   Mossmann TR, Coffman RL. Adv Immunol 1989;46:111.
9   Mossmann TR, Moore KW. Immunol Today 1991;12:A49.
10 Cher DJ, Mossmann TR. J immunol 1987;138:3688.
11 Snapper CM, Finkelman FD, Paul WE. Immunol Rev 1988;102:51.
12 Saoudi A, Kuhn J, Huygen K, DeKozak Y, et al. Eur J immunol 1993;23:3096-3103.

2. Ocular Infection: Mechanisms of Disease and Therapeutic Approaches

© 1994 Elsevier Science B.V. All rights reserved.
Advances in Ocular Immunology
R.B. Nussenblatt, S.M. Whitcup, R.R. Caspi and I. Gery, eds.

Toxin production contributes to severity of *Staphylococcus aureus* endophthalmitis

M.C. Booth[ab], R. V. Atkuri[a], S. K. Nanda[b] and M.S. Gilmore[ab]

[a]Department of Microbiology and Immunology and [b]Department of Ophthalmology, University of Oklahoma Health Sciences Center, Oklahoma City, OK, USA.

INTRODUCTION

Staphylococcus aureus is among the leading causes of both postoperative and postraumatic endophthalmitis and is associated with poor visual outcome (defined as best corrected final visual acuity of 20/200 or worse) in greater than 65% of reported cases (1-6). The recent emergence of increased antibiotic resistance among staphylococcal strains threatens to further increase the rate of treatment failure for this organism.

S. *aureus* is known to express an estimated 35 extracellular products, many of which have been implicated as virulence factors. The expression of exoproteins as well as certain cell surface proteins in S. *aureus* has been shown to be coordinately controlled by a number of global regulatory elements, one of which is *agr* (10). Mutant strains of S. *aureus* defective at the *agr* locus have been characterized at the phenotypic level. Expression of α, β, γ and δ-toxins, TSST-1, and staphylococcal enterotoxins B and C are decreased in *agr*- mutants, while coagulase, protein A and fibronectin binding protein are elevated relative to the parental strain.

The control of expression of virulence factors has been described as a virulence determinant in itself. Mutant strains defective in staphylococcal global regulators have been tested in animal infection models of endocarditis (11), septic arthritis (10) and intraperitoneal infection (9). In each of these models, mutants defective in extracellular protein expression were considerably less virulent than the wild type parental strain. To determine the role of extracellular and cell wall associated proteins in the establishment and progression of S. *aureus* endophthalmitis, we compared an *agr*- mutant strain of S. *aureus* with an isogenic *agr*+ strain in a rabbit endophthalmitis model.

MATERIAL AND METHODS

Bacterial strains, animals and media: S. *aureus* ISP479 is a derivative of NCTC 8325 (a human isolate) which has been cured of prophages (17). ISP479 expresses α, β, γ and δ-toxins, enterotoxin, acid phosphatase, serine protease, metalloprotease, lipase, hyaluronidase and staphylokinase, and low levels of coagulase and protein A (10,12). S. *aureus* ISP546 is an *agr*- derivative of strain ISP479 with a chromosomal Tn*551* insertion in the *agr* locus. ISP546 does not express α-toxin and expresses low levels of β-toxin, enterotoxin C, serine protease, nuclease and elevated levels of coagulase (9,12). Strains were propagated in brain heart infusion (BHI) broth at 37°C without aeration. Prior to intravitreal injection, cultures were serially diluted in phosphate buffered saline (PBS). Enumeration of organisms was accomplished by plating on BHI agar containing horse blood (5% v/v). New Zealand White rabbits weighing 2-4 kg were used in this study. Intraocular injections were carried out according to the procedure described by Jett *et al.* (8).

Measurement of infection parameters: ERG was performed prior to and 24, 48, 72 and 96 h post injection as described by Jett *et al.* (8). The Mann Whitney U test was used to analyze ERG results. p values of <0.05 were considered statistically significant. Infected eyes were enucleated for histopathological analysis either at 24 hours post infection or when loss of B-wave response was 100%, following standard procedures (13). Pathological interpretation was made with the investigator blinded as to the identity of the infecting organism.

Examination by slit lamp biomicroscopy at 24, 48, 72, and 96 h post infection was performed as previously described (8). Clinical observations and evaluations included presence or absence of red reflex and anterior chamber reaction. The latter was graded on a scale of 0-4+ according to the severity of pathological changes (18).

Growth of *S.aureus* in vitreous: To compare the suitability of vitreous to support growth of ISP479(*agr*+) and ISP546(*agr*-), growth rates were determined *in vitro* and compared to values obtained for organisms recovered from infected eyes. Vitreous was recovered by scleral incision into uninfected enucleated eyes. Approximately 50 ISP479(*agr*+) or ISP546(*agr*-) were inoculated into 1 ml of recovered vitreous and allowed to incubate at 37°C for 24 h. 0.1ml samples were taken at timed intervals. Growth *in vivo* was analyzed by tapping the vitreous from infected eyes at 24 h post infection . To confirm that the vitreous tap was reflective of the total number of organisms present in the eye, one eye was enucleated at 24 h post infection and the entire vitreous was removed by scleral incision. The number of colony forming units (cfu) in each sample was determined by serial dilution.

RESULTS AND DISCUSSION

Two concentrations of *S. aureus* ISP479 (*agr*+) and *S. aureus* ISP546 (*agr*-) were used to establish endophthalmitis in rabbit eyes: a low level, approximately 10 organisms per 0.1 ml, and a high level, approximately 10^3 organisms per 0.1 ml. The *agr*+ strain ISP479 caused a greater and more rapid loss of neuroretinal function at 24, 48 and 72 h postinfection compared to the *agr*- strain, ISP546, at both low and high inoculum levels (Fig. 1a and 1b).

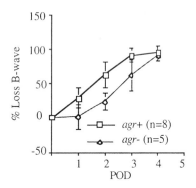 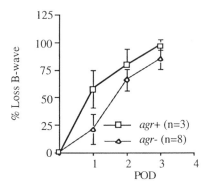

Figure 1a. Rate of loss of B-wave amplitude for eyes infected with approximately 10 cfu of *agr*- (5.6+/-3.2) and wild type *S. aureus* (12.5+/-10.9)

Figure 1b. Rate of loss of B-wave amplitude for eyes infected with approximately 1000 cfu of *agr*- (958+/-851) and wild type *S. aureus* (1080+/-452).

At the lower inoculum level, the loss of B-wave amplitude was significantly different at 24 (p<0.02) and 48 h (p<0.02), while at the higher inoculum level the difference was significant at 24 h only (p<0.02).

Similar differences were observed by slit lamp biomicroscopy. At the lower inoculum level on POD 1, ISP479 resulted in a moderate anterior chamber inflammatory reaction (mean values of 2+ cell, 2.5+ flare; n=6) whereas the *agr-* strain ISP546 elicited a mild reaction (mean values of 0+ cell, 0.4+ flare; n=5). A normal red reflex was observed in both groups. By POD 2 the inflammatory reaction had progressed to a mean of 3+ cell and flare for *agr-* and 4+ cell and flare for *agr+*. When the number of organisms was increased, both groups exhibited a more rapid onset of clinical symptoms. The *agr+* group demonstrated a greater severity of infection at the earlier time points compared to the *agr-* group (2+ cell and 3.5 + flare with diminished red reflex vs. 0.5 + cell and 2+ flare with normal red reflex respectively), but clinical symptoms equalized for both groups by 48 h (4+ cell and flare). These results show that the loss of neuroretinal function and the onset of inflammatory response is less rapid and severe in eyes infected with non-toxigenic strains and demonstrate the involvement of one or several of the toxins under the control of *agr* in the pathogenicity of *S. aureus* endophthalmitis.

Thin section histopathology demonstrated that when loss of neuroretinal response is 100%, the inflammatory response in the vitreous and anterior chamber is less severe when the infecting organism is defective in toxin production. However, there is little difference between the groups with respect to the extent of retinal damage observed. Retinal damage included infiltration of inflammatory cells into retinal layers and optic nerve head, retinal detachment, and near complete destruction of the inner limiting membrane, the nerve fiber and inner nuclear layers. Interestingly the outer nuclear layer remained largely intact. Since these eyes were examined when they no longer exhibited a B-wave response it is not surprising that the retinal damage is severe in both groups. The observed lack of red reflex in both groups at this time point supports the histopathologic results. The retinal damage observed appears to be due to the host inflammatory response to the presence of organisms in the globe. At 24 h post infection, when the greatest differences were observed by slit lamp examination and by ERG, little retinal damage is observed in either group.

The clinical differences observed between these two strains do not appear to be due to increased growth rate of ISP479 compared to ISP546, since it was found that both strains reached 2×10^8 cfu per ml *in vitro* in explanted vitreous at 24 h, with similar growth kinetics. However, vitreous recovered from enucleated eyes 24 h post infection, yielded only 10^4 cfu/ml. The low number of organisms recovered from eyes after 24 h growth *in vivo* may be due to several factors. A recent study characterized the role of complement in the host inflammatory response in *S. aureus* endophthalmitis (16). It was found that the number of organisms recovered from eyes that had been decomplemented prior to infection was significantly elevated compared to normal control eyes, indicating that complement has a role in clearance of *S. aureus* from the eye. Second, *S. aureus* may be adhering to intraocular tissues, possibly mediated by fibronectin binding protein located at the surface of *S. aureus* and are therefore not recovered in a vitreous tap. However, no increase in the number of organisms was noted in the present study when the entire vitreous body was recovered and suspended in PBS prior to serial dilution.

The results of slit lamp examination and ERG demonstrate that one or more extracellular toxins produced by *S. aureus,* and regulated by *agr,* contributes to the severity of endophthalmitis. However, the contributing toxin(s) remains to be identified. A pore forming cytolysin has been shown to contribute to the pathogenesis of *E. faecalis* endophthalmitis (8). A functionally similar pore forming toxin, α-toxin, is expressed by *S. aureus* ISP479 and has been reported to be involved in the pathogenesis of *S. aureus* keratitis (7). At sublytic levels α-toxin may stimulate the release of leukotrienes, prostaglandins and interleukin 1-β, which mediate increased vascular permeability, edema and neutrophil accumulation respectively (14). These events are consistent with the severe inflammatory response seen in *S. aureus* endophthalmitis, suggesting the possible involvement of α-toxin in the pathogenesis of *S. aureus* endophthalmitis. Gottleib *et al.* (15) assessed the role of hyaluronidase as an adjunct therapy for preretinal neovascularization in a rabbit model, and found that intravitreal injection of hyaluronidase led to extensive retinal disorganization. Therefore, hyaluronidase may also contribute to *S. aureus* virulence in the eye.

The recent emergence of multi drug resistant *S. aureus* strains has made many currently available antimicrobial agents ineffective and as a result poses a significant public health problem. The finding here and by others that inactivation of global regulatory loci leads to diminished virulence highlights the prospect that these loci, or exoproteins under their control, may be potential targets for the development of novel antimicrobial agents. Future studies in this laboratory will be directed toward identifying the toxin(s) contributing to severity in endophthalmitis.

LITERATURE CITED

1. Weber, D.J., K.L. Hoffman, R.A. Thoft, A.S. Baker. (1986) Rev. Infect. Dis. 8:12-20.
2. Kattan, H.M., H.W. Flynn, S.C. Pflugfelder, C. Robertson and R.K. Forster. (1991) Ophthal. 98:227-238.
3. Puliafito, C.A., A.S. Baker, J. Haaf, and S. Foster. (1982) Ophthal. 89:921-929.
4. Rowsey, J.J., D.L. Newsom, D.J. Sexton and W.J. Harms. (1982) Ophthal. 89:1055-1066.
5. Affeldt, J.C., H.G.W. Flynn, R.K. Forster, S. Mandelbaum, J.G. Clarkson and G.D. Jarus. (1987) Ophthal. 94:407-413
6. Phillips, W.B. and W.S. Tasman. (1994) Ophthal. 101:508-518.
7. Callegan, M.C., L.S. Engel, J.M. Hill and R.J. O Callaghan. (1994) Infect. Immun. 62:2478-2482.
8. Jett, B.D., H.G. Jensen, R.E. Nordquist and M.S. Gilmore. (1992) Infect. Immun. 60:2445-2452.
9. Smeltzer, M.S., M.E. Hart and J.J. Iandolo. (1993) Infect. Immun. 61:919-925.
10. Abdelnour, A., S. Arvidson, T. Bremell, C. Ryden, and A. Tarkowski. (1993) Infect. Immun. 61:3879-3885.
11. Cheung, A.L., M.R. Yeaman, P.M. Sullam, M. D. Witt and A.S. Bayer. (1994) Infect. Immun. 62:1719-1725.
12. Peng, H.L., R.P. Novick, B. Kreiswirth, J. Kornblum and P. Schlievert. (1988) J. Bacteriol. 170:4365-4372.
13. Sheehan, D.C. and B.B. Hrapchak. (ed.) (1980) Theory and practice of histopathology. The C.V. Mosby Co., St. Louis.
14. Bhakdi, S. and J. Tranum-Jensen. (1991) Alpha toxin of *Staphylococcus aureus*. Ann. Rev. Microbiol. 43:375-402.
15. Gottlieb, J.L., A.N. Antoszyk, D.L. Hatchell and P. Saloupis. (1990) Invest. Ophthal. Vis. Sci. 31:2345-2352.
16. Giese, M.J., B.J. Mondino, H.L. Sumner, S.A. Adamu, H.P. Halabi and H.J. Chou. (1994) Invest. Ophthal. Vis. Sci. 35:1026-1032.
17. Novick, R. (1967) Virology.33:155-166.
18. Stevens, S.X., H.G. Jensen, B.D. Jett and M.S. Gilmore. (1992) Invest. Ophthal. Vis. Sci. 33:1650-1656.

Advances in Ocular Immunology
R.B. Nussenblatt, S.M. Whitcup, R.R. Caspi and I. Gery, eds.

273

Molecular and Immunologic Mechanisms Involved in Coronavirus Induced Retinopathy

J.J. Hooks[1], Y. Wang[1], Y. Komurasaki[1], C. Percopo[1], C. N. Nagineni[1] and B. Detrick[2]

[1] Immunology & Virology Section, Laboratory of Immunology, National Eye Institute, NIH, Bethesda, MD

[2] Dept of Pathology, The George Washington University Medical Center, Washington, D.C.

INTRODUCTION

When exposed to an intravitreal inoculation of the murine coronavirus, mouse hepatitis virus (MHV), BALB/c mice develop an infection which culminates in a retinal degeneration (1-3). The disease is biphasic, consisting of an early phase and a late phase. In the early phase, 1 to 7 days post inoculation, a retinal vasculitis is observed. The late phase, day 10 to several months, is characterized by a retinal degeneration in the absence of vasculitis or inflammatory processes (4, 5). This degenerative process is associated with a reduction of the photoreceptor layer, loss of interphotoreceptor retinoid-binding protein, abnormality in the retinal pigment epithelium and retinal detachments.

There are numerous ways by which viruses trigger pathologic changes within the eye. The coronavirus - induced retinopathy model allows us to explore some of the cellular and molecular mechanisms involved in the pathogenesis of retinal tissue damage.

MATERIALS & METHODS

Animals: BALB/c mice were obtained from Harlan Sprague Dawley, Indianapolis, IN. CD-1 mice were obtained from Charles River, Raleigh, NC.

Virus: Mouse Hepatitis Virus (MHV), JHM strain, was obtained from American Type Culture Collection (ATCC) Rockville, MD and passaged 5 to 7 times in L2 cells. Stock virus was propagated in L2 cells, centrifuged at 100,000 xg for two hours and the pellet was resuspended in Delbecco Minimal Essential Medium (DMEM) with 2% fetal bovine serum (FBS). Viral infectivity titrations were performed on L2 cells propagated in 96 well microtiter plates. Infectivity was recorded as the induction of cytopathic effect (cpe) by serial 10 fold dilutions of the sample. Stock virus infectivity was $10^{5.7}$ $TCID_{50}$ / 0.1 ml.

Antibodies: Rabbit antiserum prepared against gradient-purified, NP40 disrupted MHV (strain A59) was kindly provided by Dr. Kathryn V. Holmes (Uniformed Services University of the Health Sciences, Bethesda, MD). Monoclonal antibody specific for the MHV-JHM nucleocapsid protein N was generously donated by Dr. Julian Leibowitz (Univ of Texas, Houston, TX).

Mouse Inoculations: Adult (12 week old) male BALB/c mice were injected intravitreally with $10^{4.3}$ $TCID_{50}$ / 5ul of JHM virus or with DMEM with 2% FBS. As previously described, the eyes were processed on days 1, 3, 6, 10, 20, 30-40 and 70 days after inoculation. The mice were anesthetized as described and killed by decapitation (1). They were handled according to the ARVO Resolution on the Use of Animals in Research. Eyes were fixed in 10% formalin for H&E staining, in 2.5% glutaraldehyde for electron microscopic evaluation or in OCT for frozen sections and immunocytochemical staining.

Immunoperoxidase Staining: Frozen sections were fixed in acetone for 5 min, transferred to Tris-buffered saline (pH 7.6) and then immersed in 5% normal goat serum or horse serum in buffer for 10 min. Primary antibodies were applied. After incubation in a moist chamber at room temperature for 1 hour, the slides were washed in Tris-buffered saline, then the secondary antibody, biotin-conjugated goat anti-rabbit IgG (Organon Teknica Corp., West Chester, PA) or horse anti-mouse IgG (Vector Laboratories) was layered onto the slides. After 1 hr incubation in a moist chamber, the slides were washed in Tris-buffered saline, then overlaid for 45 min with avidin-biotin-peroxidase complexes. The slides were washed again in Tris-buffered saline and developed in 0.05% 3, 3' diamino benzidine tetrahydrochloride - 0.1% nickel sulfate - 0.01% hydrogen peroxide solution. They were counterstained with methyl green (1% in methanol), dehydrated, cleared and mounted as in routine processing.

In Situ Hybridization: Clone 2-2, which contained cDNA representing MHV-A59 genes 4-6 cloned into Pst I site of pGEM-1 (Promega, Madison, WI), was provided by Dr. Susan R. Weiss (University of Pennsylvania, Philadelphia, PA) (6). The insert was excised from the vector and purified by gel electrophoresis. Then cDNA labeling with digoxigenin-11-dUTP was carried out by the random primed method using a commercially available kit (Boehringer Mannheim, Indianapolis, IN).

Mouse eyes were fixed in 10% buffered formalin and embedded in paraffin wax. All procedures were performed under RNase-free conditions. Before hybridization, the slides were dewaxed and air-dried completely. Prehybridization mixture in a volume of 25 µl that consisted of 50% deionized formamide, 1XDenhardt's solution, 4XSSC, 10% dextran sulfate and 100 µg/ml denatured salmon sperm DNA was placed on each section, and the slides were incubated for one hour at room temperature. Five µl of the labeled probe was added onto the slides (final concentration of labeled cDNA was 100ng/ml). The probe DNA was denatured at 90°C for 10 minutes. The slides were immediately cooled on ice, and hybridization was carried out for 16 hours at 37°C in a humidified box. The resultant hybridized probe was identified with anti-digoxigenin antibody conjugated to alkaline phosphatase.

RESULTS:

In order to evaluate virus expression in JHM virus infected BALB/c mice, four parameters were evaluated: infectious virus, viral protein expression, viral mRNA and anti-virus neutralizing antibodies. Infectious virus was detected by inoculating 10% suspensions of normal and infected retinas onto L-2 cells. Development of a cpe consisting of the typical JHM virus induced syncytial formation was considered a positive isolate. Each isolate was identified by neutralization of the virus with specific anti-JHM virus neutralizing antibody. As is seen in Table 1, infectious virus could be identified in the retina tissue from day 1 to day 5. Infectious virus could not be detected after this time.

The presence of viral proteins was evaluated by immunocytochemical staining. Frozen eye sections from normal and JHM virus infected BALB/c mice were tested with anti-virus antibodies. Positive reactivity was observed only in the JHM virus infected mice and not in the control, uninfected mice. Staining was observed throughout the retina and the RPE for the first 6 days post inoculation. After day 8, virus proteins could not be detected by immunocytochemical staining.

Table 1
Virus Expression in Coronavirus Induced Retinopathy in BALB/c Mice

Detection	Method	Results	
		Day 1 - 7	Day 8 - 70
Infectious Virus	Isolation & Passage	Positive	Negative
Virus Proteins	Immunocytochemistry	Positive	Negative
Virus mRNA	in situ Hybridization	Positive	Positive
Anti-Virus Antibody	Neutralization	Negative	Positive

The presence of virus mRNA was evaluated by in situ hybridization.To verify the specificity of the probe for hybridization, the labeled probe was first hybridized to MHV-JHM infected and uninfected L2 cells. The virus cDNA probe hybridized to virus RNA in the infected cultures. In contrast, no reactivity was noted in the untreated L2 cells. Moreover, plasmid cDNA probe did not hybridize to either infected or untreated L2 cells. Using this method, we found that virus mRNA was present within the retina of virus infected mice and not within the retina of normal, uninfected animals. Although infectious virus and virus proteins could not be detected beyond day 6 after infection, virus mRNA could be detected within the retina from day 1 to day 60 post inoculation.

The presence of anti-virus antibody was evaluated by neutralization assays. Neutralizing antibody to JHM virus was first detected at day 7 post inoculation and was continuously present through day 160 post inoculation.

The development of autoantibodies during murine coronavirus induced retinopathy was studied by immunocytochemical staining of mouse sera on frozen normal rat eye sections. As is seen in Table 2, sera from normal, uninfected BALB/c mice did not react with rat eye, liver, kidney or brain. In contrast, sera collected from JHM virus infected BALB/c mice did react with the rat retina and brain. This sera from virus infected animals did not react with rat liver or kidney.

DISCUSSION

These studies demonstrate that murine coronavirus can induce a biphasic disease. During the early phase, infectious virus and virus proteins are readily identified in conjunction with retinal vasculitis and perivasculitis. The development of anti-virus antibodies occurs at approximately the same time that infectious virus and virus proteins are no longer detected (day 6). During the later phase of the disease, retinal degenerative changes occur in the presence of anti-retinal autoantibodies. Interestingly, virus mRNA is detected throughout both phases of the disease induced by this positive sense RNA virus.

Table 2
Development of Autoantibodies during Murine Coronavirus Retinopathy in BALB/c Mice

BALB/c Mouse Sera	Autoantibody Staining on Normal Rat Tissue				
	EYE		Liver	Kidney	Brain
	Anterior Pole	Posterior Pole			
Normal	0 / 15	0 / 15	0 / 5	0 / 5	0 / 3
JHM virus infected	0 / 22	22 / 22	0 / 5	0 / 5	2 / 3

In conclusion, these studies on an animal model of postvirus retinopathy indicate that the virus establishes a persistent infection within the retina which is associated with the production of anti-retinal autoantibodies. It is tempting to speculate that the activation of the immune system, antibodies and cytotoxic T cells, limit the spread of the virus within the retina. Nevertheless, the persistent infection and the consequential immune and autoimmune reactivity together play a role in the degenerative process. These studies provide insight into approaches to evaluate human retinal diseases.

REFERENCES

1. Robbins S G, Hamel CH, Detrick B, and Hooks JJ. Lab. Invest. 1990; 62: 417-426.

2. Hooks JJ, Robbins SG, Wiggert B, Chader GJ, and Detrick B. In Anderson RE, Hollyfield JG and LaVail MM, eds. In "Retinal Degenerations" Boca Raton, FL: CRC Press, 1991; 529-534.

3. Robbins S G, Wiggert B, Kutty G, Chader GJ, Detrick B, and Hooks JJ. Invest. Ophthalmol. Vis. Sci. 1992; 33: 60-67

4. Hooks JJ, Percopo C, Wang Y and Detrick B. J. Immunol. 1993; 151: 3381-3389.

5. Wang Y, Detrick B, and Hooks JJ. Virology 1993; 193: 124-137.

6. Gombold J L and Weiss SR. Microbiol Pathogenesis 1992; 13: 493-502.

Advances in Ocular Immunology
R.B. Nussenblatt, S.M. Whitcup, R.R. Caspi and I. Gery, eds.

Immunization or Adoptive Transfer of Immune Cells Protects Against Retinitis following Supraciliary Inoculation of Murine Cytomegalovirus (MCMV)

Y. Lu and S.S. Atherton

Department of Cellular and Structural Biology, University of Texas Health Science Center at San Antonio, San Antonio, Texas 78284

INTRODUCTION

Cytomegalovirus retinitis is the most common infectious ocular complication observed in patients with AIDS.[1] Cytomegalovirus retinitis has been described in euthymic BALB/c mice following supraciliary inoculation of 5 x 10[4] PFU of MCMV.[2] After supraciliary inoculation, 60 to 80% of the mice develop necrotizing retinitis characterized by virus-infected cytomegalic cells in the retina and retinal pigment epithelium, zones of transition between involved and uninvolved retina, and optic neuritis. Following supraciliary inoculation of virus, virus appears to spread along the retinal pigment epithelium and replication of virus and virus-infected cytomegalic cells in the posterior segment correlate with development of retinitis. The role of virus-specific immune cells in MCMV infection has been examined using nude mice, and adoptive transfer of MCMV-specific immune CD4[+] T cells reduced the titer of virus in the adrenal glands but did not affect the titer of MCMV in either the salivary glands or the lungs.[3] In general, cell transfer studies have been done in immunodeficient mice, irradiated, or specifically immunodepleted mice[4-6] and have not looked at the effect of virus-specific cells in virus-infected, but otherwise immunologically normal, animals. In AIDS patients, strategies to augment the anti-CMV response such as in vitro amplification of virus-specific T cells which could then be reinfused into the patient might efficacious either in controlling systemic virus spread or in preventing further ocular damage in an eye with CMV retinitis. In these studies, we used immunization before ocular inoculation of virus and adoptive transfer of virus immune cells to determine if either approach conferred protection against MCMV retinitis in the euthymic BALB/c mouse.

METHODS

Animals: Adult female euthymic BALB/c mice between 7 and 11 weeks of age were obtained from Taconic, Inc. (Germantown, NY) and were housed in accordance with National Institutes of Health Guidelines. All animal treatments in this study conformed to the ARVO Resolution of the Use of Animals in Research.

Virus: The Smith Strain of MCMV was used for all experiments. Virus stocks were prepared from the salivary glands of MCMV-infected BALB/c mice as described previously.[2] Virus stocks and experimental samples were titered in duplicate by plaque assay on monolayers of mouse embryo fibroblast (MEF) cells grown in tissue culture medium containing 10% fetal calf serum; the minimum level of virus detection in all plaque assays was $0.7 \log_{10}$ PFU/ml. The titer of virus stocks was between 10^6 and 10^7 PFU/ml; a new aliquot of stock virus was thawed and diluted (if necessary) to the appropriate concentration for ocular and intraperitoneal injections.

Ocular Inoculation: Mice were anesthetized with pentobarbital (0.65 mg/10 g body weight) and inoculated with 5 x 10⁴ PFU of MCMV in a volume of 2 µl via the supraciliary route as previously described.[2]

Experimental Plan: This study consisted of two experiments. Experiment One - to determine if prior intraperitoneal immunization with MCMV confers protection against MCMV retinitis, BALB/c mice were injected with 5 x 10⁴ PFU of MCMV intraperitoneally. Two weeks after intraperitoneal inoculation, one half of the mice were injected with 5 x 10⁴ PFU of MCMV via the supraciliary route. The eyes of the remaining mice were not injected. Ten animals were sacrificed from each group on day 5, 9 and 14 PI. The eyes of 5 mice of both groups were fixed, sectioned, stained with hematoxylin and eosin and examined microscopically for retinitis. The eyes of the remaining 5 mice in each group were homogenized and plated on MEF cells for infectious virus. Experiment Two - to determine whether adoptive transfer of MCMV-immune cells (MICs) protects against retinitis, donor mice were injected intraperitoneally with 5 x 10⁴ PFU of MCMV. Two weeks later, the donor mice were sacrificed, the spleens were removed, and a single cell suspension was prepared. Five million freshly-isolated MICs were injected intravenously into naive BALB/c mice; control mice received an equal volume of PBS (0.1 ml) intravenously. Mice in both the adoptive transfer group and the control group were then injected with 5 x 10⁴ PFU of MCMV via the supraciliary route. Ten mice from each group were sacrificed on day 5, 9, 14, and 21 PI, and the eyes, salivary glands, and lungs were removed. Five eyes of each group at each time were homogenized and titered for infectious virus by plaque assay on MEF cells, and five eyes were examined microscopically for retinitis. The salivary gland and lungs of all animals in both groups were homogenized and assayed by plaque assay. The significance of plaque assay results between the control group and the experimental group was determined by Mann-Whitney U test.

RESULTS

Experiment One: None of the eyes of mice immunized with MCMV and injected two weeks later with MCMV via the supraciliary route had microscopic evidence of retinitis in the injected eye. No mouse in the control group (intraperitoneal injection of MCMV only) developed retinitis. No virus was recovered by plaque assay from virus-injected eyes collected at days 5, 9 and 14 PI (data not shown). Taken together with the histopathologic results, the results of the virus titrations demonstrate that intraperitoneal injection of MCMV two weeks prior to supraciliary inoculation of 5 x 10⁴ PFU of MCMV prevents retinitis in the injected eye.

Experiment Two: The results of virus recovery plaque assays from the injected eye, salivary glands, and lungs of control mice and of mice treated with freshly-isolated MICs immediately prior to injection of MCMV via the supraciliary route are shown in Figures 1, 2 and 3. There was significantly less virus (p<0.05

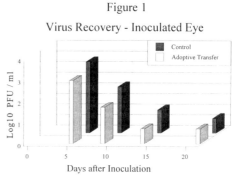

Figure 1

Virus Recovery - Inoculated Eye

or better, Mann-Whitney) recovered from the eyes of the mice in the adoptive transfer group than from the control group before day 21 PI (Figure 1 - preceding page).

In the salivary gland, there was significantly less virus in MIC-treated mice than control mice at day 14 and day 21 PI (Figure 2). In the lungs, significantly less virus was recovered from the mice in the adoptive transfer group at day 5, 9 and 14 PI (Figure 3).

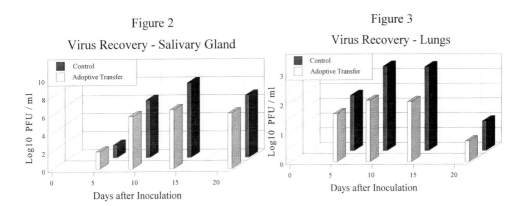

Figure 2

Virus Recovery - Salivary Gland

Figure 3

Virus Recovery - Lungs

A summary of the results of the microscopic examination of the eyes from MIC-treated mice and from control mice is presented in Table 1. At all time points, the percentage of eyes with retinitis in the MIC-treated group was significantly lower than the percentage of eyes with retinitis in the control group inoculated with virus but not given MICs.

Table 1

Mice with Retinitis

	Day 5 PI	Day 9 PI	Day 14 PI
Adoptive Transfer	1/5*	0/5*	0/5*
Control	4/5	3/5	3/5

*significantly different than control group, p<0.05, Student's t test

DISCUSSION

The results of this study demonstrate that immunization by intraperitoneal injection of live MCMV two weeks prior to injection of virus via the supraciliary route prevents retinitis. The results that there was no histopathologic evidence of retinitis and that no virus could be recovered from the inoculated eyes at any time after infection suggests that prior immunization with MCMV confers protection by preventing virus replication in the eye. Since other studies have demonstrated roles for both CD4[+] and CD8[+] T cells[3-9] as well as NK cells[10] in preventing systemic MCMV infection or preventing virus replication and disease at selected sites, it is likely that protection afforded by intraperitoneal inoculation is also mediated by T cells. Confirmation of this idea will depend on the results of future studies to look at virus replication in the eye after transfer of MCMV-immune CD4[+] and CD8[+] T cells separately.

The results of the adoptive transfer studies suggest that transfer of MCMV immune cells reduces but does not prevent virus replication in the eye, salivary gland and lungs. Since only 1 of a total of 15 mice in the adoptive transfer groups and 10 of a total of 15 mice in the control groups developed retinitis, these results suggest that virus recovery from the eye of the MIC-treated mice represents only virus from the anterior segment. Furthermore, the results of virus recovery assays from the salivary gland and lungs in experiment two suggest that transfer of immune cells may accelerate clearance of virus from these sites.

Alternatively, transfer of immune cells may prevent virus replication and in turn reduce the virus titer in the eye, salivary glands and lungs. The findings in this study seem to support the latter explanation since the salivary glands and lungs of MIC-treated mice generally contained less virus and for example, the titer of MCMV in the salivary glands at day 14 PI was approximately 50-fold lower in MIC-treated mice. The role, if any, of MICs in accelerating clearance of virus will need to be examined in studies lasting longer than 21 days in order to allow for clearance of virus from all sites. In our studies, in vitro restimulation of the adoptively-transferred cells with viral antigen prior to transfer was not required for protection; protection with freshly-isolated cells has also been observed in irradiated mice with MCMV pneumonia.[4] Although preliminary, the results of studies in this communication demonstrate that both prior immunization with virus and adoptive transfer of MCMV immune cells prevent retinitis in euthymic BALB/c mice after supraciliary inoculation of 5 x 10[4] PFU of MCMV.

Supported by NIH grant EY09169

REFERENCES

1. Jabs DA, Enger C, Bartlett JG. Arch Ophthalmol 1989;107:75-80.
2. Atherton SS, Newell CK, Kanter M, Cousins SW. Curr Eye Res 1991;10:667-677.
3. Shanley JD. J Virol 1987;61:23-28.
4. Reddehase MJ, Weiland F, Münch K, Jonjić S, Lüske A, Koszinowski UH. J Virol 1985;55:264-273.
5. Reddehase MJ, Mutter W, Münch K, Bühring H-J, Koszinowski UH. J Virol 1987; 61:3102-3108.
6. Reddehase MJ, Jonjić S, Weiland F, Mutter W, Koszinowski UH. J Virol 1988;62:1061-1065.
7. Ho M. Infect Immun 1980;27:767-776.
8. Erlich KS, Mills J, Shanley JD. J Gen Virol 1989;70:1765-1771.
9. Atherton SS, Newell CK, Kanter MY, Cousins SW. Invest Ophthalmol Vis Sci 1992;33:3353-3360.
10. Welsh RM, Brubaker JO, Vega-Cortes M, O'Donnell CL. J Exp Med 1991;173:1053-1063.

Advances in Ocular Immunology
R.B. Nussenblatt, S.M. Whitcup, R.R. Caspi and I. Gery, eds.

ORAL IMMUNIZATION INDUCES PROTECTIVE IMMUNITY AGAINST ACANTHAMOEBA KERATITIS

J.Y. Niederkorn[a], H. Alizadeh[a], W. Taylor[a], Y-G. He[a], J.P. McCulley[a], G.L. Stewart[b], E. Haehling[b], Marc Via[a], and F. van Klink[c]

[a]U.T. Southwestern Medical Center, Dallas, Texas, U.S.A.

[b]University of Texas at Arlington, Arlington, Texas, U.S.A.

[c]Leiden University Hospital, Leiden, The Netherlands

INTRODUCTION

Acanthamoeba keratitis is a progressive and potentially blinding infection of the cornea produced by pathogenic/free-living amoebae of the genus *Acanthamoeba* which are widely distributed in the environment[1]. It is generally accepted that contact lens wear is the leading risk factor in *Acanthamoeba* keratitis. However, in spite of the ubiquitous distribution of *Acanthamoeba* in the environment and the more than 24,000,000 contact lens wearers in the United States, the incidence of *Acanthamoeba* keratitis is rare. Subclinical exposure to pathogenic/free-living amoebae is probably a common occurrence because *Acanthamoeba spp.* have been isolated from nasopharyngeal cultures of healthy, asymptomatic individuals.[2] Serological surveys of normal subjects have shown that antibodies against *Acanthamoeba* were found in 52-100% of those tested[3]. Thus, the low incidence of *Acanthamoeba* keratitis might be the result of immunity acquired by environmental exposure.

We have recently established a pig model of *Acanthamoeba* keratitis that satisfies Koch's postulates and which utilizes parasite-laden contact lenses as the vector for transmitting the infectious amoebae, thereby mimicking the human disease. Using this model, we determined the efficacy of systemic and local immunization with *Acanthamoeba* antigens in preventing *Acanthamoeba* keratitis.

MATERIALS AND METHODS

Corneas of domestic pigs were infected with trophozoites of *Acanthamoeba* transmitted via contact lenses and clinical observations performed as described previously[4].

Crude aqueous extracts of trophozoites were prepared as described earlier and conjugated to cholera toxin[5]. Immunization was performed by administering 0.3 mg of protein antigen, either conjugated with cholera toxin or not conjugated, via the subconjunctival (SC), intramuscular (IM), or by combined topical and oral routes. Animals were immunized a total of four times at seven-day intervals.

Serum IgG antibody titers were measured by conventional enzyme-linked immunosorbent assay (ELISA). Peripheral blood lymphocyte blastogenic responses to trophozoite antigens were measured after in vitro incubation of lymphocytes with 100

μg/ml of *Acanthamoeba* antigen for 72 hr. Results were recorded as "blastogenic index"[6].

RESULTS

Initial experiments examined the efficacy of a commonly utilized route of antigen administration (i.e., intramuscularly) for inducing immunity to ocular challenge with *Acanthamoeba* trophozoites. Seven days after the fourth IM injection, pigs were challenged with parasite-laden contact lenses. Slit lamp examination revealed that IM immunized and control pigs developed severe keratitis which followed the same time course and which was of the same intensity (Table 1). Control animals challenged with sterile contact lenses did not develop keratitis (data not shown).

Since nonocular immunization failed to protect against corneal challenge, we considered the possibility that local immunization via the conjunctival route might be effective. Accordingly, pigs were immunized subconjunctivally with the same dose of antigen given on the same time course as the previous experiment. Unlike the previous groups, subconjunctival immunization resulted in total protection of three of the six pigs.

The association between the subconjunctival route of immunization and protective immunity suggested that local immunity (e.g., mucosal immune system) was involved. To test this, pigs were immunized orally and topically with *Acanthamoeba* antigen conjugated to cholera toxin, a strategy which is known to stimulate mucosal immune responses to various antigens. The results summarized in Table 1 show that none of the animals immunized by the oral/topical protocol developed signs of keratitis during the entire observation period. Moreover, all five animals were culture negative for *Acanthamoeba*.

Table 1
Immunization against *Acanthamoeba* keratitis

	Incidence of keratitis	
Experimental group	Primary infection	Secondary infection
Non-immunized	5/5	5/5
Immunized IM	4/4	4/4
Immunized SC	3/6	3/6
Immunized Orally/topically	0/5	0/5

The frequent recrudescence of *Acanthamoeba* keratitis in patients suggests that ocular infection does not induce long-lived immunity. Resistance to second challenge infections was examined next. Pigs were challenged with parasite-laden contact lenses seven days after the primary corneal infections cleared (usually 30-35 days post infection). In all cases, pigs that developed primary ocular infections were susceptible to re-infection. By contrast, animals immunized via the SC route or by oral/topical route resisted second challenge infections (Table 1). Thus, ocular infection fails to elicit protective immunity.

Since serum antibody titers often correlate with protective immunity to many infectious agents, IgG antibody titers were determined by conventional ELISA using serum collected at the time of each immunization and at weekly intervals after ocular challenge on day 28. Surprisingly, the most impressive antibody response was found in pigs immunized IM (Figure 1). Only feeble antibody responses were found in the other groups, including pigs that were protected against corneal infection (i.e., oral/topical immunization group).

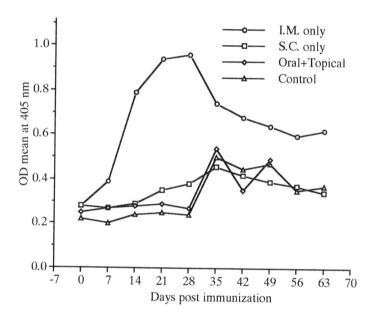

Figure 1. Serum IgG antibody responses determined by ELISA. Pigs were immunized on days 0,7,14, and 21. Corneas were infected on day 28.

Additional experiments examined cellular immune responses to parasite antigens. Peripheral blood lymphocytes were evaluated for in vitro blastogenic responses to *Acanthamoeba antigens*. Antigen-specific responses were clearly demonstrable in all four categories of immunized animals, including groups that were not protected against ocular challenge (blastogenic indices = 30 to 42). However, ocular infection alone did not induce cellular immune responses since significant blastogenic responses to *Acanthamoeba* antigens were not found at any time points after infection (data not shown). Thus, systemic immunization, but not ocular infection, elicits cellular immunity to *Acanthamoeba* antigens.

DISCUSSION

The results indicate that it is possible to confer solid protection against *Acanthamoeba* keratitis by immunizing the host with *Acanthamoeba* antigens. However, the route of antigen administration has a profound effect on the nature of the immunity. Although immunization via the IM route stimulates both humoral and cell-mediated immune responses, the hosts are not protected against corneal infection. By contrast, subconjunctival immunization totally protected 50% of the hosts. The efficacy of SC immunization suggested that a local immune mechanism, perhaps via the common mucosal immune system, was activated. The thorough immunity produced by oral immunization suggests that the mucosal immune system, namely IgA antibody in the tears, provided immunity to *Acanthamoeba* keratitis. This conclusion is based on the observation that oral administration of antigens conjugated to cholera toxin preferentially activates the mucosal immune system and stimulates the synthesis of IgA antibodies[5]. Likewise, topical application of antigen onto the corneal surface is an effective method for stimulating the mucosal immune system[7]. Thus, combined oral and topical administration of antigen should activate the common mucosal immune system in which mucosal-associated lymphocytes sensitized via the gastrointestinal tract, migrate to distant mucosal tissues, including the lacrimal gland, and elaborate secretory IgA antibodies, which appear within the tears. We propose that parasite-specific antibodies present in the tears would inhibit binding of the parasites to the corneal surface. This is plausible since IgA antibodies effectively inhibit binding of other infectious agents to epithelial surfaces. Moreover, previous studies have shown that the susceptibility of various experimental animals to *Acanthamoeba* keratitis is intimately associated with the capacity of the parasites to bind to corneal epithelium. However, the role of tear IgA in protection against *Acanthamoeba* keratitis awaits confirmation.

The inability of a primary ocular infection to elicit effective immunity to re-infection is consistent with clinical observations in which patients fail to develop long-lasting immunity and frequently suffer recrudescence. This is supported by the results in which ocular infections elicited only feeble serum antibody responses and no detectable cellular immune responses to *Acanthamoeba* antigens.

The absence of a positive correlation between parasite-specific serum IgG antibodies and immunity suggests that examining patient serum is of limited usefulness for either diagnosing or predicting risk of *Acanthamoeba* keratitis.

REFERENCES

1. Auran JD, Starr MB, Jakobiec FA. Cornea. 1987;6:2-26.
2. Wang SS, Feldman HA. N Engl J Med 1967;277:1174-1179.
3. Cursons RT, Brown TJ, Keys EA, Moriarty KM, Till D. Infect Immun 1980;29:401-407.
4. He YG, McCulley JP, Alizadeh H, et al. Invest Ophthalmol Vis Sci 1992;33:126-133.
5. Liang X, Lamm ME, Nedrud JG. J Immunol 1988;141:1495-1501.
6. Urban JF, Alizadeh H, Romanowski RD. Exp Parasitol 1988;66:66-77.
7. Murray ES, Charbonnet LT, MacDonald BA. J Immunol 1973;110:1518-1525.

Advances in Ocular Immunology
R.B. Nussenblatt, S.M. Whitcup, R.R. Caspi and I. Gery, eds.

285

Effect of genetically engineered vaccine on *Pseudomonas aeruginosa* infection in mice

M. Nishio[1], S. Nakamura[1], N. Ishii[2], S. Tanaka[3], K. Okuda[4] and S. Ohno[1]

Departments of [1]Ophthalmology, [2]Dermatology, [3]Internal Medicine and [4]Bacteriology, Yokohama City University School of Medicine, 3-9 Fukuura, Kanazawa-ku, Yokohama 236, Japan

INTRODUCTION

Infection caused by *Pseudomonas aeruginosa* (*P. aeruginosa*) is genetically restricted to compromised hosts and a common cause of bacterial keratitis, characterized by severe corneal ulceration and extensive dissolution of the stroma. One of the most virulent components of *P. aeruginosa* is elastase [1]. The present study investigates the genetic influence on the fatal effects of *P. aeruginosa* in several inbred mouse strains, as well as the sensitivity to intracorneal challenge with *P. aeruginosa* with or without vaccination. A vaccine was successfully developed against elastase by a bioenginnered technique using site-directed mutagenesis method described elsewhere [2].

MATERIALS AND METHODS

Mice: We used the congenic mice, 8-15 weeks old. These strains and their H-2 haplotypes are given in Table1.

Bacterial strains: We used *P. aeruginosa* IFO3455 which is a strain that produces elastase and alkaline protease.

Vaccine: Two amino acids (Glu-141, His-223) are the key residures for catalytic activity of the Pseudomonas elastase. The vaccine used in this study was developed by the site-directed mutagenesis (His-223→Gly-223).

Method-1: The mice were given a single intraperitoneal injection of $83\mu g/0.2$ ml vaccine on day 0. Seven days later, they were anesthetized and the corneal surface was incised with a sterile 30-gauge needle. One drop of the *P. aeruginosa* cell suspension (10^8/ml, 10^7/ml) was placed and the eyes were massaged for 15 s after injection. Seven days later, we observed the corneal response (grade0: no damage, 1: corneal opacity in the wound or corneal area only, 2: opacity over the entire cornea (possible to observe anterior chamber), 3: opacity over the entire cornea(impossible to observe anterior chamber in the central area), 4: opacity over the entire cornea (impossible to observe anterior chamber), 5, ring abscess or perforation in the cornea.))

Method-2: The mice were given a single intraperitoneal injection of 83 $\mu g/0.2$ml vaccine on day 0. Seven days later, they were anesthetized and 30% of the total body surface was burned. Immediately afterwards they were injected subcutaneously with *P.aeruginosa* (10^7/0.1 ml, 10^6/0.1 ml). Seven days later the survival rate was recorded.

Method-3: The mice were given a single intraperitoneal injection of $83\mu g/0.2$ml vaccine on day 0. Seven days later paraaortic lymph node and spleen were extracted and the lymph node cells and spleen cells were separated. By the methods of flowcytometry (EPICS Profile Analizer, Argon laser: 488nm, monoclonal antibodies: Thy1.2(FITC), Ly-5(PE), L3T4(FITC), Lyt-2(PE)), CD4/CD8 ratio was examined.

RESULTS

1. Intracorneal challenge model :
   The corneas of vaccinated mice of strains B10.MBR, B10.D2, B10.M, B10.GD, B10.A(2R), B10.A(4R), B10.BR, BALB.K, C3H/He, and A.TL were virtually all protected against the Pseudomonas infection at concentration of 10^8/ml at 7 days. However, the corneas of C57BL/10, B10.A(5R), A.SW, and B10.HTT showed little difference between vaccinated and control mice. B.10.G showed a moderate protective effect of the vaccine. The same data were observed at a concentration of 10^7/ml (Table 1).

Table 1
Genetic control of effectiveness of vaccination against 10^8/ml P. aeruginosa

Strain	H-2 region KAESD	Number of mice	Mean of corneal responce vaccinated	non-vaccinated
C57BL/10	bb0bb	31	4.6±0.3	4.2±0.3
B10.MBR	bkkkq	12	1.4±0.3	3.8±0.2
B10.D2	ddddd	22	2.3±0.2	4.6±0.2
B10.M	ff0ff	6	0.3±0.2	1.9±0.5
B10.GD	dd0bb	12	3.6±0.4	5.0±0.0
B10.A(2R)	kkkdb	7	0.4±0.2	2.8±0.2
B10.A(4R)	kk0bb	24	4.0±0.0	5.5±0.0
B10.A(5R)	bbbdd	24	4.0±0.2	4.0±0.0
B10.BR	kkkkk	26	2.2±0.4	4.3±0.3
BALB.K	kkkkk	9	1.0±0.3	2.2±0.4
C3H/He	kkkkk	10	1.1±0.3	2.3±0.3
B10.G	qq0qq	7	2.5±0.3	3.9±0.7
A.SW	ss0ss	11	3.4±0.4	2.5±0.6
A.TL	skkkd	10	1.6±0.2	4.0±0.6
B10.HTT	ssskd	8	2.5±0.3	3.1±0.3

The results obtained in strains C57BL/10, B10.MBR, and B10.BR indicate that an Ir control gene maps to the right side of the I-A region (Table 2). The results obtained in strains B10.A(2R), B10.A(4R), and B10.BR suggest that an Ir control gene maps to the left side of the A region. The E region did not regulate the effect of vaccination because mice of strains B10.A(2R) and B10.A(4R) were protected by the vaccine.

These results show that the effects of the *P. aeruginosa* vaccine were controlled by the genes within the A region of H-2, and that A^d, A^f, and A^k are protected by vaccination against *P. aeruginosa*, but A^b and A^s are not.

2. Thermal burn model :
   Vaccinated mice of strains B10.MBR, BALB/c, B10.D2, B10.A(2R), B10.A(4R), B10.BR, C3H/He, BALB.K, B10.DA(80NS), B10.R III, A.TL, and B10.AQR survived following administration of concentrations of 10^6 and 10^7 *P. aeruginosa* at 7 days. However, strains A.BY, C57BL/10, B10.A(5R), A.SW, and B10.HTT showed no beneficial effect of vaccination.

These results show that the effects of the *P. aeruginosa* vaccine were controlled by the genes within the A region of H-2, and that A^d, A^k, A^q, and A^r are protected by vaccination against *P. aeruginosa*, but A^b, and A^s are not.

Table 2
Genetic mapping

Strain	H-2 haplotype	Effect of vaccination	H-2 region KAESD
C57BL/10	b	-	bb0bb
B10.MBR	bq1	+	bkkkq
B10.(2R)	h2	+	kkkdb
B10.(4R)	h4	+	kk0bb
B10.BR	k	+	kkkkk

3. Flowcytometory :
Flowcytometorical analysis showed that CD4/CD8 ratio was increased in the paraaortic lymph node cells and spleen cells of vaccine-effected B10.BR mice after vaccination, compared with vaccine-noneffected C57BL/10 mice (Fig.1).

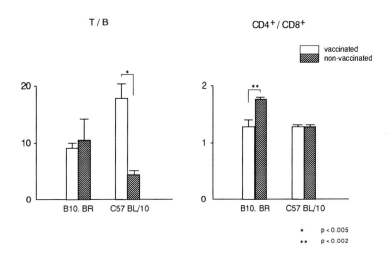

Figure 1 Flowcytometory (T / B: T cell / B cell ratio, CD4 / CD8: helper T cell / supressor T cell ratio).

DISCUSSION

The intracorneal challenge of mice with *P. aeruginosa* is used in ophthalmological research [3], and is suitable for the observation of toxigenicity. Elastase is able to inactivate a variety of biologically important proteins or phenomena[4], and plays a role in the pathogenesis of *P. aeruginosa* infections.

In this study, we used the engineered vaccine. The advantage of this vaccine is its safety,

288

as well as its feasibility for mass production.

A genetic influence in the response to the vaccine was observed in mice subjected to intracorneal challenge with *P. aeruginosa*, or in mice subjected to thermal burn and *P. aeruginosa* exposure. Mice with A^d, A^f, A^k, A^r injected with the vaccine resisted infection by *P. aeruginosa*, whereas mice with A^b, A^s remained susceptible to the infection. These results indicate that the effectiveness of the engineered vaccine against *P. aeruginosa* is associated with the A region of H-2. Moreover, flow cytometorical analysis showed that CD4/CD8 ratio was incresed in the paraaortic lymph node cells and spleen cells of vaccine-effected B10.BR mice after vaccination,compared with vaccine-noneffected C57BL/10 mice. These results indicate that $CD4^+$ helper T cells are increased in the vaccine-effected mice, and immunological responsiveness against *P. aeruginosa* may have been strengthened.

REFERENCES

1 Morihara K, Tsuzuki H, Oka T, Inoue H, Ebata M. J Biol Chem 1965; 240: 3295-3304.
2 Kawamoto S, Shibano Y, Fukushima J, Ishii N, Morihara K, Okuda K. Infect Immun 1993; 61: 1400-1405.
3 Berk RS, Hazlett LD. Infect Dis 1983; 5: 3936-3940.
4 Morihara K, Homma J. Bacterial Enzymes and Vilulence. CRC Press, Boca Raton, 1985; 41-79.

© 1994 Elsevier Science B.V. All rights reserved.
Advances in Ocular Immunology
R.B. Nussenblatt, S.M. Whitcup, R.R. Caspi and I. Gery, eds.

Induction of stromal keratitis by recombinant *Onchocerca volvulus* proteins Ov33, RAL 2 and RAL 6

Eric Pearlman[a,b], James W. Kazura[b], David S. Bardenstein[a], Thomas R. Unnasch[c], Francine Perler[d], Eugina Diaconu[a], Fred E. Hazlett, Jr.[b], and Jonathan H. Lass[a].

a Department of Ophthalmology, Case Western Reserve University, Cleveland, OH.

b Department of Medicine, Case Western Reserve University, Cleveland, OH.

c Department of Medicine, University of Alabama, Birmingham, AL.

d New England Biolabs, Cambridge, MA.

INTRODUCTION

Onchocerciasis is a major cause of blindness in the world with approximately 20 million people infected with the causative agent, *Onchocerca volvulus*. It is estimated that a total number of 336,000 individuals are blinded as a result of this disease and many more are sight impaired (1). Keratitis is believed to occur after microfilariae migrate to the cornea, die and release multiple parasite antigens. The host immune system, which has been sensitized to parasite antigens as a result of chronic exposure, elicits an inflammatory response which ultimately results in central stromal scarring and permanent visual loss (2). Eosinophils, mast cells and interleukin- (IL) -4 were present in conjunctival biopsies of infected individuals, and IgE was detected in the aqueous humor (3, 4).

The immune mechanisms which lead to onchocercal keratitis are not well understood. We therefore developed a murine model which resembles the human disease both clinically and histologically (5, 6). BALB/c mice are immunized subcutaneously with a soluble extract of *O. volvulus* antigens (OvAg) and injected intrastromally with the same. The clinical symptoms which develop following intrastromal injection of OvAg include a diffuse opacification which can completely obscure the iris, and pronounced corneal neovascularization. Histologically, there is stromal oedema and a significant infiltration of eosinophils into the stroma. Onchocercal keratitis in this model has been observed only after prior sensitization to OvAg, demonstrating that, like the human disease, keratitis is mediated as a result of the host immune response rather than as a result of parasite toxicity. Furthermore, onchocercal keratitis did not develop in athymic nu/nu mice following sensitization and intrastromal injection of OvAg, thereby demonstrating a requirement for a cellular response. OvAg stimulation of peripheral lymph node cells from immunized mice induced production of the CD4+ cytokines IL-4 and IL-5, but not interferon (IFN) - g. This pattern of cytokine production is indicative of a predominant T helper (Th) type 2 subset response (7). In the current study, we determined if a similar keratitis could be induced by recombinant *O.volvulus* proteins.

METHODS

O.volvulus recombinant proteins

Recombinant *O.volvulus* proteins were isolated from cDNA libraries prepared from adult parasites after screening with rabbit hyperimmune sera to either adult worms (Ov 33) or infectious larvae (RAL2, RAL6). Ov 33 (clone 5B), is a 33kD protein (isolated by F.P.) having homology with aspartyl protease inhibitor (8); RAL 2 (isolated by T.R.U.) (9) is a 17kD protein; RAL 6 (isolated by T.R.U.) is an 18kD protein, having homology with protein disulfide isomerase. Each protein was expressed as a soluble fusion protein with *E.coli* maltose binding protein (MBP). MBP was used as control protein in all experiments.

Immunization and determination of keratitis

BALB/c mice received 3 weekly subcutaneous injections of 10 µg protein in squalene adjuvant. One week after the final immunization, 10 µg protein in 10 µl saline were injected intrastromally. Animals were examined by slit lamp microscopy 3, 7, and 10 days later, and graded 0-3+ for stromal disease as follows: 0: no pathology; 1+:slight opacity; 2+:moderate opacity; and 3+:severe opacity. Neovascularization scores were scored 0-3+ based on the number of vessels and the distance from the limbus. Mice were then sacrificed, and inguinal lymph nodes were removed for cytokine determination.

Cytokine analysis

Lymph node cells (5×10^6 cells/ml) were incubated with either culture medium alone or medium containing 10 µg/ml antigen. After 72 h incubation, secretion of IFN-g, IL-4 and IL-5 was determined by two site ELISA using monoclonal antibodies specific for each cytokine.

RESULTS

The clinical scores for animals immunized subcutaneously and injected intrastromally with either Ov33 or MBP alone are shown in Figure 1. Five of five mice given Ov33 developed moderate to severe keratitis with scores between 2.0 and 3.0. Neovascularization progressed centrally over the 10 days until vessels reached the center of the eye. In contrast, mice treated with MBP showed no signs of corneal disease at any time during ther study. Animals given RAL 2 or RAL 6 had similar stromal disease and neovascularization scores to Ov33 - treated mice (data not shown). Furthermore, intrastromal injection of unsensitized mice did not induce keratitis, demonstrating a role for the host immune response.

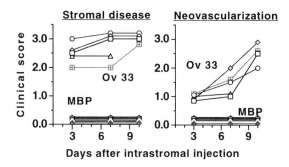

Figure 1. BALB/c mice were sensitized to either Ov33 or MBP, and injected intrastromally with the homologous protein. Clinical scores for each group were significantly different (p<0.01) at each time point.

To determine the Th response induced by Ov33, lymph node cells from Ov33 - sensitized mice were stimulated in vitro with Ov33, and cytokine production was determined as described in Methods. As shown in Figure 2, IFN-γ and IL-4 were secreted by all five mice, and IL-5 was produced by three of the five mice. Stimulation with MBP rather than Ov33 did not induce cytokine production in these cells (data not shown), indicating that the *O.volvulus* portion of the fusion protein is immunodominant. These data are consistent with the notion that Ov33 induces both a Th1- and a Th2- type response. Cells from animals immunized with MBP control protein proliferated in response to antigen stimulation, but did not induce production of these cytokines , whereas cells from RAL 2 - and RAL 6 - sensitized animals secreted all three cytokines (data not shown).

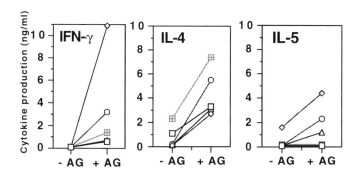

Figure 2. Ov33 - specific cytokine production. Lymph node cells from Ov33 - immunized mice were incubated with either culture medium alone (- AG) or with medium containing 10 µg/ml Ov33 (+ AG). IFN-γ, IL-4 and IL-5 production was determined in the supernatants. Data points represent five individual mice.

DISCUSSION

Intrastromal injection of recombinant *O.volvulus* proteins Ov33, RAL2 or RAL6 into sensitized mice induced clinical signs which closely resembled the keratitis observed after similar treatment with total parasite extract (6). Injection of a control protein, MBP, did not induce keratitis, thereby demonstrating the specificity of *O.volvulus* proteins in mediating the inflammatory response. The cytokine profile of sensitized lymph node cells is consistent with activation of both Th1- and Th2- subsets (7). As both the current and previous work (5, 6) demonstrate that activation of the host immune response is required for induction of keratitis, future studies will determine more precisely the role of Th subsets in the development of onchocercal keratitis.

REFERENCES

1 World Health Organization Expert Committee on Onchocerciasis. Third Report. WHO, Geneva. 1987; 8-21.
2 Taylor H. Int Ophthalmol 1990; 14: 189-196.
3 Chan CC, Ottesen EA, Awadzi K, et al. Clin Exp Immunol 1989; 77:367-372.
4 Chan CC, Li QiAn, Brezin AP et al. Ocular Immunol 1993; 1:71-77.
5 Chakravarti B, Lass JH, Bardenstein DS et al. Exp. Eye Res 1993; 57:21-27.
6 Pearlman E, Bardenstein D, Lass JH et al. Invest Ophthalmol Vis Sci 1993; 34 (suppl):3329.
7 Mosmann TR, Coffman RL. Ann Rev Immunol 1989; 7: 145-162.
8 Lucius R, Erondu N, Kern A, Donelson JE. J Exp Med 1988;168:1199-1204.
9 Gallin MY, Tan M, Kron MA et al. J Infect Dis 1989; 160: 521-529.

Advances in Ocular Immunology
R.B. Nussenblatt, S.M. Whitcup, R.R. Caspi and I. Gery, eds.

Expression of Vβ T cell receptor (TCR) transcripts in eyes, lymph nodes, and spleen in experimental murine keratitis.

M. Pedroza-Seres MD, Stephanie Goei MD, J. Merayo-Lloves MD, James E. Dutt BA, V. Arrunategui-Correa PhD and C. Stephen Foster MD, FACS.

Rhoads Molecular and Hilles Immunology Laboratories, Massachusetts Eye and Ear Infirmary, Harvard Medical School, Boston, MA, USA.

Introduction

Host immune mechanisms directed toward the elimination of herpes simplex virus (HSV) play a major role in the pathogenesis of HSK. Studies in Igh-1 disparate BALB/c congenic mice, C.AL-20 (H-2^d, Igh1^d) HSK-susceptible, and C.B-17 (H-2^d, Igh1^b) HSK-resistant mice, have led to the notion that CD4+ T cells are involved in the induction of HSK and CD8+ T cells in the protection from HSK.[1] Most of the CD4+ T cells infiltrating the corneas of susceptible mice were Vβ8.1,2+, and some Vβ3+ were also detected. When C.AL-20 susceptible mice were rendered CD4+ Vβ8.1,2+ or Vβ3+ T cell deficient through in vivo monoclonal antibody therapy, a dramatic reduction was found in both the incidence and the severity of keratopathy following HSV corneal inoculation as compared to controls.[2] In this report we have analyzed the TCR repertoire in both strains of mice using polymerase chain reaction technique.

Material and methods

Corneal inoculation and clinical scoring. C.AL-20 and C.B-17 mice were anesthetized, and the right cornea of each mouse was scratched in a crisscross pattern· Five ul of an HSV-1 (KOS strain) suspension containing 2.5×10^5 p.f.u. of virus were instilled in the cul-de-sac. The corneas were examined under binocular microscopy for 21 days after inoculation to determine the severity of keratitis.

Oligonucleotide primers and PCR amplification. Sequence specific primers for 19 Vβ families and a primer antisense for the constant region of TCR β chain (Cβ) were chosen from the Gene Bank and synthesized using an automated DNA synthesizer (Pharmacia LKB, Piscataway, NJ).

RNA isolation, cDNA synthesis, and PCR amplification. Inoculated eyes, spleens, and regional lymph nodes were harvested both before, and at various time points after corneal HSV infection (4, 7, 11, 14 and 21 days p.i.). Total RNA was extracted from each organ.[3] cDNA was synthesized and its confirmed using primer specific β-actin, a housekeeping gene that is expressed at a relatively constant level in all cells. PCR was performed by using a wax pellet hot-start technique. The amplification was performed in a Perkin Elmer thermal cycler model 9600 (Perkin Elmer Cetus, Norwalk, CT) with the following profile: 30 cycles of 1' at 94ºC, 1' at 55ºC, and 2' at 72ºC.

Southern blot analysis and scanning densitometry. PCR products were electrophoresed in 1.5% agarose gels, visualized with ethidium bromide and blotted onto nylon membrane (Boehringer). Densitometry was used to determine the differences between Vβ TCR transcripts of the same family members in HSK-susceptible and HSK-resistant mice.

Results

TCR Vβ mRNA expression in spleen. In the spleen more Vβ tanscripts were seen in C.B-17 resistant mice as compared with C.AL-20 mice. The pattern of Vβ transcripts expressed was different from that seen in eyes and LN. (data not shown).

TCR Vβ mRNA expression in LN. At later time points (11, 14 and 21), more Vβ transcripts were found in regional LN of C.AL-20 mice as compared to C.B-17 (data not shown). Only at day 14, densitometer analysis showed differences in the Vβ/Cβ ratios for Vβ8.1, Vβ8.2 and Vβ8.3; greater intensity in the message was detected for Vβ8.1 and Vβ8.2 in LN of C.AL-20 mice, while C.B-17 mice showed a greater intensity for Vβ8.3. (Fig. 1).

TCR Vβ mRNA expression in eyes. As was seen in LN, at day 11, 14 and 21 more Vβ transcripts were expressed in the inoculated eyes of C.AL-20 mice as compared to C.B-17 mice. Vβ8 family members were seen in both strains of mice at the later time points (Table 1). At day 11, in C.AL-20 mice Vβ8.2 and Vβ8.3 showed a significantly greater intensity in the message, when compared to C.B-17 mice. (Fig. 2). At day 11, Vβ 8.1 was expressed only in C.B-17 mice. At day 14, both strains of mice showed mRNA gene expression of the three family members with not significantly different densitometer ratios (data not shown).

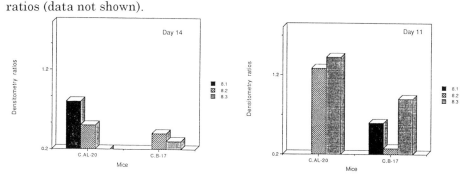

Fig. 1 and 2. Densitometry ratios of Vβ/Cβ in LN (left) at day 14, and inoculated eyes (right) at day 11 after corneal inoculation with HSV.

Table 1. TCR Vβ transcripts in eyes. A) C.AL-20 mice (Igh-1d), and B) C.B-17 mice (Igh-1b).

A

D	1	2	3	4	5.1	5.2	6	7	8.1	8.2	8.3	9	10	11	12	13	14	15	16	17	18	19
0										+								+				
4			+			+	+			+	+						+	+				
7	+	+	+				+		+	+	+	+					+	+	+			
11	+	+		+	+		+	+	+	+	+	+	+	+	+	+	+	+	+			+
14	+	+	+			+			+	+	+	+				+	+	+	+			+
21	+	+		+	+		+	+	+	+	+	+	+	+	+	+	+	+				+

B

D	1	2	3	4	5.1	5.2	6	7	8.1	8.2	8.3	9	10	11	12	13	14	15	16	17	18	19
0			+							+	+						+	+				+
4	+		+						+	+	+						+					
7	+	+		+				+	+	+	+						+	+	+			+
11	+								+	+	+						+					+
14									+	+	+				+			+				+
21						+	+	+		+	+		+			+		+				+

Transcription of Vβ genes in congenic mice at several time points as detected by PCR and Southern blot. "+" signifies Vβ mRNA detected, while blank means absence. D=day.

Discusion

Attempts to define the participation of different Vβ T cell receptor families have been made in many experimental diseases.[4] The interpretation of the data obtained has not been conclusive. We found that BALB/c congenic Igh-1 disparate mice, differentially HSK susceptible have different TCR usage kinetics in response to HSV corneal inoculation. In general, more diverse Vβ mRNA expression was detected in eyes and LN from HSK-suscpetible mice as compared to HSK-resistant mice. Densitometry readings showed evident differences in the intensity of the message in Vβ8 family members at several, later time points. Our findings at the level of gene expression correlate with our previous results regarding the probable participation of Vβ8+ T cells in the pathogenesis of HSK.

Bibliography

1.- Doymaz M, Rouse B. Herpetic stromal keratitis. An immunopathologic disease mediated by CD4+ T lymphocytes. Invest Ophthalmol Vis Sci. 1992;33:2165-2173

2.- Foster CS, Rodriguez Garcia A, Pedroza-Seres M, Berra A, Heiligenhaus A, Soukiasian S, Sundararajan Jayaraman. Murine herpes simplex virus keratitis is accentuated by CD4+, Vβ8.2+ Th2 T cells. Trans Am Ophthalmol Soc. 1994;91:325-350.

3.- Chomczynski P, Sacchi N. Single step method of RNA isolation by acid guanidinium thiocynate-phenol-chloroform extraction. Anal Biochem. 1987;162:156-159.

4.- Vandenbark AA, Hashim G, Offner H. TCR peptide therapy in autoimmune diseases. Intern Rev Immunol. 1993;9:251-276.

© 1994 Elsevier Science B.V. All rights reserved.
Advances in Ocular Immunology
R.B. Nussenblatt, S.M. Whitcup, R.R. Caspi and I. Gery, eds.

Genetics of the Virus Determines Retinal Tissue Damage Induced by Coronaviruses

Y. Wang[a], C.M. Percopo[a], M.N. Burnier[b], B. Detrick[c] and J.J. Hooks[a]

[a] Immunology and Virology Section, Laboratory of Immunology, National Eye Institute, NIH, Bethesda, MD, USA

[b] Department of Ophthalmology, Royal Victoria Hospital, Montreal, Quebec, Canada

[c] Department of Pathology, The George Washington University Medical Center, Washington, DC, USA

INTRODUCTION

The coronavirus, murine hepatitis virus (MHV), induces central nervous system disease characterized by both acute infections and chronic demyelinating disease (1,2). We have recently described a retinal disease induced by MHV which is biphasic in nature. The early phase consists of a retinal inflammation and the late or chronic phase consists of a retinal degeneration (3,4).

Numerous inflammatory and degenerative processes in man and animals are frequently associated with genetic factors, such as virus serotype, genetic constitution of the host, age or developmental stage of the host and route of inoculation (5). The purpose of this study was to evaluate the possible role of virus genetics in murine coronavirus induced retinal disease.

MATERIALS AND METHODS

Virus: JHM, A59 and MHV-3 strains of MHV were obtained from American Type Culture Collection (ATCC) and passaged 3 to 8 times in L2 cells. Viral infectivity titrations were performed on L2 cells propagated in 96 well microtiter plates. Infectivity was recorded as the induction of cytopathic effect by serial 10 fold dilutions of the sample. Stock virus infectivity was $10^{5.25-5.75}$ $TCID_{50}/0.1ml$.

Animals: BALB/c mice were obtained from Harlan Sprague Dawley, USA.

Mouse Inoculation: Adult (12-15 week old) male BALB/c mice were injected intravitreally with virus or DMEM (5μl/eye). At 0, 1, 3, 6-7, 10, 20 and 45 days after inoculation, the mice were sacrificed, and the eyes and livers were fixed in 10% formalin for H&E staining.

RESULTS

BALB/c mice were inoculated with 3 strains of MHV (JHM, A59 and MHV-3) by the Intravitreal route. The virus concentration inoculated into the vitreous ranged from $10^{4.0}$ to $10^{4.5}$ $TCID_{50}/eye$. As is seen in table 1, there is a striking difference in the mortality rate induced by these virus strains. Following intravitreal inoculation with JHM or A59 virus strain, a 3 to 9% mortality rate was noted in BALB/c mice. In contrast, MHV-3 inoculation resulted in 100% mortality rate within 5 days in BALB/c mice.

Table 1
Comparative Mortality Following Intravitreal Inoculation of BALB/c Mice with 3 MHV Strains

Virus Strain	Infectivity Titer (TCID$_{50}$/eye)	Dead / Total	% Dead
JHM	$10^{4.5}$	4 / 45	9
A59	$10^{4.2}$	1 / 37	3
MHV-3	$10^{4.0}$	21 / 21	100

We next evaluated the retinal tissue damage induced by the three virus strains. Retinal inflammation was noted in eyes harvested from JHM and A59 virus infected mice. This was noted from 3 to 7 days post inoculation. In contrast, only minimal or no inflammation was seen within the retinas from MHV-3 inoculated mice. Retinal degeneration was noted in eyes harvested from JHM and A59 virus infected mice. This was observed in eyes collected from 10 to 45 days post inoculation. `

Both JHM and A59 strains of MHV induced similar retinal disease. The early phase (day 3-7) was characterized by a retinal vasculitis with infiltrating cells surrounding the retinal vessels. The late phase (day 10-45) was characterized by retinal degenerative changes in the absence of infectious virus and inflammation. The degenerative changes consisted of a disorganization of the inner nuclear layer and photoreceptors, abnormality in the retinal pigment epithelium, and retinal detachments.

Table 2
Comparative Pathology in BALB/c mice Infected with 3 MHV strains

Virus Strain	Time	Pathology	
		Retina	Liver
JHM	Early	Inflammation	Inflammation
	Late	Degeneration	Regeneration
A59	Early	Inflammation	Inflammation
	Late	Degeneration	Regeneration
MHV-3	Early	Minimal Inflammation	Fulminant Acute Hepatitis (death)

MHV-3 inoculated animals were evaluated further in order to determine the cause of death. The brains harvested from these animals 3 to 5 days post inoculation had a normal appearance. In contrast, the liver was grossly enlarged and yellow in color. Pathologically , the liver changes were consistent with fulminant acute hepatitis including hepatocellular vacuolization, lack of cord pattern, and necrosis. In contrast, both JHM and A59 strains of MHV resulted in liver changes, which consisted of minor focal inflammation in the early phase and regeneration in the later phase (Table 2).

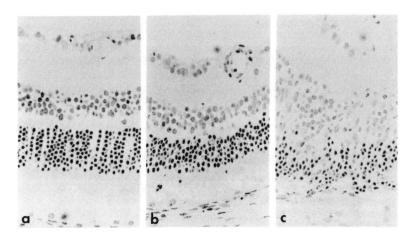

Figure 1. Biphasic retinal alteration induced by A59 virus in BALB/c mice (H&E, 400X). a) normal retina, b) A59 virus infected retina at day 7 (vasculitis), c) A59 virus infected retina at day 10 (degeneration).

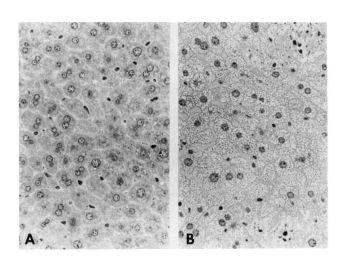

Figure 2.The liver pathology of BALB/c mouse induced by MHV-3 strain (H&E, 200X). A) normal tissue, B) infected tissue with cellular vacuolization and focal necrosis (day 5).

DISCUSSION

Numerous genetic parameters can determine the pathological alterations induced during a virus infection. MHV is a virus which has been shown to have a tropism for the liver and/or the central nervous system (6,7). We have developed a model of postvirus retinal degeneration in BALB/c mice induced by the JHM strain of MHV (8). In this report, we show that the A59 strain of MHV also is capable of inducing a biphasic retinal disease in BALB/c mice. In contrast, the inoculation of MHV-3 strain by the intravitreal route did not result in a retinal degenerative disease. Within 3 to 5 days all of the animals died. Evaluation of the brain did not reveal pathologic damage. However, the liver contained pathologic changes consistent with fulminant acute hepatitis. These remarkably different diseases are induced by different strains of the same virus.

The ability of different MHV strains to cause fatal acute hepatitis or persistent retinal diseases may help to decipher the mechanism of viral tissue tropism in this strain-specific pathogenesis. For example, the presence of viral receptors on target cells, the level of virus replication, the induction of IFN and cytokines, and the particular type(s) of immune response to the infection, may all contribute to the varied pathologies produced (5,9-11). In conclusion, these studies demonstrate that the genetics of the virus can profoundly affect the pathology generated by a virus using the eye as a portal of entry.

REFERENCES

1   Flaming JO, Trousdale MD, Bradbury J, et al. Microb Pathogen 1987; 3: 9-20.
2   Woyciechowska JL, Trapp BD, Patrick DH, et al. J Exp Pathol 1984; 1: 295-306.
3   Burnier M, Wang Y, Detrick B, Hooks JJ. Exp Pathol 1994 (in press).
4   Hooks JJ, Percopo C, Wang Y, Detrick B. J Immunol 1993; 151: 3381-3389.
5   Roos PR. Prog Med Genet 1985; 6: 241-276.
6   Barthold SW, Beck DS, Smith AL. Arch Virol 1986; 91: 247-256.
7   Lucchiari MA, Martin JP, Moldolell M, Pereira CA. J Gen Virol 1991; 72: 1317-1322.
8   Robbins SG, Hamel CP, Detrick B, Hooks JJ. Lab Invest 1990; 62: 417-426.
9   Wang Y, Detrick B, Hooks JJ. Virology 1993; 193: 124-137.
10 Holmes KV, Williams RK, Cardellichio CB, et al. In: Cavanagh D, Brown TDK, eds. Adv Exp Med Biol. New York: Plenum, 1990 (276); 37-44.
11 Massa PT, Wege H, ter Meulen V. Virus Research 1988; 9: 133-144.

II. CLINICAL PRACTICE
1. Inflammatory Disease
a. Mechanisms, manifestations and diagnosis

Advances in Ocular Immunology
R.B. Nussenblatt, S.M. Whitcup, R.R. Caspi and I. Gery, eds.

A study of cytokines in minor salivary glands in Sjogren's syndrome: Prevalence of Th2 pattern.

Karim E. Aziz, Boban Markovic, Peter J. McCluskey and Denis Wakefield.

School of Pathlology, Univ. NSW, Immunopathology Department, Prince Henry Hospital, NSW 2036, Australia.

Abstract

Cytokines may play an important role in mediating and modulating autoimmune responses. Their role in Sjogren's syndrome (SS) is not known.The aim of this study was to determine the synthetic capacity for different cytokines in minor salivary glands in SS. Minor salivary gland (MSG) biopsies were performed on twenty one patients with primary SS and ten controls. In situ hybridization with c-DNA probes for IL-1β (Interleukin-1 β), IL-2, IL-4, IL-6, IL-6R (receptor) and IFN-α (interferon alpha) mRNAs were used. Indirect immunoperoxidase staining with monoclonal antibodies to IL-2R, TNF-α (Tumour necrosis factor-alpha) and IFN-γ proteins was performed.

Although there was an increase in the number of cells producing IL-1β, IL-2, IL-4, IL-6, IL-6R m-RNAs and IFN-γ polypeptide in biopsies from patients when compared to controls, the increase did not reach statistical significance, except in the case of IL-4 ($P<0.05$). Occasional cells in patients biopsies were positive for IL-2R or TNF-α.

This pattern suggests the prevalence of Th2 lymphocytes in autoimmune lesions in SS. We conclude that IFN-γ, IL-1β, IL-2 and IL-6 may play a role in SS while IL-4 is the main cytokine present in MSGs in this disease and may be the principal regulator of the autoimmune response.

Introduction

SS is an autoimmune disorder characterized by keratoconjunctivitis sicca, xerostomia, increased incidence of autoantibodies, polyclonal hypergammaglobulinemia, a wide variety of systemic immunologic disorders and an increased risk of lymphoma[1]. Cytokines are local peptide mediators that act over small distances, either in an autocrine or paracrine fashion. Cytokines may be locally present in autoimmune lesions where they are produced by inflammatory cells or by target cells of the autoimmune attack. SS is associated with lymphocytic and monocytic infiltration of exocrine glands. The profile of cytokines in autoimmune lesions in SS is not known. The aim of this study was to examine the profile of cytokines expressed in MSG of patients with primary SS.

Materials & Methods

Patients and controls:

Twenty one patients (20F/1M, Mean age 63 years) fullfilling published criteria (1) for the diagnosis of primary SS, and 10 healthy controls were included in this study. MSGs were obtained from the lower lip beneath the mucous membrane (2). Tissue was placed immmediately into PBS (portion for immunohistology) or 10% buffered formalin (portion for ISH). The part kept in formalin was processed by a standard procedure into paraffin blocks. Sections were cut at 4 microns to be deparaffinated before the ISH procedure. The part kept in PBS was frozen and cut into 4 microns sections for immunohistology.

In situ Hybridization (ISH) procedure:

cDNA probes were used for the detection of IL-1β, IL-2, IL-4, IL-6, IL-6R and IFN-α mRNAs by in situ hybridization (3). A pBR322 plasmid was used as a negative control. A poly d(T):r(A) probe was also used as a positive control. All probes were photobiotin labelled. Tissue sections were covered with hybridization solution (including the cDNA probes) and incubated at

42^0c for 24 hrs. After washing the sections with a special procedure, detection of biotin was performed using suitable dilutions of steptavidin and biotinylated alkaline phosphatase and histochemical visualization using Naphthol AS-MX phosphate/fast red TR salt coupled reaction yielding a red stain.

Indirect Immunoperoxidase:
Frozen sections were incubated with Mouse monoclonal antibodies to IFN-γ (Genzyme), TNF-α(Behring) and IL-2R (Becton Dickinson) in tested dilutions. A biotinylated secondary antibody (horse anti mouse) (Vector) was used. Avidin and biotinylated peroxidase (Vector) was added to detect the binding of antibodies with a peroxidase reaction yielding a brown colour.

Analysis and grading of the sections:
Cells producing positive cytoplasmic signals were counted within a total of 400 cells and the result expressed as a percentage. The counting was carried out twice as a percentage of the total present cells and as a percentage of the mononuclear infiltrating cells. Mean±SES was calculated for each group. Student (t) test was used for statistical comparison.

Table 1

Comparison between the number of cytokine producing cells in patients and control biopsies as a percentage of total cells.

Cytokine	Patients	Controls	(t)test
IL-1βmRNA	6.8+1.6%	3.4+1.3%	P>0.05
IL-2mRNA	3.6+1.03%	1.6+0.64%	P>0.05
IL-4mRNA	25.7+3.4%	9.3+5.3%	P=0.0261
IL-6mRNA	3.95+0.99%	1.3+0.26%	P>0.05
IL-6RmRNA	3.62+0.89%	1.4+0.42%	P>0.05
IFN-amRNA	6.92+2.7%	7.5+2.9%	P>0.05
IFN-γ	14.6+3.2%	5.1+1.83%	P>0.05
TNF-α	Rare (<1%)	Rare (<1%)	
IL-2R	Rare (<1%)	Absent	

Results

Histological examination of the biopsies revealed that fourteen of the patients had grade IV minor salivary gland changes with >2 lymphocytic foci/4mm^2. The levels of expression of IL-1β, IL-2, IL-4, IL-6, IL-6R and IFN-α mRNAs, IFN-γ, IL-2R and TNF-α antigens as a percentage of total present cells is shown in table (1) and as a percentage of mononuclear infiltrating cells in table (2). Several other cellular elements demonstrated evidence of cytokine production (table 2). We compared the number of cells producing those cytokines in both patients and controls MSGs, there was an increase in the number of cells producing IL-1β, IL-2, IL-4, IL-6 mRNAs and IFN-γ polypeptide (table 1), but did not reach statistical significance except in the case of IL-4 (P<0.05).

Table 2

Cytokine producing cells in MSG bioposies from patients with SS.

Cytokine	% Infiltrating mononuclear cells (monocytes/ lymphocytes)	Other cell types
IL-1βmRNA	10%	Rarely epithelial
IL-2mRNA	7%	None
IL-4mRNA	33%	Very rarely endothelial
IL-6mRNA	4%	Rare epithelial and rare endothelial
IL-6RmRNA	5%	Rare epithelial and rare endothelial
IFN-αmRNA	12%	Epithelial & endothelial
IFN-γ	13%	Epithelial
TNF-α	Rare	Few epithelial cells
IL-2R	Rare	Absent

Discussion

Although IL-1β and IL-6 have been reported to play an important role in Rheumatoid arthritis (4,5), only few IL-1β producing cells were detected in MSGs in SS. Despite the fact that the majority of the infiltrate is formed of T-cells (mainly CD4 helper inducer subtype) and expressing the activation markers HLA-DR and ICAM-1, only 4-10% of these cells were involved in IL-1β or IL-2 or IL-6 mRNA synthesis. While only about 13% of them were positive for IFN-γ. This finding demonstrates that a distinct immune response is involved in this disease. IL-1β, IL-2, IL-6 and IFN-γ expression can not explain the state of activation seen in such an autoimmune situation, though they may contribute to the immunopathogenesis in certain stages of the disease.

We demonstrated that IL-4 was the predominant cytokine expressed in MSGs of patients with primary SS. IL-4 has been shown to stimulate class II MHC molecule expression, increase adhesion molecule expression, upregulate cytotoxic activity of T-cells and stimulate IgG synthesis (6,7). All are phenomena repeatedly demonstrated in patients with Sjogren's syndrome. IL-4 was found to reduce IFN-α production (8). IL-4 inhibits IL-1β, IL-6 and IFN-γ synthesis (9). This pattern suggests the prevalence of a Th2 lymphocyte profile (10) in autoimmune lesions in SS.

References

1 Fox, RI, Robinson, CA, Curd, JG, Kozin, F, and Howell, FV. Sjogren's syndrome, proposed criteria for classification. Arthritis Rheum 1986, 29:577-585.

2 Daniels, TE. Labial salivary gland biopsy in Sjogren's syndrome. Arthritis Rheum 1984, 27:147-156.

3 Akhtar, N, Rupair, A, Pringle, JH, Lauder, I, and Durrant, ST. In situ hybridization detection of light chain mRNA in routine bone marrow trephines from patients with suspected myeloma. Brit J Haematol 1989, 73:296-301.

4 Rooney, M, Symons, JA, Duff, GW. Interleukin-1β in synovial fluid is related to local disease actyivity in rheumatoid arthritis. Rheumatol Int 1990, 10:217-219.

5 Tan, PL, Farmiloe, S, Yeoman, S, Watson, JD. Expression of the IL-6 gene in rheumatoid synovial fibroblasts. J Rheumatol 1990, 17:1608-1612.

6 Paul, WE and Ohara, J. B-cell stimulatory factor-1/ Interleukin-4. Ann Rev Immunol 1987, 5:429-459.

7 Thornhill, MH, Kyan-Aung, U and Haskard, DO. IL-4 increases human endothelial cell adhesiveness for T-cells but not for neutrophils. J Immunol 1990, 144:3060-3065.

8 Gobl AE & Alm GV. Interleukin-4 down regulates Sendai virus induced production of interferon-γ and β in human peripheral blood monocytes in vitro. Scand J Immunol 1992, 35:167-175.

9 de Waal Malefyt, R, Abrams, J, Bennett, B, Figdor, CG, and de Vries, JE. Interleukin-10 (IL-10) inhibits cytokines synthesis by human monocytes: an auto regulatory role of IL-10 produced by monocytes. J Exp Med 1991, 174: 1209-1220.

10 Mosmann, TR and Coffman, RL. Two types of mouse helper T-cell clones. Immunol Today 1987, 8:223-226.

Advances in Ocular Immunology
R.B. Nussenblatt, S.M. Whitcup, R.R. Caspi and I. Gery, eds.

Adhesion molecule expression in minor salivary glands from patients with primary Sjogren's syndrome

Karim E. Aziz, Peter J. McCluskey & Denis Wakefield.

School of Pathology, Univ. NSW, Immunopathology Department, Prince Henry Hospital, Little Bay, 2036, Australia.

Abstract

The aim of this study was to examine the pattern of distribution of different adhesion molecules in minor salivary glands in Sjogren's syndrome (SS). Thirty one patients with primary SS and twenty one normal subjects were studied. Minor salivary gland biopsies were examined with monoclonal antibodies to adhesion molecules using an indirect immunoperoxidase technique. There was an increased expression of ICAM-1 (31% total cells), class I MHC, HLA-DR (59% total) & HLA-DQ on endothelial cells, lymphocytes, fibroblasts and salivary epithelial cells (DR>>ICAM-1 for epithelial cell expression). ELAM-1 and VCAM-1 were demonstrated over some of the endothelial cells in patients, but not controls. Many of the endothelial cells expressing ICAM-1, HLA-DR, DQ, ELAM-1 were high endothelial venules. CD44 was strongly expressed over epithelial, endothelial and infiltrating mononuclear cells, while LFA-3 was expressed on epithelial cells and faintly on infiltrating cells. There was no differences between patients and controls with regard to CD44 or LFA-3 expression. The ligands for the above mentioned molecules, namely: LFA-1α (68% infiltrating cells), LFA-1β (73%), CD4 (44%), CD8 (17%), LECAM-1 (18%), VLA-4α(CD49d) (38%), CD2 (56%), CD44 (77%), ICAM-1 (55%) and HLA-DR (72%) were demonstrated on the surface of infiltrating lymphocytes. CD11b and CD11c were detected over monocytes/macrophages. A proportion of lymphocytes expressed VCAM-1 (14%) and CD11c (21%) and in some biopsies they were localized at the centre of lymphoid follicles, with the appearance of dendritic cells. We conclude that adhesion molecules play a major role in the pathogenesis of SS.

Introduction

Sjogren's syndrome (SS) is a common autoimmune disorder, characterized by chronic inflammatory destruction of exocrine glands (1,2,3). The mechanism responsible for the lymphocyte infiltration of exocrine glands is unknown. Lymphocyte migration from the blood stream to sites of tissue inflammation requires specific adherence to specialized post capillary high endothelial venules (HEV)(4,5). Such migration is not random, and distinct populations of lymphocytes can be selectively directed to sites of local immune responses (6,7,8). The aim of this study was to examine the pattern of distribution of different adhesion molecules in minor salivary glands in primary Sjogren's syndrome (SS).

Material & Methods

Thirty one patients fulfiling published criteria for the diagnosis of primary Sjogren's syndrome were included in this study (1). Twenty one age and sex matched controls were also included. Minor salivary gland biopsy was performed on all subjects. Tissue specimens were embedded in OCT compound (Bayer, Miles laboratories) and cryostat sections 4 microns thick were cut. Sections were stored at -70^{0}c until examined for adhesion molecule (Table 1) expression.

Table 1

Main adhesion molecules and their ligands

Molecule	Specific ligand
ICAM-1 (Intercellular adhesion molecule-1)	LFA-1 (Lymphocyte Function. Ag-1)
CD44 (Hermes-1)	CD44, Hyaluronic acid
LFA-3 (Lymphocyte Function. antigen-3)	CD2 (E-rosette receptor)
ELAM-1 (Endoth. Leuk. adhesion molecule-1)	LECAM-1, Sailyl Lewis[x]
VCAM-1 (vascular cell adhesion molecule-1)	VLA-4 (Very late antigen-4)
Class I MHC + Antigen	CD8+TCR.
Class II MHC + Antigen	CD4+TCR.

Indirect immunoperoxidase staining with mouse monoclonal antibodies: anti CD3, CD4, CD8, CD14, CD19, CD18, CD11a, CD11b, CD11c, CD49d (VLA-4α), LECAM-1, HLA-DR, HLA-DQ, Class I MHC, CD54 (ICAM-1), ELAM-1 (E-Selectin), VCAM-1, CD58 (LFA-3), CD44 (Hermes-1), CD25 (IL-2Rα) and a biotin labelled polyclonal anti mouse IgG (Vector) prepared in horse was performed as previously described (3). Direct immunoperoxidase with peroxidase labelled anti VW factor (Von Willebrand factor, factor VIII) polyclonal antibody (DAKO). Positive cells were counted and results expressed as mean percentage±S.E.S. (standard error of sample).

Results

Monocytes/Macrophages as defined by CD14 expression formed a minority (4.7±1.6%) of infiltrating cells. The majority of the infiltrating cells were T-cells. CD2 and CD3 positive cells formed 56.2±4.2% and 52.4±6.1% of the infiltrate respectively. In some focal structures CD2 or CD3 +ve cells formed over 90% of the lymphocytes. The majority of these T- cells were CD4 +ve (43.7±3% of infiltrating cells), while CD8 (16.8±1.6%) and CD19 (12.9±2.9%) formed only a small proportion of the infiltrate. The proportion of the infiltrating cells expressing different adhesion receptors is shown in (Table 2).

Table 2

Adhesion receptors and activation markers expressed by infiltrating mononuclear cells in the salivary glands from patients.

Adhesion receptor	% infiltrating mononuclear cells (Mean%±SES)
CD18	73.1±5.3%
CD11a	67.95±4.7%
CD11b	13.3±2.6%
CD11c	21.4±3.2%
CD49d	37.6±4.8%
Leu-8 (LECAM-1)	17.9±2.6%
CD58 (LFA-3)	13.3±2.21%
CD44 (Hermes-1)	76.5±4.8%
CD54 (ICAM-1)	54.6±6%
HLA-DR	72.4±4.1%
HLA-DQ	41.6±7.2%
CD25 (IL-2R)	≤1%

The variable cellular elements expressing each of those adhesion molecules in minor salivary glands from patients with SS is shown in (Table 3).

There was a significant increase in the number of cells expressing ICAM-1, HLA-DR, HLA-DQ and class-I MHC in biopsies from patients when compared to controls (Table 4), but not CD44 or LFA-3 antigens. When acinar or ductal epithelial cells were considered separately a significant increase in ICAM-1, HLA-DR, HLA-DQ and Class I MHC molecules was demonstrated in the patients. Table (5) shows ductal epithelial cells expression of these molecules in both patients and controls.

Table 3
Cellular elements expressing different adhesion molecules in MSGs from patients with primary SS

	Lymphocytes	Monocytes	Epithelial	Endothelial
CD18	++++	++++	Negative	Negative
CD11a	++++	++	Negative	Negative
CD11b	+	++	Negative	Negative
CD11c	+	+++	Negative	Negative
Class I MHC	+++	+++	++	++
HLA-DR	++++	++++	++	++
HLA-DQ	++	++	+	+
ICAM-1	+++	+++	+	+
LFA-3 (CD58)	+	+	++	++
Hermes-1(CD44)	++++	++++	+++	+++
ELAM-1	Negative	Negative	Negative	+++
VCAM-1	+	Negative	Negative	+
VLA-4 (CD49d)	++	++	Negative	Negative
LECAM-1	+	+	Negative	Negative
V. W. F.	Negative	Negative	Negative	++++

Table 4
Comparison of the percentage of positive cells in minor salivary glands in patients & controls

Adhesion receptor	Patients (Mean%±SES)	Controls (Mean%±SES)	(t)
ICAM-1(CD54)	31.3±4.7%	7.8±1.7%	P<0.0001
HLA-DR	59.3±5.1%	18.9±2.4%	P<0.0001
HLA-DQ	22.9±4.9%	8.6±1.8%	P<0.03
CD44(Hermes-1)	65.9±4.2%	61.4±7.1%	P=0.6
CD58(LFA-3)	24.1±3.2%	22.1±5.2	P=0.7
Class-I MHC	66.3±6.1%	33.3±11.5%	P<0.01

Anti VWF (factor VIII) stained all endothelial cells in both patients and normal subjects. Many morphologicaly identifiable high endothelial venules were present in patients MSGs, but not those from normal subjects. The total number of endothelial markings expressing ICAM-1 (22.5±2.2/hpf) or HLA-DR (30.1±3/hpf) was significantly increased in patients (P<0.05) as the controls counts were ICAM-1 (11.6±2.4/hpf) or HLA-DR (20.2±2.2/hpf). None of the vascular markings from controls expressed ELAM-1 or VCAM-1, while 32.2% and 7% of them expressed ELAM-1 or VCAM-1 in MSGs from patients with SS, respectively.

Table 5
Expression of adhesion molecules by ductal epithelial cells in patients with primary SS

Adhesion receptor	Patients (Mean%±SES)	Controls (Mean%±SES)	(t)
ICAM-1(CD54)	6.6±2.1%	0.21±0.14%	P<0.007
HLA-DR	58±6.4%	5.9±2.02%	P<0.0001
HLA-DQ	11.1±5.8%	2±0.8%	P<0.001
CD44(Hermes-1)	57.1±5.6	60.6±7.5	P=0.7
CD58(LFA-3)	29.8±4.6%	23.4±4.3%	P=0.35
Class-I MHC	73.7±5.7%	40.9±15.3%	P<0.02

Discussion

This study clearly demonstrates the enhanced expression of adhesion molecules in minor salivary glands of patients with SS. The presence of high endothelial venules strongly expressing adhesion molecules such as ICAM-1 HLA-DR , HLA-DQ, ELAM-1 and (to a lesser extent) VCAM-1 suggests that these molecules may play a role in the homing of lymphocytes and monocytes to the salivary glands (2,4,8,9). The presence of LFA-1, LECAM-1, VLA-4, CD44 and CD2, the ligands of the previously mentioned adhesion molecules expressed over endothelial cells, on the surface of a considerable proportion of infiltrating lymphocytes also supports the possibility of an interaction between each receptor/ligand during the process of infiltration.

The interaction of adhesion molecules expressed on infiltrating cells with their ligands expressed on a variety of cells in the microenvironment of salivary glands in Sjogren's syndrme may be necessary for the different immune responses and functions mediated by infiltrating lymphocytes and monocytes (4,9). These interactions may play a role in retaining the infiltrating lymphocytes in the salivary glands in such an autoimmune exocrinopathy.

References

1 Fox RI, Robinson CA, Curd JG, Kozin F and Howell FV. Sjogren's syndrome. Proposed criteria for classification. Arthritis Rheum 1986; 29: 577-585.
2 Aziz KE, Montanaro A, McCluskey PJ and Wakefield, D. Sjogren's syndrome: review with recent insights into immunopathogenesis. Aust NZ J Med 1992, 22:671-678.
3 Fox RI, Carstens SA, Fong S, Robinson CA, Howell F and Vaughan JH. Use of monoclonal antibodies to analyse peripheral blood and salivary gland lymphocyte subsets in Sjogren's syndrome. Arthritis Rheum 1982, 25: 419-426.
4 Patarroyo M, Makgoba MW. Leukocyte adhesion to cells: molecular basis, physiological relevance and abnormalities. Scand J Immunol 1989,30:129-164.
5 Patarroyo M, Makgoba MW. Leukocyte adhesion to cells: molecular basis, physiological relevance and abnormalities. Scand J Immunol 1989,30:129-164.
6 Patarroyo M, Makgoba MW. Leucocyte adhesion to cells in immune and inflammatory responses. Lancet 1989, Nov 11;1139-1141.
7 Shimizu Y, Shaw S, Graber N et al. Activation-independent binding of human memory T cells to adhesion molecule ELAM-1. Nature 1991, 349:799-802.
8 Shimizu Y, Newman W, Tanaka Y and Shaw S. Lymphocyte interactions with endothelial cells. Immunology today 1992, 13:106-112.
9 Springer, TA. Adhesion receptors of the immune system. Nature 1990, 346: 425-434.

Advances in Ocular Immunology
R.B. Nussenblatt, S.M. Whitcup, R.R. Caspi and I. Gery, eds.

311

P-36, A Novel Circulating Protein in Active Pars Planitis.

N.S. Bora[a], N.H. Kabeer[a], M.T. Tandhasetti[a], S. Amin[a], T.P. Cirrito[a], J.B. Fleischman[b] and H.J. Kaplan[a].

[a]Department of Ophthalmology and Visual Sciences and [b]Department of Molecular Microbiology, Washington University School of Medicine, St. Louis, MO, USA.

INTRODUCTION

Pars planitis is a relatively common clinically well defined form of uveitis whose etiology is unknown. Without a definite etiologic diagnosis the patient can only be treated and not cured. The disease takes its name from the fact that inflammation in this entity involves an area of the eye, the pars plana, that is intermediate between the anterior and posterior uvea - thus, it is a type of intermediate uveitis. It is a chronic inflammatory disease whose onset is generally insidious [1,2]. The present study was undertaken to understand the etiology and pathogenesis of pars planitis. During the course of this study we have identified a novel protein in the plasma/serum of patients with active pars planitis. Furthermore, when these patients entered the inactive state of their disease, the circulating plasma protein disappeared [3]. The role of this protein in pars planitis is unknown, but its correlation with disease activity may provide an important marker for diagnosis and therapy. The present investigation reports the quantitative estimation of P-36 levels in pars planitis patients and various controls.

MATERIALS AND METHODS

(a)   Patient groups:
Uveitis patients included in our study were divided into groups 1, 2 and 3 and were evaluated by history, clinical examination and diagnostic testing as described [4]. Group 1 had 30 patients with active pars planitis (i.e. chronic cyclitis and peripheral uveitis); Group 2 had 13 patients with acute idiopathic anterior uveitis (HLA-B27+ and B27-); and Group 3 included 9 patients with chronic idiopathic panuveitis. Group 4 included 18 normal control subjects who had no previous history of eye disease. Plasma or serum

samples were obtained from the individuals in all the above-mentioned groups.

(b)   Identification and quantitation of P-36:
        250 microliters of plasma or serum was treated with the polyethylene glycol-8000. The resulting precipitate was resuspended in borate buffer and incubated at 37^0C for 30 minutes, followed by incubation with protein A beads at 4^0C. The beads were heated to 80^0C in the elution buffer to elute the bound proteins. The bound proteins were analyzed by 10% sodium dodecylsulfate-polyacrylamide gel electrophoresis, SDS-PAGE [3] and the gels were silver stained. Quantitative estimation of the P-36 levels was done by the densitometric tracing of the stained gels. Paired and unpaired student's t-test were used for the statistical analyses.

RESULTS

The results are presented in the Table 1. The levels of P-36 were quantitatively estimated in pars planitis patients and various controls by the densitometric tracing of the stained gels. We observed high levels (statistically significant; $p<0.05$) of P-36 in all 30 patients in Group 1. The levels of P-36 were very low in all the patients in Groups 2 and 3 and normal controls (Group 4). Six pars planitis patients in the Group 1 who then entered the inactive state of the disease showed very low levels of P-36 [Table 1].

Table 1. P-36 in plasma/serum of patients with different subsets of uveitis and normal healthy controls.

Group	Disease	Disease Activity	P-36 Levels mean $\pm$SD
1	Pars planitis (30)	Active	10 ± 0.7*
	Pars planitis (06)	Inactive	2.0 ± 0.1
2	Acute anterior uveitis (13)	Active	2.1 ± 0.6
3	Chronic panuveitis (09)	Active	1.4 ± 0.5
4	Normal controls (18)		1.2 ± 0.4

Number in parentheses indicates the number of subjects in each group.
*$p<0.05$

DISCUSSION

In the present study we report the quantitative estimation of P-36 levels in the patients with pars planitis (both active and inactive), acute anterior uveitis, chronic pan uveitis and normal control. The levels of P-36 in active pars planitis are six to eight fold higher in concentration than in the control groups used in our study and these differences are statistically significant ($p < 0.05$). Furthermore, there is no overlap in the concentration of P-36 with either normal or other controls. These results suggest a correlation between P-36 levels and disease activity in pars planitis. It appears that this protein is uniquely associated with active pars planitis since it is not present in other forms of intraocular inflammation. The biological function of P-36 is still unknown. However, even in the absence of a known role for the molecule, quantitative assessment of its levels in the patient's blood might be of importance in the evaluation and management of patients with pars planitis.

FINANCIAL SUPPORT

This work was supported in part by grant from Research to Prevent Blindness, Inc., N.Y. and NIH grants 1R01-EY10543 and 1R01EY09730.

REFERENCES

1.   Bloch-Michel E, Nussenblatt RB: International uveitis study group recommendations for the evaluation of intraocular inflammatory disease. Am J Ophthalmol. 1987; 103:234-235.
2.   Kraus-Mackiw E, O'Connor GR (eds): Uveitis: pathophysiology and therapy. Intermediate uveitis (pars planitis). Georg Thieme Verlag, New York, pp. 98-100.
3.   Bora NS, Bora PS, Kabeer NH, Fleischman JB and Kaplan HJ. Identification of a distinct 36 kD protein (P-36) in active pars planitis. Reg   Immunol. 1994 (In Press).
4.   Kaplan HJ, Waldrep C, Nicholson JKA, Gordon D: Immunologic analysis of intraocular mononuclear cell infiltrates in uveitis. Arch Ophthalmol 1984; 102:572-573.

© 1994 Elsevier Science B.V. All rights reserved.
Advances in Ocular Immunology
R.B. Nussenblatt, S.M. Whitcup, R.R. Caspi and I. Gery, eds.

Flow Cytometry of Diagnostic Vitrectomy Specimens

J. Davis, [a] P. Ruiz, [b] A. Viciana, [b] W. S. Thompson, [a] and T. Murray [a]

aDepartment of Ophthalmology, bDepartment of Pathology, University of Miami School of Medicine, Miami, FL, USA

INTRODUCTION

Expert cytopathologic examination of vitreous cells is standard for establishing a diagnosis of intraocular lymphoma, but success depends heavily on the skill of the observer and adequate morphologic preservation of cells. [1–5]

Immunohistochemical staining may improve the diagnostic yield by exploiting the predominance of B-cell lineage in intraocular lymphomas which usually have monoclonal expression of kappa or lambda surface immunoglobulin light chains. [6] Immunohistochemical staining is also useful to identify activated T-lymphocytes which supports a diagnosis of immunologically-mediated uveitis rather than lymphoma. [6–9] Interpretation of immunohistochemical staining, like cytology, is highly dependent on the experience and skills of the observer.

Recently, flow cytometry has been described as a technique of immunophenotyping of vitreous cells useful to a lesser [5] or greater extent. [10] We became interested in flow cytometry because we could not routinely obtain immunohistochemical staining. We also thought that flow cytometry might prove an easier, more rapid, and more objective technique than immunocytochemistry.

METHODS

Eight consecutive patients undergoing diagnostic and therapeutic vitrectomies had undiluted vitreous aspirated manually from the outflow line of the vitreous cutter. Vitrectomy then proceeded with infusion turned on and the cutter tip constantly within vitreous. Twenty to 30 cc of dilute vitreous were obtained. Vitrectomy was then completed in standard fashion. The specimens were kept at room temperature and analyzed within 45 minutes of collection.

Cells were pelleted by centrifugation at 1100 to 2500 RPM, resuspended in tissue culture medium, counted, and stained with antibodies from a leukemia and lymphoma panel developed for blood and solid lymphoid tumors. Lymphocyte-sized cells were gated for dual-color display using a Becton-Dickinson FACSort. Various antibodies were used according to initial diagnosis and the number of cells present. At least one histologic smear was made in each case.

RESULTS

Cases 1–3 carried a diagnosis of lymphoid malignancy; surgery was carried out principally to improve vision. Cases 4, 6, 7 and 8 had vitreous specimens removed in part to rule out intraocular lymphoma. Case 5 had vitreous analyzed coincident with pars plana lensectomy and vitrectomy for active ocular inflammatory disease. Clinical characteristics are given in Table 1.

Table 1
Clinical Characteristics of Patients and Diagnoses

Patients	Clinical Diagnosis		Pathologic Diagnosis	
Age, gender	Initial	Final	Flow Cytometry	Cytology
1)52, male Cutaneous lymphoma	Mycosis fungoides	Large granular cell lymphoma	Large granular cell lymphoma	None
2)62,female CNS lymphoma	Recurrent B-cell lymphoma post radiation	Recurrent B-cell lymphoma	B-cell lymphoma	None
3)38, male Cerebellar lymphoma	B-cell lymphoma	B-cell lymphoma	No diagnosis	None
4)81,female Aphakic	Toxoplasmosis R/O lymphoma	Uveitis	Heterogeneous T-cell, T-helper	None
5)50, male Increased lysozyme	Panuveitis	Panuveitis	Heterogeneous T-cell, T-helper	None
6)88,female Post IOL	Vitritis R/O lymphoma	Uveitis	Heterogeneous T-cell	None
7)81, male CLL	Vitritis R/O ALL	Cryptococcal endophthalmitis	Heterogeneous Neutrophils	Fungal forms
8)43, male HIV+	Vitritis R/O lymphoma	HIV-related uveitis	No diagnosis	None

Antibodies were selected for each case according to individualized strategies intended to make maximum use of the cells available. The bulk of the cellular material was diverted to flow cytometry rather than to cytology. Only Case 7, with a previous diagnosis of chronic lymphocytic leukemia (CLL), had sufficient material to permit a complete panel of markers to be tested as well as a cytospin preparation. CD10 (CALLA) was chosen because of its association with acute leukemia (ALL) but fortuitously confirmed neutrophils in the vitreous infiltrate. In Case 2, known to have large cell lymphoma, only 150,000 viable cells were obtained and pan B-cell, early B-cell, kappa and lambda markers were chosen. Case 1 had a large number of cells and was thought to have a T-cell lineage cutaneous lymphoma (mycosis fungoides). T- and B-cell markers were selected along with CD4, a surface marker for mycosis cells. CD4, CD8 and activation markers (HLA-DR) were also used in the inflammatory cases when cell number permitted. The per cent expression of specific markers is listed in Table 2.

Table 2. Cytofluorographic Analysis of Vitreous Specimens

Marker	Cell Type	Percentage of Cells Expressing Marker							
		Case 1	2	3	4	5	6	7	8
CD45	Pan leukocyte	98	89	--	54	94	--	30	--
CD14	Mono/macrophage	0	5	--	0	2	--	0	--
CD11c	Monocyte	--	--	--	0	--	0	3	--
CD2	Pan T-cell	1	7	--	--	91	--	0	--
CD7	Pan T-cell	99	--	--	63	--	--	0	--
TCR	Pan T-cell	99	--	--	50	--	--	0	--
CD3	Pan T-cell	80	--	--	47	--	54	0	--
CD5	Pan T-cell, some B	1	--	--	53	--	--	0	--
CD19	Pan B-cell	71	91	--	11	8	0	0	--
CD20	Pan B-cell	0	--	--	16	--	--	0	--
CD10	B-cell, ALL, neutrophil	--	--	--	--	--	--	34	--
CD4	T helper/inducer	0	--	--	31	78	--	0	--
CD8	T suppressor	98	--	--	12	14	--	0	--
CD25	Activation marker	38	--	--	--	--	--	0	--
HLA-DR	MHC Class II	1	--	--	7	--	14	3	--
	HLA-DR on T-cells	--	--	--	14	--	6	--	--
CD56	Natural killer	97	--	--	--	--	--	0	--
IgG	B-cell	--	--	--	--	--	--	9	--
IgM	B-cell	--	--	--	--	--	---	7	--
IgA	B-cell	--	--	--	--	--	--	5	--
Kappa	B-cell	--	14	--	12	--	0	--	--
Lambda	B-cell	--	5	--	10	--	0	--	--
CD22	Early B-cell	--	88	--	0	--	0	--	--

CONCLUSION

Any technique of examination of vitreous cells is judged first on its ability to confirm the diagnosis of intraocular lymphoma. In this series, cytofluorographic examination was highly informative in Case 1 in which precise immunophenotyping led to reclassification of the patient's cutaneous malignancy as a large granular cell lymphoma rather than mycosis fungoides based on aberrant expression of CD56, CD25, CD19 on a homogeneous T-cell population, and absence of CD4. In Case 2, previously confirmed as lymphoma, loss of kappa and lambda markers and aberrant early B-cell marker expression on a homogeneous cell population confirmed the diagnosis of recurrent B-cell lymphoma. In both cases, immunohistochemical staining as typically performed for the diagnosis of B-cell lymphoma would have failed to confirm the diagnosis since kappa and lambda markers were poorly expressed by the immature neoplastic B cells in Case 2 and the T-cell lymphoma in Case 1 would have been indistinguishable from a uveitic T-cell infiltrate if multiple markers showing aberrant expression had not been employed. Case 3, in which lymphoma was also highly suspected, had too few viable cells for diagnosis by either flow cytometry or histology.

Two other cases (4 and 6), finally diagnosed as ocular inflammatory disease, underwent vitrectomy in part to exclude intraocular lymphoma. Flow cytometry revealed a heterogeneous cell population in both cases, the majority of which were T-cells, typical of the pattern reported for uveitis. Case 4 had a large percentage (31%) of cells expressing T-helper/inducer phenotype (CD4). This pattern was also seen in Case 5, who had bilateral, active panuveitis and 90% T-cells, the great majority of which were T-helper/inducers. Case 7, confirmed by vitreous culture to be cryptococcal endophthalmitis, also had a heterogeneous infiltrate but with many neutrophils rather than a T-cell predominance. Case 8, an HIV positive patient with chronic vitritis and decreased retinal function by electroretinography, yielded no viable cells to help elucidate this previously reported disorder. [11]

Cases 1, 2, 4, 5, and 6 most clearly demonstrate the power of flow cytometry to provide information useful in discriminating between malignant and inflammatory vitreous infiltrates. Although this series was not designed to formally compare cytology with cytofluorography, it is our impression that more markers can be tested more rapidly and perhaps more objectively than with immunohistochemical staining techniques.

One of the major problems in immunophenotyping of vitreous cells is to obtain adequate cell numbers for study. Case 3 may have had poor yield because of recent corticosteroid use, sparing of the vitreous skirt to make surgery quicker and safer, or a 45 minute delay in delivery of specimen. Optimization of specimen collection may improve yield. We tried enzymatic digestion of specimen with hyaluronidase [10] in Case 1 and had poor results. We could not discern any clear advantage of diluted versus undiluted specimens.

Despite difficulties inherent in any method of immunophenotyping of vitreous cells, flow cytometry may be an alternative to cytology with immunocyto-chemistry and may be easier for clinicians in some institutions to obtain. Success in the interpretation of vitreous specimens requires dedication on the part of both ophthalmologists and cytopathologists to improve yield and maximize information. Immunophenotyping should be employed in the context of a comprehensive diagnostic approach including cytology and culture in most cases.

REFERENCES

1. Scroggs MW, Johnston WW, Klintworth GK. Acta Cytol 1990: 34: 401-408.
2. Michels RG, Knox DL, Erozan YS, Green WR. Arch Ophthalmol 1975: 93: 1331-1335.
3. Parver LM, Font RL. Arch Ophthalmol 1979: 97: 1505-1507.
4. Engel HM, Green WR, Michels RG, Rice TA, et al. Retina 1981: 1: 121-149.
5. Char DH, Ljung BM, Deschênes J, Miller TR. Br J Ophthalmol 1988: 72: 905-911.
6. Davis JL, Solomon D, Nussenblatt RB, Palestine AG, et al. Ophthalmology 1992: 99: 250-256.
7. Belfort RJ, Moura NC, Mendes NF. Arch Ophthalmol 1982: 100: 465-467.
8. Toledo de Abreu M, Belfort RJ, Matheus PC, Santos LM, et al. Am J Ophthalmol 1984: 98: 62-65.
9. Deschênes J, Char DH, Freeman W, Nozik R, et al.. Trans Ophthalmol Soc UK 1986: 105: 246-251.
10. Wilson DJ, Braziel R, Rosenbaum JT. Arch Ophthalmol 1992: 110: 1455-1458.
11. Brodie SE, Friedman AH. Br J Ophthalmol 1990: 74: 49-51.

© 1994 Elsevier Science B.V. All rights reserved.
Advances in Ocular Immunology
R.B. Nussenblatt, S.M. Whitcup, R.R. Caspi and I. Gery, eds.

Infectious agents as trigger factors in intermediate uveitis

J.P. Dernouchamps[a] and M.J. Tassignon[b]

[a]Lambert Foundation Eye Clinic, rue Baron Lambert, 35, B-1040 Brussels, Belgium

[b]Eye Clinic and Laboratory, University of Antwerp, Wilrijkstraat, 10, B-2650 Edegem, Belgium

INTRODUCTION

Intermediate uveitis (IU) is a well-known clinical entity often of unknown etiology and its pathogenesis still remains an enigma. It is actually considered that IU is an immune disease caused by an escape of the regulatory control of helper T cells. These T cells could be directed against ocular antigens, e.g. vitreo-retinal antigens. However, the question may be raised whether the target antigen could be an exogenous viral or bacterial antigen. Active borreliosis has been found as the cause of some cases of IU responsive to antibiotic therapy (1). Moreover an association between IU and a focal extraocular infection has been reported earlier by Offret and Saraux (2), Bec et al. (3), Stanojevic-Paovic et al. (4) and by Daus and Krauss-Mackiw (5), where *Streptococcus*, *Mycobacterium tuberculosis* and virus were the most frequently found infectious agents.

The aim of this study is to present four patients with an intermediate uveitis associated with extraocular infectious diseases where antibiotic treatment of the extraocular infection resulted in a remission of the uveal inflammation.

CASES REPORT

Case 1

A 9-year-old caucasian boy complained of blurred vision at his right eye. The examination of this eye showed (a) in the anterior segment, some cells in the aqueous humor, but no keratic precipitates, no synechiae and no cataract, and (b) in the posterior segment, cells 2+ in the vitreous with snowballs located inferiorly, but no snowbank, no peripheral retinal vascular abnormalities and no cystoid macular edema. The left eye was normal. Except for his intraocular inflammation, the patient enjoyed a good health. The serological tests disclosed no inflammatory reaction, no antibodies against toxoplasmosis, streptococcus, syphilis and virus. Chest X-ray was normal. The treatment consisted in three or four periocular injections of corticosteroids which resulted in the remission of the uveal inflammation.

Five months later there was a recurrence of the intermediate uveitis at the same right eye. At that time, the parents of the patient drew our attention to the presence of an ingrowing nail at the big toe with recurrent infections since one year. The young boy was sent immediately to a general surgeon for treatment and a microbiological analysis of the pus revealed the presence of *Staphylococcus aureus*. In addition to the surgical treatment of the nail and systemic antibiotherapy, three periocular injections of steroids were administrated with remission of the intraocular inflammation as a result.

Six months later, the young patient was complaining again of blurred vision at the same right eye due to a recurrence of the intermediate uveitis with, once again, an ingrowing nail at the big toe and infection due to *Staphylococcus aureus*. After a larger surgical treatment of the nail, systemic antibiotherapy and three periocular injections of steroids, the eye quieted down. Actual follow-up is of five years without any recurrence of the uveal inflammation.

Case 2

This case concerns a 24-year-old caucasian male, who was suffering from intermediate uveitis at his right eye since one year when examined by us for the first time. At the time of the examination we observed (a) in the anterior segment of the eye, keratic precipitates on the whole posterior side of the cornea, cells 1+ in the aqueous humor and some posterior subcapsular opacities of the lens, and (b) in the posterior segment, cells 1+ to 2+ in the vitreous but no snowbank, no snowballs, no retinal vascular abnormalities and no cystoid macular edema. The left eye was completely normal. The serological tests performed were negative, especially for syphilis, sarcoidosis and borreliosis. As this uveitis was of low intensity we decided not to treat.

The uveal inflammation remained at the same low intensity during one year until the patient was complaining of toothache. A stomatologist diagnosed the inclusion of the left inferior wisdow teeth with signs of chronic infection. After extraction of the teeth and systemic antibiotherapy, there was a remission of the uveal inflammation and this for more than six months up to now.

Case 3

A 77-year-old caucasian male was seen at our department because of a blurred vision at his left eye since a few months. The patient was psychically dement and physically neglected. Ophthalmological examination revealed corneal edema, ciliary injection, posterior synechiae, cells 2+ in the aqueous humor and cells 1+ in the vitreous. The presence of snowballs and cystoid macular edema could not be evaluated. Laboratory findings of the anterior chamber fluid showed some Gram positive diplococcus.

Further clinical examination showed an ulcus at the level of the second toe of the left foot, which revealed to be caused by a multiresistant *Staphylococcus aureus*. Intravenous antibiotic therapy with Vancomycin® was started with marked and simultaneous improvement of the peripheral wound and of the uveal inflammation of the left eye.

Case 4

A 51-year-old caucasian male was referred to our department for bilateral recurrent uveitis. Three years before he had a severe accident with multiple fractures (ankle, pelvis, femur, elbow) and wounds requiring an intensive antibiotic therapy. A few months after the accident he started complaining of blurred vision. Ophthalmological examination at that moment revealed a bilateral anterior and intermediate uveitis with cystoid macular edema, more pronounced at the left eye. The inflammatory reaction did not respond completely to a combined therapy of local corticosteroids and oral antibiotics. Even antimycotic drugs were given without success. A vitrectomy was then performed at the left eye but remained negative for infectious organisms.

When seeing this patient three years after the initial complaints, the vision was 5/10 at the right eye and 2/10 at the left one. Slitlamp examination revealed cataractous lenses and posterior synechiae at the left eye. White snowballs were present in the right vitreous and fluoangiography showed bilateral cystoid macular edema. Anterior chamber fluid of the left eye was negative for infectious organisms.

Because of a cataract formation, a lensextraction with phakoemulsification was performed on both eyes with two weeks interval. Lens materiel as well as a sample of anterior chamber fluid were cultured. Only the fluid of the phakoemulsification was positive for *Fusarium* species. An intensive intravenous amphotericin B therapy was started as soon as the results of the cultures were known. This treatment was combined with an oral administration of itraconazol and a low dosis of corticosteroids. The vision improved to 10/10 right and 5/10 left two months after the intravenous antimycotic therapy. The post-treatment follow-up is actually of six months without any recurrence of the uveal inflammation. The way of entrance of *Fusarium* was probably the multiple wounds when the patient was lying on the street just after the accident three years before.

DISCUSSION

In this study we present four patients with an intermediate uveitis associated with extraocular infectious diseases where the treatment of the extraocular infection resulted in a remission of the uveal inflammation. The four cases of intermediate uveitis were characterized by a long lasting (between four months and three years) and relapsing intraocular inflammation. The extraocular infectious diseases consisted of a focal toe infection in two patients, a focal wisdow teeth infection in one patient and infected wounds after polytrauma in the fourth patient. Microbiological analysis of the extraocular infectious focus was positive for *Staphylococcus aureus* in the two cases with toe infection and was not available in the case with teeth infection. In the patient with polytrauma, microbiological examination of the fluid collected during phakoemulsification was positive for *Fusarium* in both eyes. After systemic antibiotherapy of the bacterial infections, both extraocular infection and intraocular inflammation regressed simultaneously. The uveal inflammation in the patient with *Fusarium* was cured with a combined systemic treatment of amphotericin B and itraconazol.

It is actually suggested that IU could be driven by an inappropriate activation of helper T cells against a vitreo-retinal antigen or another ocular antigen still to be identified. This is supported by the fact that ciclosporin, which specifically regulates helper T cells by interfering with the synthesis of interleukin-2 (6), has been reported to result in improved vision in some cases of IU (7). This activation of helper T cells could occur because of exposure of an ocular antigen previously sequestred or because of combination of ocular and exogenous infectious antigenic determinants. Moreover, it may be asked whether the initiating factor leading to immunologic reactions against ocular tissues is not the immune response against an exogenous infectious antigen whithin the eye. Supporting this point of view, infectious agents, i.e. *Fusarium*, have been found in both eyes of our case 4 and an antibiotic treatment against infectious agents resulted in remission of both extraocular infection and intraocular inflammation in all our four cases of IU.

In summary, our four cases of IU indicate that infectious agents could play a role in the pathogenesis of some cases of IU. This role, however, remains to be defined.

REFERENCES

1   Winward KE, Smith JL, Culbertson WW, et al : Am J Ophthalmol 1989; 108: 651-657
2   Offret G, Saraux H: Doc Ophthalmol 1960; 14: 247-263
3   Bec P, Ravault M, Arne JL, Trepsat C: La périphérie du fond d' oeil. Paris, Masson, 1980, p 269
4   Stanojevic-Paovic A, Blagojevic M, Micovic V, Begic V: Clinical and therapeutical aspects of intermediate uveitis: in Saari KK (ed): Uveitis Update. Excerpta Int Congr Ser 651. Amsterdam, Elsevier, 1984, pp 179-183
5   Daus W, Krauss-Mackiw E: Clinical evaluation of intermediate uveitis observed in Heidelberg: in Saari KM (ed): Uveitis Update. Excerpta Medica Int Congr Ser 651. Amsterdam, Elsevier, 1984, pp 185-188
6   Talal N: in Kahan BD (ed): Cyclosporine: Applications in Autoimmune Disease. Baltimore, Grune & Stratton, 1988, pp 11-15
7   Nussenblatt RB, Palestine AG, Chan CC: Am J Ophthalmol 1983; 96; 275-282

© 1994 Elsevier Science B.V. All rights reserved.
Advances in Ocular Immunology
R.B. Nussenblatt, S.M. Whitcup, R.R. Caspi and I. Gery, eds.

Immunoglobulin isotype usage in retinal vasculitis

B.A. Ellis[1], M.R. Stanford[1,2], Elizabeth M. Graham[2] and G.R. Wallace[1]

[1]Department of Immunology, UMDS, The Rayne Institute, St. Thomas' Hospital, Lambeth Palace RoadLondon SE1 7EH, United Kingdom.

[2]Department of Medical Ophthalmology, St. Thomas' Hospital, Lambeth Palace Road, London SE1 7EH, United Kingdom.

INTRODUCTION

Retinal vasculitis can present as a complication of systemic or extra-ocular inflammatory disease (such as Behcet's disease, sarcoidosis and multiple sclerosis) of unknown aetiology, or it can present in isolation, where the inflammation is confined to the posterior uveal tract (idiopathic disease). Furthermore, retinal damage is associated with ocular toxoplasmosis following infection, either acquired or congenital, with *Toxoplasma gondii.*
A point-prevalence study of patients with idiopathic retinal vasculits showed that 51% of patients (compared with 2% of healthy normal donors and 24% of patients with systemic inflammatory disorder without eye involvement) had substantial levels of circulating anti-retinal antibodies, and that seropositivity was associated with disease severity, particularly in isolated retinal vasculitis [1]. The anti-retinal antibody was predominantly of IgG class.
It is well known that IgG subclasses possess different biological and physicochemical properties and that the immune system selects different IgG subclasses in response to a particular antigen. Several authors have described the production of mainly IgG1 and IgG3 or IgG4 antibodies in response to protein antigens {2] whilst polysaccharide antigens induce mainly IgG2 immunoglobulins [3]. Estimation of the distribution patterns of IgG subclasses may provide insight into the immunological processes involved in the pathogenesis of retinal disease.

MATERIALS AND METHODS

Patients: Venous blood was taken from patients attending routine outpatient ophthalmology clinics at St. Thomas' Hospital, and laboratory staff as normal control donors. Serum was collected within 3 h and stored at -40°C.

Immunoglobulin levels: Serum immunoglobulin G, immunoglobulin G subclass and immunoglobulin A levels were measured by a two-stage sandwich ELISA. The results were expressed, relative to a commercially-available calibrator reagent (Binding Site), as mg/L.

Antibody isotype to retinal S-antigen: Antigen specific antibodies were measured by ELISA using microtitre plates (Nunc Maxisorb Immuno-plate) coated with bovine retinal S-antigen (SAg) at 0.5 µg/well [4]. After incubation with samples, anti-S-antigen antibodies were detected using isotype specific monoclonal antibodies conjugated with horseradish peroxidase and tetra-methylbenzidine as the substrate. Results were expressed as percentage of the absorbance (at 450 nm) obtained using a similar dilution of a pool of sera from normal donors.

Statistics: Differences between groups were assessed using the Mann-Whitney U-test; a p value of 0.05 being considered significant.

RESULTS

Various isotypes were found to be expressed in reduced quantities in different patient groups: IgG was reduced in patients with idiopathic disease compared with normal donors (p = 0.049); IgG1 was reduced in patients with both idiopathic disease (p = 0.016) and Behcet's disease (p = 0.040) compared with normal donors; whilst both IgG3 (p = 0.034) and IgG4 (p = 0.019) were reduced in patients with sarcoidosis compared with normal values.

Likewise total serum IgA levels were reduced in patients with either idiopathic disease (p = 0.045) or Behcet's disease (p = 0.019) compared with normal donors.

The amounts of retinal S-antigen specific IgG isotype antibodies were no different between normal donors and any of the patient groups with the exception of IgG3 in patients with sarcoidosis (p = 0.05). Nor were any differences found between the different subject groups for antigen-specific IgA. In contrast, antigen-specific IgM antibodies were elevated in patients with either Behcet's (p = 0.037) or ocular toxoplasmosis (p = 0.014) compared with normal donors (see Figure 1).

DISCUSSION

Within this limited study using ELISA, as opposed to the direct immunofluorescence approach applied to our earlier point prevalence study [1], anti retinal S-antigen IgG *per se* was not found to be significantly raised in any patient group compared with healthy normal donors. The possibility that S-antigen, one of three retinal proteins known to cause uveitis in experimental animal models, is not the most appropriate retinal antigen must be considered.

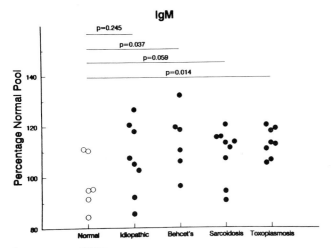

Figure 1. The levels of retinal S-antigen specific IgM in the serum of normal donors, and patients with idiopathic retinal vasculitis, or retinitis in association with Behcet's disease, disease or toxoplasmosis. Values are expressed as percentage relative to a pool of normal serum.

Whilst selective IgG subclass reactivity towards retinal autoantigens may well be a co-pathogenic feature in certain uveoretinitis syndromes the only significant difference found within this cohort of patients were increased levels of IgG3 and IgG4 directed to retinal S-antigen in patients with sarcoidosis. These differences were the only ones to be found when the usage of IgG subclasses was expressed as percentage of total IgG, i.e., compared with normal donors, patients with sarcoidosis had elevated expression of IgG3 (p = 0.005) and IgG4 (p = 0.001).
These data would be compatible with the low functional affinity of anti-S-antigen antibodies in retinal vasculitis patients [4] and with evidence that circulating immune complexes may play both a regulatory role in autoimmune uveoretinitis [5]. Patients were admitted to this study purely on the basis of diagnosis, consequently further studies are underway to evaluate whether there is a relationship between disease activity and subclass specificity towards retinal S-antigen. Additionally the effect of systemic steroid treatment will need to be evaluated in light of the evaluated production of all immunoglobulin classes induced by glucocorticoids [6].

CONCLUSIONS

There is no specific increase in total IgG in patients with retinal vasculitis
With the exception of IgG3 and IgG4 in patients with sarcoidosis, no IgG subclass was found in response to retinal S-antigen in the different patient groups.

326

There was an increased IgM response to retinal S-antigen in patients with Behcet's disease and ocular toxoplasmosis (and possibly those with sarcoidosis). This finding may be related to circulating immune complex formation in these patients.

REFERENCES

1. Kasp E, Graham EM, Stanford MR, *et al.* Br J Ophthalmol 1989; 73: 722
2. Shakib F Monogr Allergy, 1986; 19:1
3. Yount WJ, Dorner MM, Kunkel HG and Kabat EA J Exp Med 1968: 127: 633
4. Kasp E, Whiston R, Dumonde DC, *et al.* Am J Ophthalmol., 1992: 113: 697
5. Kasp E, Stanford MR, Brown E, *et al.* Clin Exp Immunol., 1992; 88: 307
6. Fischer A and Konig W. Immunology 1991; 74: 228

ACKNOWLEDGEMENTS

This work was supported by The Guide Dogs for the Blind Association, the Frances and Augustus Newman Foundation and The Iris Fund for Research into the Prevention of Blindness.

© 1994 Elsevier Science B.V. All rights reserved.
Advances in Ocular Immunology
R.B. Nussenblatt, S.M. Whitcup, R.R. Caspi and I. Gery, eds.

Elevated tear EDN levels in different conjunctival allergic disorders

V. Fuentes[1], L. Helleboid[2], E. Bloch-Michel[2], L. Prin[1].
[1]: Unité d'Immunologie, CHU Amiens; [2]: Centre d'Allergie, Hôpital Rothschild, 33 Bd. de Picpus, 75012 Paris, France (address for correspondance).

Abstract:

Eosinophil derived neurotoxin (EDN) was assayed in the tears by ELISA in different clinical types of conjunctival allergy. The mean level of EDN was increased to 123.5 ng/ml in 21 eyes with VKC, 75.6 ng/ml in 6 eyes with GPC, 271.8 ng/ml in 5 eyes with AKC, 46.9 ng/ml in 4 eyes with seasonal allergic conjunctivitis, 33.8 ng/ml in 21 eyes with perennial allergic conjunctivitis, versus 9.4 ng/ml in 28 healthy control eyes. These results reflect a varying degree of eosinophil activation for each type of disease when compared to the controls. Studies of EDN and of other eosinophil-derived mediators may provide clues on particularities of eosinophil activation mechanisms characteristic of each clinical entity.

Introduction:

It is now well established that the active contribution of eosinophils to type I hypersensitivity reactions is made possible by particular cellular features: specific membrane receptors transmit activating and modulating messages triggered by immunoglobulins (degranulation) [1], by IL5, IL3, GM-CSF (expression of functional surface markers) [2], by integrins (cell cooperation), and by PAF, LTB4, ECFA, C5A, histamine (chemotactic effect) [3]; the eosinophil's response is carried out by its proinflammatory mediators [1]: the cationic proteins MBP (major basic protein), ECP (eosinophil cationic protein), EPO (eosinophil peroxydase), and EDN (eosinophil derived neurotoxin) are best known for their cytotoxic effect; they also activate mast cells, macrophages, lymohocytes, fibroblasts, have a modulating influence on fibrinolysis, coagulation, and the complement system, and have a ribonucleasic effect [1,4,5]; Other mediators include cytotoxic oxygen metabolites (O_2^-, H_2O_2, $OH\cdot$), PAF, PGE2, LTC4, 15 HETE [1], and an array of enzymes (arylsulphatase, lysophospholipase, collagenase, histaminase).

Recent evidence has shown that during an antigen-triggered degranulation, a selective release of cationic proteins occurs, depending on the class of immunoglobulin involved [6,7]. IgE antibodies mainly determine EPO and MBP liberation, whereas ECP and EDN predominate after an IgG mediated reaction. MBP and ECP are released in the conjunctival tissue and in the tears during vernal keratoconjunctivitis (VKC) and contact lens-associated giant papillary conjunctivitis (GPC) [8,9,10]. The object of this study was to determine if high levels of tear EDN could also be found in VKC and GPC as well as in other clinical types of conjunctival allergy. Varying results between different clinical conditions may be an indication of the eosinophils' activation mechanisms in each one of them.

Materials and methods:

Tears were sampled with Schirmer paper strips in 21 eyes with active VKC, 6 eyes with GPC, 4 eyes with active seasonal allergic conjunctivitis (SAC), 4 asymptomatic eyes of 2 patients with SAC, 21 eyes with perennial allergic conjunctivitis (PAC), 5 eyes with atopic keratoconjunctivitis (AKC), 35 eyes with various non-allergic inflammatory conjunctival disorders, of which 10 had ocular rosacea, and 28 controls.

Each paper strip was removed from the eye after the tears had covered a 25 mm distance (35 μl), then dried immediately and sent for assay.

EDN was eluted from each strip in 350 μl of 0.1% PBS-Tween 20 to obtain a final estimated dilution of 1/10, then assayed with a sandwich-ELISA technique (rabbit serum anti-EDN and purified EDN kindly provided by P. Deviller, U.E.R. Alexis Carrel, Lyon, France). The standard range of EDN was 0.1 to 10 ng/ml.

Wilcoxon's test was used to compare the tear EDN levels between allergic conditions and controls.

Results:

The main tear EDN levels for each group is shown in the following table:

clinical diagnosis	EDN ± S.E. (ng/ml)	p vs. controls
controls (n=28):	9.4 ± 1.6	
VKC (n=21):	123.5 ± 20.1	0.001
GPC (n=6):	75.6 ± 33.1	0.02
AKC (n=5):	271.8 ± 36.7	0.02
SAC (n=4):	46.9 ± 21.5	0.06
extra-seasonal SAC (n=4):	8.9 ± 2.4	0.10
PAC (n=21):	33.8 ± 9.9	0.01
rosacea (n=10):	28.6 ± 7.1	0.01
other causes (n=25):	17.8 ± 3.6	0.01

Discussion:

Our results show that in VKC and GPC as well as in the other clinical forms of conjunctival allergy, eosinophils liberate EDN. The highest levels were found in AKC, although the small number of patients tested calls for a confirmation of this finding. Of greater significance was the elevated quantity of EDN in VKC, which is characterized by high levels of eosinophil-attracting and activating mediators, and by an important tissular eosinophil infiltrate. In one case, VKC lesions were present in both eyes, but only the left eye showed active inflammation: tear EDN was >260 ng/ml versus 4.3 ng/ml in the asymptomatic right eye, maybe confirming the idea that eosinophil-derived mediators reflect the intensity of an allergic reaction better than mast-cell mediators [10].

Active SAC expressed a smaller scale of eosinophil activation than VKC. The relatively low quantities of EDN found in SAC may not reflect the intensity of the reaction, because of the 24 hour or more delay between the onset of the symptoms and tear sampling. The eosinophilic infiltrate peaks at about 6 hours after contact with the allergen [11], and one would expect maximum mediator liberation at that time. Also, other eosinophil mediators such as MBP may be selectively released in SAC, resulting in a limited EDN liberation. Furthur studies using provocation tests may clarify this point.

EDN levels in PAC were also significantly increased compared to controls. An increased tear EDN level could be an important element in the frequently difficult task of distinguishing PAC from the other causes of chronic conjunctivitis. Its specificity would seem greater than that of mast cell-derived mediators, which may be liberated by a variety of non-specific degranulating agents.

The increased quantities of tear EDN during ocular rosacea, although at a relatively low level, came as a surprise. Further investigations are needed to confirm this finding, because eosinophil activation is not a classical feature of seborrhea.

According to in vitro studies, the liberation of EDN is mostly IgG-dependant, whereas MBP and EPO are mainly IgE-dependant. Most allergic eye conditions are believed to be IgE-mediated, and indeed MBP is found in VKC and GPC patients. However, tear EDN is also increased in all forms of conjunctival allergy. A possible explanation for this apparent contradiction may be that allergic conjunctivitis is not purely IgE-mediated, and may result from a mixed IgE-IgG activation. Some VKC patients have increased tear IgG, but not IgE levels. Also, in vitro studies do not take into account the possible intercellular modulation between different cell types; a better comprehension of adhesion molecules may explain the differences seen with in vivo situations. It is equally possible that other degranulating agents, lacking the potential for a selective mediator release, activate eosinophils during the reaction. We believe differences between cationic protein release patterns in the different clinical types of allergic conjunctivitis may partially explain conjunctival allergy's multiple expressions.

330

References

[1] Prin L, Capron M. Rev Prat (Paris), 1990, 40, p1866-1872.

[2] Chihara J, Gruart V, Plumas J, Tavernier J, Kusnierz J-P, Prin L, Capron A, Capron M. Eur Cytokine Netw 1992, 3, p53-61.

[3] Bruijnzeel PLB. Int Arch Allergy Appl Immunol 1989, 90, p57-63.

[4] Gleich GJ. J Allergy Clin Immunol 1990, 85, p422-436.

[5] Venge P. Agents and Actions 1990, 29, p122-126.

[6] Capron M, Tomassini M, Torpier G, Kusnierz JP, McDonald S, Capron A. Int Arch Allergy Appl Immunol 1989, 88, p54-58.

[7] Tomassini M, Tsicopoulos A, Chun Tai P, Gruart V, Tonnel AB, Prin L, Capron A, Capron M. J Allergy Clin Immunol 1991, 88, p365-375.

[8] Udell IJ, Gleich GJ, Allansmith MR, Ackerman SJ, Abelson MB. Am J Ophthalmol 1981, 92, p824.

[9] Trocme SD, Kephart GM, Allansmith MR, Bourne WM, Gleich GJ. Am J Ophthalmol 1989, 108, p57-63.

[10] Leonardi AA, Borghesan F, Smith LM, Plebani M, Secchi AG. Invest Ophthalmol Vis Sci 1994, 35, p1290.

[11] Bonini S, Tomassini M, Bonini S, Capron M, Balsano F. Int Arch Allergy Immunol 1992, 99, p354-358.

Advances in Ocular Immunology
R.B. Nussenblatt, S.M. Whitcup, R.R. Caspi and I. Gery, eds.

SYSTEMIC MORBIDITY OF PATIENTS PRESENTING WITH ISOLATED IDIOPATHIC RETINAL VASCULITIS

E M Graham, C J Edelsten, H Palmer, M R Stanford, M D Sanders

Medical Eye Unit, St Thomas' Hospital, London, United Kingdom

Introduction

Retinal vasculitis (RV) is an inflammatory disease of the retina, uveal tract and the vitreous. Although RV may be associated with infection, neoplasia, or systemic inflammatory disease, eg, sarcoidosis or Behcet's, there are a substantial number of patients in whom at presentation no systemic disease can be identified and in whom there are no specific retinal features suggestive of a systemic disease such as choroidal lesions in sarcoidosis, or retinal infiltrates in Behcet's. These patients are labelled as having idiopathic 'isolated' retinal vasculitis (IIRV). Long-term follow up of this special group of patients had suggested to us that despite the absence of overt systemic disease at presentation, these patients do have a significant systemic morbidity. This study was performed to assess how many patients who present with IIRV, that is disease apparently confined to the eye, develop systemic complications within five years of follow up.

Methods

A retrospective review was undertaken of patients attending the retinal vasculitis clinic of the Medical Eye Unit with IIRV and follow up of at least 5 years. At presentation all patients had a normal full medical history and general examination and routine investigations (full blood count, ESR, liver function tests, serum angiotensin converting enzyme, VDRL TPHA and chest x-ray) were unhelpful. All patients with pigment epithelial or choroid disease were excluded from the study. The pattern of retinal vasculitis was described as either 'leaky' or 'ischaemic'. Cells in the vitreous, peripheral vascular sheathing, cystoid macular oedema and disc or peripheral neovascularisation were seen in both ischaemic and leaky retinal vasculitis. Ischaemic retinal vasculitis was identified by the presence of capillary non-perfusion on fluorescein angiography.

Results (See Table 1)

Sixty-seven Caucasian patients fulfilled the study criteria. Forty-five patients had leaky retinal vasculitis. 31 (69%) of these were female and their mean age was 31 years. Twenty-two patients had ischaemic retinal vasculitis. 13 (53%) of these were female and their mean age was 27 years. Significant systemic disease developed

Table 1   Systemic Disease in 32 Patients with Isolated Retinal Vasculitis

Type of Systemic Disease	Leaky (45 patients)	Ischaemic (22 patients)	Total
Neurological - definite MS	13	0	13
MINUS -	1	2	3
meningoencephalitis	1	0	1
atypical optic neuritis	1	0	1
peripheral neuropathy	0	1	1
myelitis	2	2	4
Poser + systemic disease isolated episode	1	0	1
Vascular CVA	0	5	2
- myocardial infarction	0	2	2
Other - multiple abscesses	0	1	1
TOTAL	19	13	32

in 32 patients (48%): 19 with leaky RV, and 13 with ischaemic RV (Table 1). All the 19 patients with leaky RV who developed systemic disease, developed a neurological disease. However, only 13 of these (28%) of patients fulfilled the Poser criteria for definite multiple sclerosis (MS), the others suffered various Multifocal Intermittent Neurological and Uveitic Syndromes (MINUS) but a definite diagnosis could not be established. In contrast, 7 of the 22 (32%) of patients with ischaemic RV suffered a major vascular event, 5 developed MINUS, and one multiple abscesses, the latter probably secondary to immunosuppressive therapy. None of this group developed definite MS.

Vascular Disease in Patients with Ischaemic RV   (See Table 2)

All the seven patients who suffered a major vascular event did so within 5 years of presenting with their eye problems: four of them were not taking any systemic therapy at the time, two were taking prednisolone and one prednisolone in conjunction with azathioprine. None of them had hypertension, diabetes or high lipids and there was not any significant increase in risk factors in these patients compared to the group of patients with ischaemic retinal vasculitis as a whole.

Table 2   Risk Factors in Patients with Ischaemic Retinal Vasculitis

Risk Factor	CVA/MI (7 patients)	Other (15 patients)
Family history of vascular disease	2/7	0/15
Male	4/7	5/15
Smoke	5/7	10/15
*Abnormal clotting profile	4/6	2/4

* Protein C deficiency (2 patients), tissue plasminogen activator deficiency (one patient), anticardiolipin antibodies (2 patients), von Willebrand Factor increased (one patient.

Neurological Disease in Patients with Leaky RV   (See Table 3)

Eleven of the thirteen patients who developed MS were female: nine women with MS were tissue typed and seven of them carried the haptotype HLA B7 but this was also present in 8 of the patients without MS, six of whom were women. None of the six patients with MINUS had a family history of multiple sclerosis.

Table 3   Risk Factors in Patients with Leaky Retinal Vasculitis

Risk Factor	MS (13 patients)	MINUS (6 patients)	Other (17 patients)
Female	11/13	3/6	17/26
Family history MS	1/13	0/6	3/26
HLA B7	7/9	1/3	8/18

Discussion

The retrospective study has shown that 48% of patients presenting with apparently isolated retinal vasculitis developed significant systemic illness within five years of diagnosis. Approximately, one third of patients with leaky retinal vasculitis progressed to definite MS but none suffered vascular events. One third of patients with ischaemic retinal vasculitis had major vascular events, but none developed MS. A few patients in each group progressed to MINUS although in none of these could a definite diagnosis be substantiated.

334

The association between retinal vasculitis (intermediate uveitis, retinal vascular sheathing) and multiple sclerosis is well recognised, and studies show that between 5% and 22% of patients presenting with intermediate uveitis will develop MS within 5 years.[1-3]

It is most likely that the patients with MINUS have a known systemic disease which has eluded diagnosis: sarcoidosis is notoriously difficult to confirm when the disease is confined to the eye and the brain: 20% of patients with neuro-sarcoid do not have systemic features of sarcoidosis[4] and the Kveim test may be positive in only 25% of patients with normal chest x-rays[5].

The development of major vascular events in one third of our young patients with ischaemic retinal vasculitis causes concern. This association is not well recognised although Gordon et al reported a similar patient with Eales disease who suffered a stroke[6]. Our patients showed no stigmata of systemic vasculitis but a significant proportion smoked and had abnormal clotting factors. There may be a small subgroup of patients with ischaemic retinal vasculitis in whom consideration of these non-inflammatory factors may be as important as control of the ocular inflammation and for whom a different therapeutic regime from the standard immunosuppression might be beneficial. It is important to identify these patients at presentation in order to prevent vascular catastrophes.

References

1.   Arnold A C, Pepose J S, Hepler R S, Foos Y. Retinal periphlebitis and retinitis in multiple sclerosis. Ophthalmology. 1984; 91: 255-262.

2.   Malinowski S M, Pulido J S, Folk J C. Long-term visual outcome and complications associated with pars planitis. Ophthalmology. 1993; 100: 818-825.

3.   Edelsten C E, Stanford M R, Ormerod I, Welsh K, Graham E M. HLA B7 in patients with retinal vasculitis may predict the development of multiple sclerosis. Lancet. 1992; 339: 942.

4.   Cahill D W, Salcman M. Neurosarcoidosis: a review of the rarer manifestations. Surg Neurology. 1981; 15: 204-211.

5.   Scadding J G, Mitchell D N. Sarcoidosis. London. Chapman and Hall 1985.

6.   Gordon M F, Coyle P K, Golub B. Eales disease presenting as stroke in young adults. Ann Neurol. 1988; 24: 264-266.

Advances in Ocular Immunology
R.B. Nussenblatt, S.M. Whitcup, R.R. Caspi and I. Gery, eds.

HLA Class II Genotypes in Vogt-Koyanagi-Harada Disease

S. M. M. Islam[a], J. Numaga[a], Y. Fujino[a], R. Hirata[b], H. Maeda[b] and K. Masuda[a]

[a]Department of Ophthalmology, University of Tokyo School of Medicine, 7-3-1/ Hongo, Bunkyo-ku, Tokyo 113, Japan

[b]Blood Transfusion Services, Saitama Medical Center, Saitama Medical School, 1981 Kamoda, Saitama 350, Japan

INTRODUCTION

Vogt-Koyanagi-Harada Disease (VKH) is a systemic disorder that especially affects the individuals of pigmented races. The disease causes a bilateral diffuse granulomatous uveitis often with associated alopecia, vitiligo, poliosis, tinnitus, dysacousia and meningeal symptoms. Clinically, VKH is classified into prolonged and non-prolonged types. The exact cause of the disease has not yet been clearly demonstrated but strong association of human leukocyte antigens (HLA) with VKH have already been reported.[1, 2] HLA specificities are originally determined by serology and each of the specificities is now considered to include many genotypes (variants) at the DNA level.[3] In our previous study we reported that HLA-DRB1 *0405 and/ or *0410 genotypes were responsible for the development of the prolonged type of the disease.[2] In this study we analyzed all HLA class II genotypes in Japanese VKH patients by the recently developed techniques of molecular biology to demonstrate the immunogenetic backgrounds of the disease.

MATERIALS AND METHODS

Fifty-seven (29 males and 28 females) Japanese patients with VKH were included in this study. The diagnosis was determined according to the criteria proposed by Sugiura.[4] Serological tissue typing for HLA-DR and -DQ antigens were performed in all patients while typing for class I antigens were carried out in only 44 patients. Controls were 461 healthy Japanese blood donors. Serological HLA tissue typing was performed by the modified two-stage complement-dependent microcytotoxicity method.

DNA analyses for all HLA class II genotypes were carried out in all the patients and in 122 healthy controls. Genomic DNA was extracted from the peripheral white blood cells by the phenol-chloroform extraction method.[5] After extraction, DNA was subjected to group-specific amplification by polymerase chain reaction (PCR). Genomic DNA (approximately 200 ng) was mixed with 49 µl of reaction mixture containing 2.5 units Taq DNA polymerase 200 µmol dNTPs, 10 mmol Tris/HCl (pH 8.3), 50 mmol KCl, 1.5

mmol $MgCl_2$ with 20 pmol of each (forward and reverse) of the group-specific PCR primers. PCR reactions were performed by automated DNA thermal cycler (Perkin Elmer). After PCR amplification single strand conformation polymorphism and restriction fragment length polymorphism analyses were performed according to the methods we described previously.[2]

Chi-square test or Fisher's exact test was employed to obtain P values between patients and controls.[6] Corrected P values (Pc) were calculated as: $Pc = 1 - (1-P)^n$ where n stands for the number of antigens examined or the number of detected gene variants of the particular specificity observed in the compared groups. Relative risk values were calculated according to Woolf's method and we applied Haldane's modification when it was necessary.[6]

RESULTS

In serological tissue typing of the patients, among HLA class I antigens only -B54 showed a significant increased frequency with a relative risk value of 2.7 (Pc< 0.01). Among class II antigens, the frequencies of HLA-DR53, -DR4 and -DQ4 were significantly increased in the patients. The relative risk for -DR53 was 27.0 (Pc< 0.0001), for -DR4 and -DQ4 were 17.4 and 9.9, respectively (Pc<1.0×10^{-9}). On the other hand, a significant decrease in the frequencies of -DR52, -DQ1 and -DQ3 was observed in the patients (serological data is not shown).

The Table shows the results of DNA analyses. All patients had HLA-DQA1*0301, while only 67.2% of the controls had this genotype. Relative risk for -DQA1*0301 was 56.5 (Pc<1.0×10^{-5}), the highest of all the genotypes. Fifty-six of the 57 patients had -DRB4*0101 genotype (relative risk: 30.5; Pc< 0.001). The frequencies of -DRB1*0405 and -DQB1*0401 were also significantly increased among the patients. Relative risks for -DRB1*0405 and -DQB1*0401 were 9.5 and 10.4, in respective order (Pc<1.0×10^{-9}). The frequencies of HLA-DQB1*0601 and -DQA1*0103 were decreased; -DQB1*0603 and *0604 were not detected in the patients.

DISCUSSION

In our previous paper we investigated only the HLA-DRB1 gene variants. We discussed the strong associations of -DRB1*0405 and/ or *0410 genotypes with the prolonged type of VKH in Japanese patients.[2] In that paper we also discussed the strong association of HLA-DR53, -DR4 and -DQ4 with the disease. In this study we performed a complete DNA typing for all HLA class II genotypes in Japanese VKH patients.

In serological typing for class I antigens, the increased frequency of HLA-B54 among patients could be due to the increased frequency of -DR4 since there is a strong linkage disequilibrium between -DR4 and -B54 among the Japanese.[7] For class II antigens the increased frequencies of HLA-

DR53, -DR4 and -DQ4 with higher relatives risks for them reconfirm our previous findings.[1,2]

Table

Genotype frequencies in the patients and controls

Genotypes	Patients n=57		Controls n=122		Relative risk
	n	(%)	n	(%)	
DRB1*0403	4	(7.0)	6	(4.9)	
DRB1*0405	44	(77.2)	32	(26.2)	9.5[†]
DRB1*0406	5	(8.8)	8	(6.6)	
DRB1*0410	4	(7.0)	4	(3.3)	
DRB4*0101	56	(98.2)	79	(64.8)	30.5[‡]
DQB1*0401	44	(77.1)	30	(24.6)	10.4[†]
DQB1*0601	8	(14.0)	51	(41.8)	0.2[‡]
DQB1*0603	0		3	(2.5)	
DQB1*0604	0		19	(15.6)	0.04[‡]
DQA1*0103	9	(15.8)	52	(41.6)	0.2[‡]
DQA1*0301	57	(100)	82	(67.2)	56.5[§]

†: Pc<1.0x10^{-9} ‡: Pc<0.001; §: Pc<1.0x10^{-5};

At the DNA level, one-hundred percent association of HLA-DQA1*0301 genotype was detected among the patients and the relative risk for this genotype was the highest of all genotypes. This indicates the primary association of -DQA1*0301 might be necessary for the development of VKH disease in the Japanese. From the viewpoint of relative risk, the second important genotype was HLA-DRB4*0101 (relative risk 30.5). HLA-DRB4*0101 is serologically defined as HLA-DR53. However, it is unlikely that -DR53 confers the susceptibility because -DR53 is known to be tightly linked with -DR9 & -DR7 and the frequencies of -DR7 and -DR9 were not increased in the patients. Two other genotypes were significantly increased in the patients. These genotyoes were HLA-DQB1*0401 (relative risk 10.4) and -DRB1*0405 (relative risk 9.5). The increase of -DRB1*0405 would be secondary to the -DQA1*0301 increase because of the strong linkage disequilibrium between -DQA1*0301 and -DRB1*04 variants in the Japanese.[8] HLA-DRB1*0405 / -DQB1*0401 is the most frequently detected haplotype in the Japanese population.[9] So, the increase of -DQB1*0401 frequency in the patients could be secondary to the increase of -DRB1*0405 genotype frequency among them. Considering the above facts the hypothesis of HLA-DRB1*0405 or -DQB1*0401 genotype as the primary factor for the development of the disease looses validity.

The exact mechanism in the pathogenesis of VKH has not been clearly demonstrated so far. At the protein level, it is known in autoimmune diseases that some endogenous or foreign peptide binds with the HLA protein, and the HLA protein presents it to T cells causing T cell activation as the initial mechanism in the pathogenesis of autoimmune diseases.[10] Based on the association pattern of different genes it can be postulated that the amino acid sequence of HLA-DQA1*0301 genotype binds with a putative pathogenic peptide and presents it to T cells for T cell activation as the initial mechanism in the pathogenesis, thereby confering suseptibility to VKH.

Some of the HLA class II genes were decreased in frequency among the patients. The decreased frequency of -DQB1*0601 and absence of -DQB1*0603 among the patients could be secondary to the decrease of -DQA1*0103, because both the -DQB1 genes are very tightly linked with -DQA1*0103 genotype in the oriental population.[11] Although the decreasd frequency of -DQA1*0103 among the patients was significant, yet 9 patients had this genotype. In contrast to -DQA1*0103, -DQB1*0604 was completely absent among the patients. This absence was more significant. From this negative association we propose HLA-DQB1*0604 might act as a suppressive factor in the development of VKH by interfering in the binding with the pathogenic peptide and presentation of it to T cells. Thus the individuals having HLA-DQB1*0604 genotype can be considered to be relatively resistant to VKH.

REFERENCES

1. Numaga, J, Matsuki, K, Tokunaga, K, Juji, T. et al. Invest Ophthalmol Vis Sci. 1991; 32: 1958-1961.
2. Islam, S.M.M, Numaga, J, Matsuki, K, Fujino, Y. et al. Invest Ophthalmol Vis Sci. 1994; 35: 752-756.
3. Marsh, S.G.E & Bodmer, G. Hum. Immunol. 1991; 31: 207-227.
4. Sugiura, S. Jpn J Ophthalmol. 1978; 22: 9-35.
5. Kimura, A. & Sasazuki, T. 1992; in HLA 1991; (eds. Tsuji, K, Aizawa, M. & Sasazuki, T.) 397-419 (Oxford University Press, Oxford).
6. Thompson, G. Theor. Popul. Biol. 1981; 20: 168-206.
7. Tokunaga, K, Omoto, K, Fuji, Y. & Juji, T. Ishoku. 1983; 18: 179-189.
8. Albert, E, Sierpe, G, Keler, E, Bettinotti, M.D.L.P. et al. 1992; in HLA 1991; (eds. Tsuji, K, Aizawa, M. & Sasazuki, T) 454-457 (Oxford University Press, Oxford).
9. Stastny, P. & Kimura, A. 1992; in HLA 1991; (eds. Tsuji, K., Aizawa, M. & Sasazuki, T) 465-470 (Oxford University Press, Oxford).
10. Fremont, D.H, Matsumura, M, Stura, E.A, Peterson, P.A. et al. Science. 1992; 257: 919-927.
11. Noreen, H, Hors, J, Ronningen, K.S, Busson, M. et al. 1992; in HLA 1991; (eds. Tsuji, K, Aizawa, M. & Sasazuki, T) 477-484 (Oxford University Press, Oxford).

© 1994 Elsevier Science B.V. All rights reserved.
Advances in Ocular Immunology
R.B. Nussenblatt, S.M. Whitcup, R.R. Caspi and I. Gery, eds.   339

Ocular manifestations of Takayasu's arteritis in Brazil

Myung K. Kim [1], Iracema A. Nishie [2], Renata E.Hirata [1], Jorge E.
Amorim[3], Francisca S. Hatta [3], Emilia I. Sato [2] ·

Ophthalmology Department [1], Rheumatology Department [2] and
Vascular Surgery Department[3] at Paulista School of Medicine -
São Paulo, Brazil.

Av. Aclimação, # 39   São Paulo, Brazil   CEP 01531-001

Takayasu disease is a chronic, inflammatory, idiopathic arteriopathy involving
the aorta and its major branches. Ocular manifestations such as arteriovenous
shunts are common in Japan and is considered to occur due to hypotension in
the central retina artery.   In our group of 23 patients we observed arteriovenous
shunt in only one patient and vessel dilation in another. The majority of patients
presented normal fundus.

Our findings are different from japanese experience in Takayasu disease, and
this may have occurred in fact on the different type of the disease and severity.

Takayasu disease, or pulseless disease, is a life threatening
inflammatory process that affects the aorta and its major branches.   Asian
women in their second to third decades are most commonly affected.

Common symptoms include headaches, claudication, visual
disturbances and syncopes. The various clinical manifestations of the disease
are mainly due to insufficient arterial blood supply to the tissue. Attenuation or

obliteration of the carotids would result in cerebral ischemia and in arterial hypotension in the eye.

Takayasu disease is classified in type I (aortic arch involvement), type II (abdominal aorta involvement), type III (mixed aortic arch and abdominal aorta occlusion) and type IV (I, II or III with pulmonary artery involvement).

Ophthalmic manifestations were described by Takayasu in 1908 [1] . Uyama and Asayama [2] classified the retinopathy of a common variant which involves the aorta arch and branches into the following stages. Stage 1 (dilation of vessels), stage 2 (microaneurysm formation), stage 3 (arteriovenous anastomoses) and stage 4 (vitreous hemorrhage and proliferative retinopathy).

In our group of 23 patients, 22 were female and 1 male. The age ranged from 22 to 58 and we had 6 family cases.

Clinical manifestations were weight loss, fever, claudication of arms and legs, periphery pulse diminished or absent, systemic hypertension. The vascular alteration were confirmed by digital pan arteriography and classified in type I (7 patients), type II (4 patients), type III (10 patients) and IV (2 patients).

We observed only one patient with arteriovenous anastomose confirmed by angiography, and was not severe as was demonstrated by japanese authors elsewhere [3]. One patient presented vessel dilation and the others remaining patients did not have retinopathy. We did not have bilateral carotid artery occlusion.

The ocular manifestations described by Takayasu are uncommon in hyspanic patients [4]. We observed the same result in our group of patients.

The difference in ocular findings may indicate the variation in the type of the disease with different pattern of vascular occlusion and retinal perfusion observed in our patients when compared with the japanese patients.

References

1.   Takayasu, S. Nippon Ganka Gakkai Zasshi 1908; 12:554-555.

2.   Uyama, M., Asayama, K. Doc. Ophthalmol. Proc. Ser. 1976;9:549-554.

3.   Tanaka, T.,Shimizu, K. Ophthalmology 1987;94(11):1380-1388.

4.   Bodker, F.S., Tessler, H.H., Shapiro, M.J. 1993;115(5):676-677.

Advances in Ocular Immunology
R.B. Nussenblatt, S.M. Whitcup, R.R. Caspi and I. Gery, eds.

Humoral Immune Response to Porcine Retinal S Antigen in Filipino Patients with Uveitis and Normal Volunteers.

A. Mamaril [1], J. Lopez [2] and R. Noche [2]

[1] Consultant, Calamba Medical Center, Calamba, Laguna, Philippines

[2] Faculty, University of the Philippines, Philippine General Hospital, Manila, Philippines

INTRODUCTION

Uveitis, its pathogenesis is still an enigma up to the present. Several authors have developed animal models to help elucidate the different types of uveitis. The first is endotoxin-induced uveitis (EIU),[1,2] which is a model for human endogenous acute anterior uveitis. Another model called experimental autoimmune anterior uveitis (EAAU),[3] represents a delayed type of anterior uveitis. The third and most understood model is the experimental autoimmune uveitis or EAU, which is a delayed-type of posterior uveitis that can be induced by different retinal proteins.

Retinal S antigen, the most studied uveitogen, is a soluble 48 KDalton protein. It is located mainly in the disc membrane of the rod outer layer. EAU induced by retinal S antigen is a T-lymphocyte mediated disease. Retinal S antigen contains multiple uveitogenic sites including peptide M. Molecular mimicry to peptide M exists and that these peptides or antigens can also incite a EAU response providing a basis for human autoimmune inflammatory disease.

Studies on humans have demonstrated specific cellular immune responses to S antigen. [4,5] In these studies, both the normal and uveitis group had similar percentages of responders. Anti-S antigen antibodies, likewise, were found with equal frequency in patients and controls in a study by Forrester et al. [6] However, another study showed a higher incidence of retinal S antibodies in patients than in healthy blood donors.[7]

These findings indicate that the immune response to S antigen varies from one type of uveitis to another. Most previous studies involved mostly patients with Behcet's disease, VKH, SO, or Birdshot choroidopathy. Since uveitis in Filipinos are mostly due to tuberculosis and idiopathic causes, the immune response may be different. It was therefore the aim of this study to determine the humoral immune response to porcine retinal S antigen in Filipino patients with uveitis and those of normal individuals.

METHODS AND MATERIALS

I. SUBJECTS

Sixteen patients with uveitis were included in the study. Sixteen healthy volunteers of similar age range and sex distribution served as controls. None of these controls had any present or past uveoretinal or systematic disease. Peripheral whole blood was extracted and the serum collected.

II. PURIFICATION OF PORCINE RETINAL S ANTIGEN

Fifty fresh porcine retinas were suspended in phosphate buffer and completely homogenized. The homogenized suspension was centrifuged and the clear supernatant was collected. The supernatant was saturated with ammonium sulfate. The precipitates were collected and redissolved and then introduced into the Sepharose column. Standard bovine S antigen (from Alcon Laboratories) was run into the column first to determine the elution time before running the extract. The porcine extract was further purified with DEAE column.

Samples of porcine retinal extracts were taken from each purification step and checked against the standard S antigen by electrophoresis. To determine the ability to induce experimental autoimmune uveitis, Balb-C mice were inoculated with extracted porcine S antigen in complete Freund adjuvant (CFA). Control mice were inoculated with CFA only. The eyes were harvested after 14 days and underwent histopath examination.

III. ENZYME LINKED IMMUNOSORBANT ASSAY

Both the standard and porcine extracted S antigen were tested by ELISA. Checkerboard analysis was done to determine the best concentration of both antigen and antisera. Microtitre plates were coated with purified S antigen, serum, and anti-human IgG. Serum samples were tested in triplicates. Substrate for the enzyme peroxidase was added. The color reaction was stopped with sulfuric acid and read at 490 nm. Control wells were those without any antigen but underwent the same steps as mentioned. A value above the mean of the control wells plus three times its standard deviation was considered to be significant. The means of the uveitis group and of the normal individuals were compared using chi-square. The mean computed from patients with tuberculosis uveitis was also compared with the mean computed from the rest of the patients.

RESULTS AND DISCUSSION

There was an equal number of males and females in both the uveitis and normal groups, with ages ranging from 20 to 70 years old. Out of the 16 patients with uveitis, 8 had a history of pulmonary tuberculosis and/or positive with PPD.

The isolation of porcine retinal S antigen has not yet been reported. Using SDS-PAGE electrophoresis, the porcine S antigen migrated together with the standard bovine retinal S antigen at about the 50,000 MW marker, which is similar to retinal S antigen isolated from other species. Likewise, porcine S antigen was serologically similar to bovine S antigen when both exhibited similar color reactions with ELISA. Furthermore, porcine retinal S antigen was to able to induce an experimental autoimmune   uveitis in Bald-C mice with lymphocytic infiltration of the retina and uvea. The control mice did not show any cellular infiltration at all.

All patients, irregardless of etiology and activity, and 87% of normal volunteers showed significant levels of antibodies to S antigen. The mean absorbance for normal individuals was slightly higher but not statistically different from that of the uveitis group. Furthermore, patients with tuberculosis uveitis, did not have significantly higher antibody titers compared to the rest of the patients. These results indicate that autoantibodies to S antigen occurs within the normal population.

Table # 1. Humoral response to retinal S antigen of each clinical category as measured by the mean absorbance after ELISA.

Clinical Category	Absorbance at 490 nm *
All Uveitis Patients	0.530 -/+ 0.084
Tuberculous Uveitis	0.555 +/- 0.093
Non-TB Uveitis	0.500 +/- 0.070
Normal Individuals	0.544 +/- 0.115

* accumulative mean absorbance of all patients
+/- standard deviation

The presence of natural autoantibodies is well established in normal adults [8] as well as in certain disease processes like SLE and myasthenia gravis. In the eye, antiretinal antibodies may have a protective role. Cohen and Cooke [9] suggested that the autoantibodies act as a "blind to the immune system" by filtering out invading uveitogenic foreign antigens before they could be processed by the immune system. Since EAU is predominantly a T-cell mediated inflammation, lymphocytes must first be challenged by uveitogenic antigens that have been processed by antigen presenting cells (APC). Therefore, several alternative processes can occur when autoantibodies confront invading organisms or antigen. In one situation, there are enough antibodies to screen-out all the invading antigens, thus preventing the occurrence of uveitis. However, if there is not enough antibodies, some invading antigens may escape, allowing for its presentation to T-lymphocytes, which will result to a T-cell mediated uveitis. Uveitis can also occur if the antigen load is too large for the amount of antibodies present which may be the case in SO and chronic intractable uveitis. An ocular Arthus reaction occurs with high levels of sensitizing antigen giving rise to circulating Ag-Ab complexes. The presence of severe uveoretinal inflammation caused by T-cell mediated immune processes will lead to continuous release of more uveitogenic antigens and further aggravate the disease process. This can explain the difficult in treating certain chronic progressive uveitis like VKH and SO.

In support of the previous statements: Dua [10] has shown inhibition of induction of EAU by pretreating Lewis rats with a monoclonal antibody against an epitope in S antigen. The antibody completely destroys the epitope and dramatically prevents the occurrence of uveitis. Based on Anterior Chamber Associated Immune Deviation or ACAID, Mizuno et al [11] was able to suppress EAU by injecting the antigen into the anterior chamber.

In summary, retinal S antigen was purified from pigs eyes and found to be similar to bovine S antigen. Autoantibodies to porcine retinal S antigen was found to be present in both Filipino patients and normal individuals. A theoretical model of the role of autoantibodies in uveitis was presented.

BIBLIOGRAPHY

1. Bhattarcherjee, P., Williams, R.N. and Eakins, K.E. (1983). An evaluation of ocular inflammation following the injection of bacterial endotoxin into the rat footpad. Investi Ophthalmol. Vis. Sci. 24: 196-202.

2. Rosenbaum, J.T., McDevitt, H.O., Guss, R.B. and Egbert, P.R. (1980) Endotoxin induced uveitis in the rat as a model for human disease. Nature (London) 286: 611-613.

3. Broekhuyse, R.M., Kuhlmann, E.D., Winkens, H.J. and Van Vugt, H.M. (1991). Experimental Autoimmune Anterior Uveitis (EAAU), a new form of Experimental Uveitis. Induction by a detergent-insoluble, intrinsic Protein Fraction of the Retinal Pigment Epithelium. Vol. : 320-324.

4. Hirose, S., Tanaka, T., Nussenblatt, R.B., et.al. (1988). Lymphocyte responses to retinal-specific antigen in uveitis patients and healthy subjects. Curr Eye Res. 7 : 393.

5. Nussenblatt, R.B., Gery, I., Ballintine, E.J., (1980). Cellular immune responsiveness of uveitis patients to retinal S-antigen. Am J Ophthalmology.

6. Forrester, J.V., Stott, D.I., Kercus, K.M. (1989). Naturally occuring antibodies to bovine and human retinal S-antigen : a comparison between uveitis patients and healthy volunteers. Br. J. Ophthalmol 73 : 155-159.

7. Klass M., Bohnke, M., Damms, T., Knospe, V. (1991) Humoral immune response to retinal S-antigen in patients with uveitis. Fortschr - Ophthalmology. 88: 450-454.

8. Pfister, C., Dorey, C., Vadot, E.< et.al. (1984). Identification of the so-called 48 K protein that interact with illuminated rhodopsin in retinal rods, and the retinal S-antigen, indicator of experimental autoimmune uveitis. CR Acad. Sci. 299 : 261-265.

9. Dumonde, D.C., Kasp-Grochoasko, E., Graham, E., et.al. (1982). Antiretinal autoimmunity and circulating immune   complexes in patients with retinal vasculitis. Lancet. ii: 787-792.

10. Dua, H.S., Hossain, P., Brown, P.A., Mckinnin, A., et.al. (1991). Structure Function studies of S-antigen : Use of proteases to reveal a dominant uveitogenic site. Autoimmnunity. 10 : p. 153-167.

11. Mizuno, K., Clark, A.F., Streilen, J.W. (1989). Ocular injection of retinal S-antigen : Suppression of Autoimmune uveitis. Invest. Ophthalmol. Vis. Sci. 30 : 772-774.

Advances in Ocular Immunology
R.B. Nussenblatt, S.M. Whitcup, R.R. Caspi and I. Gery, eds.

Psychosomatic aspects of uveitis in the context of working life

H. Mayer, E. Kraus-Mackiw[a], E. Arocker-Mettinger, T. Barsani[b], T. Tischner and H. Tischner[c]

[a] Ergophthalmological and Stress Research Units, University of Heidelberg, P.O.Box 10 23 69, D-69013 Heidelberg, Germany

[b] Uveitis Clinic, Eye Hospital, University of Vienna, Währinger Gürtel 18-20, A-1090 Vienna, Austria

[c] Ophthalmic Surgery, Linienstr. 83a, D-10119 Berlin, Germany

INTRODUCTION

In 1735 the mathematician Leonhard Euler was confronted with the task of mastering a calculation in the briefest possible time. To quote contemporary experts, others would have needed months, yet he managed it in three days. The result was "hot fever and an abcess of the right eye", from which the affected eye never properly recovered. Euler commented in 1740, "it cost me an eye" [1].

It is not known whether uveitis develops on the basis of specific psychodynamic configurations, or even of a certain "risk personality". As in the case of other chronic inflammatory diseases, however, psychic, social and ecological factors often exert a considerable influence on the course of the disease. Emotional reasons were raised by Mackenzie [2], and also by O'Connor [3]. The role of "stress" in uveitis development was taken up by Kumar, Nema and Thakor [4], along with Wolintz and Miller [5]. We began to explore the significance of working life for uveitis patients in a qualitative pilot study. This is part of a multicentric cohort study of uveitis [6]. Spontaneously and on direct questioning, patients of different ages reported on "typical" trigger situations. Parallel to that we inquired about recent life experience. 21 patients agreed to cooperate on this (questionnaire 1994; average age: 47; range: 25-82;). The breakdown of patients according to the recommendations for the evaluation of intraocular inflammatory diseases of the International Uveitis Study Group [7] was as follows: 8 men - 7 anterior uveitis, 1 posterior uveitis; 13 women - 7 anterior uveitis, 3 intermediate uveitis, 3 posterior uveitis. Four of them were pensioners and three unemployed. Of the remaining 14 in work, four had a job requiring a degree, three were business people, four were office staff, one was a skilled worker and two were semi- or unskilled workers.

RESULTS

Asked about their recent life events [8], the patients naturally first mentioned health problems (6.5 points). This was followed by problems of working life (4.9 points), followed by those in partnership relationship (3.3 points). Specifically, the top seven items of the most important individual changes all have to do with working life. The other areas follow.

No distinction is made here as to whether these are situations to be regarded as consequences of the disease or not. However, in assessing the actual potential of the person, "accompanying diseases" are also important. 14 of these 21 patients had such a disease. Seven of them had rheumatism, mostly Morbus Bechterew. Five others had rheumatic symptoms and conditions, one patient had encephalitis disseminata and one had psoriasis. Seven patients had chronic skin diseases. Seven of these patients had at least two other diseases besides uveitis. In such a situation , it is only natural to expect further loss of performance with the corresponding psychic, social and labour-law consequences. Apart from this, it is known that in clinical samples of patients suffering from chronically recurrent inflammatory processes, the results of questionnaires concerning quality of life have a tendency towards higher values in all kind of items contributing to negative descriptors of life. Since we do not have a statistical basis, these rises in life change scores are not to be evaluated here. They are merely to serve as qualitative data and be compared with the qualities of the data of trigger situations. Five of the 21 patients gave no information. They were, moreover, patients who were not particularly compliant in filling out the whole questionnaire. Another one reported that her illness was not intermittent. So the following statements relate to the remaining 15 patients. They expressly confirmed the existence and importance of trigger situations. Nine patients exclusively reported on psychic and/or social triggering factors. Three reported physical triggers and three claimed that both levels had come into play. This means that with 12 out of 15 patients the episodes were triggered by psychic or social factors and with six patients by physical ones.

Table 1
Life change units in 21 uveitis patients*

Changes	Points
Changes in working hours and/or working conditions	12
Less competence and responsibility	11
Other work	10
Holidays	9
Problems with superiors	8
Other problems at work:	8
disqualification	
reduced communication	
threatened or real job loss	
Financial losses	8
Necessary decisions regarding the immediate future	8
Deterioration of relations with partner	8

*Life Change Scale by R.H. Rahe from Stress and Coping Inventory (SCI),
Nevada Stress Research Center, University of Nevada, Reno

A total of 39 different replies were given here. 14 of them related to working life; too much work and too little time, "stress", job changes, overly hard work and problems with superiors. Outside the world of work there were problems with their life partners, and often the anticipation of a supposedly insurmountable situation.

Two patients reported that worried thoughts about uveitis had sufficed to trigger an episode. If you compare these statements on episodes with those on the above biographical events, 16 of the latter come under the heading of "classical major/minor life events": separation from near and dear ones, their falling ill or dying. Social rites of passage are particularly frequent, like moving cities or house, changing jobs, exams etc. One patient reported an episode triggered by his own wedding. However, their own illness and operations are of crucial importance. About a third of the patients report that e.g. arthritic joint symptoms may herald an episode. The list of these trigger events and the general biographical life changes naturally have many identic semantic modules. The situations are often located on both sides of the processes: consequences and origin.

Neuro-pineo-thymo-lymphatic chain reactions come to mind here, for example. As a rule however, we will have to endorse Schlaegel's reference to "predisposing factors such as external stress or internal psychopathology" [9]. Quite a few questionnaire reply patterns reveal the special complexity of the psychophysical interdependence, i.e. the transactional dimension when it comes to uveitis episodes. The pathogenicity of negative results of processes of cognitive appraisal in the present life situation of the patients is reinforced and accelerated by the deterioration in performance of the most important control and adjustment system of our inner world in relation to the outside world, i.e. the eyes.

CONCLUSIONS

This study shows that - besides the partner relationship - working life is of considerable prognostic significance for uveitis patients. If it is possible here to absorb the loss of performance through work organisation and ergonomic means, and if the patient receives the necessary support from colleagues, superiors and family - with the result that there are no changes in status relationship, or even financial losses - then it may be expected that many a negative "reinforcement loop" will disappear. The supportive function of a job that is sustainable in its relationship structures is of crucial importance for uveitis patients. However, we are not of the opinion that one should recommend e.g. part-time work in every case. As a rule, this is felt, at least subjectively to be a social comedown, and thus has a pathological effect. At most a better type of job - often making lower visual demands and with a greater degree of freedom - could be organised as flexible part-time work. This should be anchored in a strict regime of breaks, rest and sleep. In addition, it seems advisable to us for uveitis patients to be given protective psychosomatic guidance, or at least therapeutic supervision, at the earliest possible point in time, i.e. as a rule on establishment of the diagnosis. This guidance must be geared to anticipating problems of human relationship and work performance and must be concerned to avoid stress and to deal with conflicts in a very cautious and careful manner. Even if it is generally not very helpful to trace disease phenomena back to "stress" in a reduced sense [10], in the case of uveitis the psycho-neuro-immunological effect mechanisms can at least be sensed. This is where the clinical psychophysiologist comes into play, as an ergo-psychosomatic doctor and empiricist. Even if uveitis does not seem to be a problem of significance to the whole economy, at least the points it has in common with rheumatic illness suggest a need for interdisciplinary, more extensive research activities into the psychoimmunology of work stress [11].

352

At any rate, we should give the following advice to our patients regarding life-changing events [12]:

Τοῦτον οὖν χρὴ τὸν χρόνον τὰς παραινέσιας ποιέεσθαι τοῖσιν
ἀνθρώποισιν τοιάσδε. Τὰ μὲν διαιτήματα μὴ μεταβάλλειν, ὅτι γε
οὐκ αἴτιά ἐστι τῆσ νούσου ....ἤν γὰρ μεταβάλλῃ ταχέως τὴν
δίαιταν, κίνδυνος καὶ ἀπὸ τῆς μεταβολῆς νεώτερόν τι γενέσθαι ἐν
τῷ σώματι. .....

This was written over 2000 years ago by Hippocrates. Translated for our day it could run: "At such a point in time (he means in the case of actual or threatened illness) one should give people the following instructions: not to change their life habits, because they are not in themselves the cause of the disease .... If they do suddenly change their habits there is a risk of some new phenomenon appearing in the body as a consequence."

Even if the joint efforts of the patient and the doctor do not succeed in healing uveitis, such a procedure will improve its course and the chances of a cure. As a rule, this will at least lead to a reduction in medication.

ACKNOWLEDGEMENTS

We are grateful to Jochen Wahl, M.D., Elaine Griffiths, B.A., and John Webster, B.A., University of Heidelberg, for the careful preparation of the manuscript.

REFERENCES

1 Bernoulli R. Julius Hirschberg Gesellschaft Nuntia Documenta Annotationes (in press).
2 Mackenzie W. London, Longmans, 1854
3 O'Connor GR. Am J Ophthalmol 1983; 96:577-599.
4 Kumar A, Nema HV, Thakur V. Ann Ophthalmol 1981; 13:1077-1080.
5 Wolintz AH, Miller CF. Mount Sinai J Med 1987; 54:78-85.
6 Kraus-Mackiw E, Mayer H, Arocker-Mettinger E, Tischner T, Tischner H. In: Dernouchamps JP, Verougstraete C, Caspers-Velu L, Tassignon MJ, eds. 3rd International Symposium on Uveitis. Amsterdam/New York: Kugler, 1993; 139-143.
7 Bloch-Michel E, Nussenblatt RB. Am J Ophthalmol 1987;103: 234-235.
8 Rahe RH, Arthur RJ. In: Lolas F, Mayer H, eds. Perspectives on Stress and Stress-Related Topics. Berlin/Heidelberg/New York/London/Paris/Tokyo: Springer 1987; 108-125.
9 Schlaegel TF. Int Ophthalmol Clin 1968; 8:409-485.
10 Lazarus RS. In: Filipp SH, ed. 2nd edition Kritische Lebensereignisse. München: Psychologie Verlags-Union, 1990; 198-232.
11 Schwarz-Eywill M, Breitbart A, Pezzutto A, Krastel H. Immun Infekt 1991; 19: 90-91.
12 Littré MPE. Oeuvres complètes d'Hippocrate, Vol VI. Paris: Libraire de L'Academie Nationale de Médecine, 1849; 54-56.

Advances in Ocular Immunology
R.B. Nussenblatt, S.M. Whitcup, R.R. Caspi and I. Gery, eds.

The value of combined serum angiotensin converting enzyme and gallium scan in the diagnosis of ocular sarcoidosis

R. A. Neves, A. Rodriguez, W. J. Power, M. Pedroza-Seres, C. S. Foster

Immunology Service, Massachusetts Eye and Ear Infirmary, Harvard Medical School, 243 Charles St. Boston MA, 02114, USA

Introduction

The diagnosis of ocular sarcoidosis is usually suspected in a patient with granulomatous uveitis with or without systemic manifestations and radiologic and laboratory abnormalities. However a definite diagnosis is only established when non caseating granulomas are found in tissue specimens of affected organs (1). Serum angiotensin converting enzyme (ACE) is probably a marker of macrophage activity within granulomatous inflammation (1) and Gallium scanning of parotid and lacrimal glands and pulmonary tissues may reflect cellular infiltration in these tissues (2). Both these tests may be abnormal in a series of circumstances, including inflammatory and tumoral diseases. Special attention to these tests in the most recent diagnostic approach for patients suspected of having sarcoidosis has been mainly because of the difficulties in obtaining good sample biopsies of involved sites and unavailability of the Kveim skin test reagent.

We analyzed the value of combined elevated serum ACE levels and abnormal gallium scan in the diagnosis of ocular sarcoidosis.

Patients and Methods

Twenty-two patients with active intraocular inflammation and (ultimately) biopsy-proven sarcoidosis, were studied (sarcoid group). A second group (control group) consisting of 70 patients with uveitis of definitive non sarcoid etiology was also analyzed for ACE and gallium scan abnormalities. Concurrent with their clinical evaluation, all of these patients had a serum ACE determination and a gallium-scan performed. Significant gallium uptake in any of the tissues evaluated 72 hours after intravenous injection of 4mCi of gallium citrate was considered to be abnormal. ACE values above the limits of normal for our laboratory (50U/ml) were considered abnormal.

The sensitivity and the specificity of the tests were calculated and compared between the two groups.

Results

Table 1 lists the prevalence of abnormal gallium scan and elevated angiotensin converting enzyme level in the sarcoid and control groups. In the sarcoid group, 16 patients (73%) had both an abnormal serum ACE and gallium scan and all patients had either a positive gallium or an elevated ACE. The sensitivity of an elevated ACE in the diagnosis of sarcoidosis was 82% and the specificity was 60%. Using the combination of a positive gallium and an elevated ACE the specificity for diagnosis of sarcoidosis was 100% and the sensitivity was 73%. On the contrary, twenty-three patients (33%) from the control group had either an elevated angiotensin converting enzyme or an abnormal gallium scan, but even more importantly, none of these patients had both an abnormal ACE and gallium scan. Other uveitic entities giving abnormal results for ACE or gallium scan are listed on Table 2.

Table 1
Results of abnormal gallium (Ga) scan and elevated ACE

Test	Biopsy-proven Sarcoidosis (n=22)		Control group Non-sarcoid uveitis (n=70)	
	No.	%	No.	%
Abnormal Ga scan	20	(91)	11	(16)
Elevated ACE	16	(73)	12	(17)
Either test abnormal	22	(100)	23	(33)
Both tests abnormal	16	(73)	0	(0)

Discussion

Sarcoidosis is a multisystemic granulomatous inflammation, that most frequently affects the lungs, parahilar lymph nodes, skin and eyes. Ocular involvement in systemic sarcoidosis is common (25-50%) and may precede, by several years, the systemic involvement. However only 3% of uveitis patients in a large survey have systemic manifestations of sarcoidosis (3). As there is no pathognomonic ophthalmologic feature for sarcoidosis uveitis, the clinical suspicion has to be supported by laboratory tests. Serum lysozyme and calcium levels, skin anergy and pulmonary function tests can be abnormal in the disease but the use of these tests is limited due to low specificity and sensitivity (4,5).

ACE and gallium scan, on the other hand, are the most frequently used tests for the diagnosis of sarcoidosis. Both tests, although sensitive, are not specific for sarcoidosis (5,6). The pulmonary uptake of gallium is increased in lymphomas, carcinomas, tuberculosis and silicosis, and other diseases in which T cell and macrophage infiltration occurs. In a similar fashion, ACE, which is normally produced by pulmonary capillary endothelial cells and alveolar macrophages, is normally increased in children (6) and may be elevated when large amounts are produced by epithelioid cells in any granulomatous disease. Using the combination of ACE and gallium scan in patients with biopsy proven sarcoidosis the specificity was increased to 100% and the sensitivity decreased to only 73%. Furthermore, no patients with uveitis of different etiology had both increased ACE level and abnormal gallium scan.

These results indicate that the combination of two non invasive methods such as serum ACE and Gallium scan uptake increases diagnostic specificity without affecting the sensitivity and are of a great value in cases of limited ocular sarcoidosis where no tissue biopsy is available.

Table 2
Patients with diagnosis of non sarcoidosis uveitis presenting with abnormal gallium scan or elevated ACE.

Diagnosis	Abnormal Ga Scan* N Patients	Elevated ACE* N Patients
Systemic Lupus Erytematosus	5	2
Tuberculosis	2	1
Juvenile Rheumatoid Arthritis	0	2
Intraocular Lymphoma	1	1
Acute Retinal Necrosis	0	1
Behçet's Disease	1	1
HLA B27 associated uveitis	1	1
Toxoplasmosis	0	1
Birdshot retinochoroidopathy	0	1
Fuchs heterochromic iridocyclitis	0	1
Vogt-Koyanagi-Harada syndrome	0	1
Total	11(16%)	12(17%)

*Each patient only contributed once to an abnormal test.

References

1   Nosal A, Schleissner LA, Mishkin FS, Lieberman J. Angiotensin converting enzyme in noninvasive evaluation of sarcoidosis. Ann Int Med 1979; 90:328-331.

2   Karma AA, Poukkula AAZ, Ruokonen AO. Assessment of activity of ocular sarcoidosis by gallium scanning. Brit J Ophthalmol 1987; 71,361-367.

3   Foster CS. Ocular manifestations of sarcoidosis proceeding systemic manifestations. Exerpta Medica 1988: 177-81

4   Weinreb RN, Kimura SJ. Uveitis associated with sarcoidosis and angiotensin converting enzyme. Am J Ophthalmol 1980; 89:180-185.

5   Weinreb RN, Barth R, Kimura SJ. Limited gallium scans and angiotensin converting enzyme in granulomatous uveitis. Ophthalmol 1980; 87:202-209.

6   Baarma GS, LaHey E, Glasius E, Vries J, Kijlstra A. The predictive value of serum angiotensin converting enzyme and lysozyme in the diagnosis of ocular sarcoidosis. Am J Ophthalmol 1987; 104:211-217

Advances in Ocular Immunology
R.B. Nussenblatt, S.M. Whitcup, R.R. Caspi and I. Gery, eds.

The proliferative response of γδ[+]CD8 dull positive T cells of patients with Behçet's disease to streptococcal antigen (*S. sanguis*) *in vitro*

T. Nishida[1,2], K. Hirayama[2], S. Nakamura[1], E. Hori[2] and S. Ohno[1].

1. Department of Ophthalmology, Yokohama City University School of Medicine, 3-9 Fukuura, Kanazawa-ku, Yokohama, Kanagawa, 236, Japan.

2. Department of Medical Zoology, Saitama Medical School, 38 Moroyama, Iruma, Saitama, 350-04, Japan.

INTRODUCTION

Behçet's disease (BD) is characteristic for its systemic inflammatory lesions including uveoretinitis, recurrent aphtha, inguinal ulcer and sometimes inflammations of bowel and central nervous system. The etiology is unclear, but the strong association with HLA-B51 has been reported in different ethnic groups (1) indicating host genetic factor is essential in the etiology.

Although this strong association with HLA-B51 observed, it is difficult to find multiple families suggesting that some environmental factor plays an important role to develop the disease.

Two microbial agents have been implicated. The herpes simplex virus type 1 genome were found in circulating leukocytes (1). *Streptcoccus sanguis* (*S. sanguis*) has also been proposed as a possible agent (3). Especially, uncommon strains KTH-1, KTH-3, ST-3 and H·83 are thought to be involved in BD (4). Isogai, E. et al. (3) reported that whole cells of *S. sanguis* significantly stimulated delayed type hypersensitivity (DTH) of the patients with BD wheareas no response occured in the normal control group.

Here, we found a unique subset of T cells of the patients with BD, γδ+CD8 dull positive T cells showed a good proliferative response *in vitro* against *S. sanguis* in an antigen specific manner.

MATERIALS AND METHODS

Subjects

Nine patients with BD were examined for their T cell reactivity to *S. sanguis* *in vitro*. As a control, 9 healthy individuals were used (Table1).

Table 1. Subjects

	BD	Healthy controls
Mean age	41.3	35.2
Male	7	6
Female	2	3
Complete type	7	-
Incomplete type	2	-

In vitro culture of mononuclear cells (MNC)

MNC were separated by Ficoll paque gradient centrifugation. One million / ml of MNC were suspended in RPMI-1640 supplemented with 10% human AB male serum and antibiotics and were cultured for 9 days with 20μg/ml of *S. sanguis* antigen or with 5μg/ml of purified protein derivatives (PPD). Two color analysis was performed using PE anti-CD3 monoclonal antibody (mAb) or PE anti-CD8 mAb and FITC anti-TCR γ/δ-1 mAb (Becton Dickinson) before and after the stimulation culture. At the same time, whole viable cell count of each culture was obtained by trypan blue staining to calculate absolute number of each subset of 2 color analysis as follows : Absolute number = whole viable cell count X percentage of the subset.

T cell line and proliferation assay

After the first stimulation culture, specific subset of T cells were purified by the negative selection using anti-CD4 mAb alone or anti-CD4 plus anti-γδTCR (TCRδ 1) coupled with iron beads coated with sheep anti mouse IgG (Dynal inc. Sweden). Purified T cells were re-suspended in the culture medium containing 5ng/ml of human recombinant IL-2 (Roche), antigen and autologous feeder cells (3000R) and were cultured for more 7 days. The expanded T cells were examined for their proliferative response to various antigens in the presence of antigen presenting cells (APC), EBV-transformed B cell line AKIBA, as previously described(5).

Antigen

S. sanguis (ATCC: 49298) was provided through Behçet's Disease Reserch Comittee of Japan, described in details elsewhere (4).

RESULTS AND DISCUSSION

There was no significant difference observed between BD and controls in γδ⁺CD8⁺T cells percentage on day0. But, after 9 days culture with *S. sanguis*, proportion of γδ⁺CD8⁺T cells significantly increased in BD group compared with healthy control group. Absolute number of this specific subset, γδ⁺CD8⁺T cells, was calculated as described. On day0, there was no significant difference by Student's t test between BD and healthy control group (Table 2). But, on day9, the cell number of this subset of BD significantly elevated compared with healthy controls (P<0.05). The mean stimulation index (SI) of BD was 78.40 and SI of BD was significantly increased (P<0.05) (Table 2).

Table 2. γδ⁺CD8⁺Tcell percentage before and after *S.sanguis* stimulation

	Day 0	Day 9	SI
BD	1.28 ± 0.32	17.83 ± 4.83	78.40 ± 22.28
Healthy controls	1.07 ± 0.31	7.62 ± 2.86	35.84 ± 16.82

mean ± S.E.

The next question is whether this specific γδ⁺T cell subset is derived from memory T cells specific for *S. sanguis* or just proliferated by some non-specific mechanisms such as LAK cells. In order to answer this question, we tried to produce long term cultured T cell lines from the patients to see their reactivity to the antigen. After repeated stimulation with the antigen and elimination of CD4$^+$ cells and/or γδ$^+$T cells, we produced two different T cell lines. Whose surface markers are αβ$^+$CD8$^+$, γδ$^+$CD8dull$^+$, γδ$^+$CD4$^-$CD8$^-$ (mixture line) and αβ$^+$CD8$^+$ (αβ line).

The proliferative response of the T cell lines is shown in Figure 1. Only the mixture line specifically responded to *S. sanguis* in the presence of APC indicating that this γδ$^+$T cell line is derived from memory T cell population reactive to original bacterial antigen. But, it is still not clear which subset is responsible for this specific response, γδ$^+$CD8dull$^+$T cells or γδ$^+$CD4$^-$CD8$^-$T cells.

Figure 1. Immune response of the T cell lines

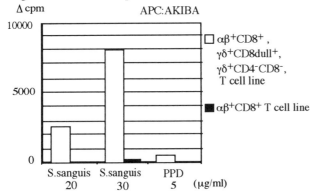

Now we are producing a number of γδ$^+$CD8dull$^+$ T cell clones from the patients for further analysis of this unique subset of γδ$^+$T cells.

REFERENCES

1 Ohno, S. , Ohguchi, M. , and Hirose, S. 1982. Close association of HLA-Bw51 with Behçet's disease. Arch. Ophthalmol. 100: 1455-1458.

2 Bonass, W.A. , J. A. Bird-Stewart, M. A. Chamberlain, and I. W. Halliburton. 1986. Molecular studies in Behçet's syndrome. 181-186. *In* T. Lehner and C.G. Barnes (eds.), Recent advances in Behcet's disease, Royal Society of Medicine Services, London and New York.

3 Isogai, E. , Ohno, S. , Takeshi, K. , Yoshikawa, K. , Tsurumizu, T. , Isogai, H. , Yokota, K. , Kotake, S. , Sasamoto, Y. , Hashimoto, T. , Shimizu, H. , Matsuda, H. , Fujii, N. , Yamaguchi, M. , and Oguma, K. 1990. Close Association of *Streptococcus sanguis* uncommon serotypes with Behçet's Disease. Bifidobacteria Microflora 9(1) : 27-41.

4 Mizushima, Y. 1989. Skin hypersensitivity to streptcoccal antigens and the induction of systemic symptoms by the antigens in Behçet's disease - a multicenter study. J. Rheumatol. 16(4): 506-511.

5 Mochizuki, M. , K, Hirayama. , S, Yamamoto. , and T, Sakane. 1994. Streptcoccal antigen specific γδ T cell lines and clones were blocked by anti HLA-class I monoclonal antibody. Eur. J. Immunol. in press.

© 1994 Elsevier Science B.V. All rights reserved.
Advances in Ocular Immunology
R.B. Nussenblatt, S.M. Whitcup, R.R. Caspi and I. Gery, eds.

SMALL AMOUNTS OF TNF-α IN VITREOUS SPECIMENS OF PATIENTS WITH INTERMEDIATE UVEITIS

B. Nölle, R.S. Gordes, and B. Wiechens
Department of Ophthalmology, University Eye Hospital,
Hegewischstr.2, D-24105 KIEL, FRG

ABSTRACT

Chronic forms of uveitis often show vitreous inflammation. Most of the vitreous inflammatory cells consist of T lymphocytes. A considerable number of monocytes/macrophages infiltrates the vitreous too. The latter cells are able to synthesize various cytokines, among them TNF-α. We are interested in the detection of TNF-α, because of its known uveitogenic capacity. For this reason we analyzed vitreous specimens for TNF-α by an ELISA-method. Fourteen patients suffering from intermediate uveitis underwent pars plana vitrectomy for therapeutic reasons. Vitreous specimens could be obtained undiluted in 16 eyes. Serum samples were analyzed in parallel. Only 2 of the 16 serum samples had detectable amounts of TNF-α (10 and 30 pg/ml). However, in 5 out of 16 vitreous samples TNF-α could be measured (range: 5 - 35 pg/ml). Although about one quarter of vitreous inflammatory cells expresses surface markers of the monocyte/macrophage type in the patients tested so far, only small amounts of TNF-α could be measured in their vitreous. Therefore in the vitreous TNF-α seems to play no uveitogenic role during late but active stages of intermediate uveitis. Whether other cytokines are produced and are pathologically relevant in uveitis awaits for further clarification.

INTRODUCTION

Uveitis is still an enigmatic disease, although the knowledge of inflammatory mechanisms involved has rapidly grown during the last years. Several studies suggest a role for cytokines in the mediation of inflammatory ocular diseases (for review see [1]). Tumor necrosis factor α (TNF-α) is one of the cytokine candidates, which may contribute to inflammation during uveitis. Its main biological functions are (1) activation of polymorphonuclear cells, (2) induction of cell surface molecules (e.g. HLA class I and II, ICAM-1), and (3) induction of prostaglandin- and leucotriene-synthesis (e.g. PGE, LTB4). TNF-α is mainly produced by macrophages/monocytes and to lesser amounts by T cells or NK cells [2]. Soluble TNF-receptors can inhibit TNF and, therefore, act immunoregulatorily [3].

Experimental studies suggest a role for TNF-α in uveitis. Intravitreal application of TNF-α in rabbits induces acute anterior uveitis [4,5,6], in addition a synergism between TNF-α and IL-1α has been observed in an equivalent setup [7]. TNF-α may be an initiating factor in experimental endotoxin uveitis in rats and possibly mediate its effect through IL-6 [1].

TNF-α in human uveitis has been detected in macrophages of retinal tissue sections from patients with AIDS-related retinal disease and gliosis [8].

Intermediate uveitis is a clinical defined uveitis entity primarily affecting the peripheral retina and pars plana region in young people [9]. Besides benign and prolonged courses of the disease, a chronic smoldering course may be difficult to treat. During the last years pars plana vitrectomy has become an accepted surgical intervention in patients suffering from intermediate uveitis and relevant vitreous opacifications [10].

Previous studies in intermediate uveitis show a considerable number of inflammatory cells within the vitreous bearing cell surface markers characteristic for monocytes/macrophages [11]. Therefore, we were interested in vitreous TNF-α levels during intermediate uveitis.

METHODS

In 16 eyes of 14 patients pars plana vitrectomy was performed because of vitreous opacities, recurrent uveitis relapses, recurrent or persistent cystoid macula edema and/or necessity for long lasting systemic immunosuppression. The clinical patients' characteristics are outlined in table 1. During surgery 0.5 to 1.0 ml of vitreous and a 10 ml blood sample were taken undiluted. The vitreous specimen and serum sample were stored frozen at -80°C within 2-12 hours after surgery.

Table 1
Clinical characteristics of study patients

No.	Age	Sex	Duration of disease	Affected eye	Previous systemic therapy	Systemic therapy prior to surgery	Previous surgery	Associated findings
1	15	f	6mo.	OS	steroids	yes	no	no
2	26	f	36	OU	no	no	no	no
3	"	"	42	"	steroids	no (3 mo.)	"	"
4	32	m	24	OU	no	no	no	no
5	"	"	26	"	"	no	"	"
6	7	f	15	OU	no	no	cryo	no
7	21	m	23	OD	steroids	no (3 mo.)	no	Tbc
8	46	m	48	OS	no	no	no	
9	2	f	6	OU	steroids,azathiopr.	no (3 mo.)	cat.	JCA
10	44	m	30	OU	steroids,azathiopr.	yes	cryo	HLA-B27
11	6	m	17	OU	steroids	no (3 mo.)	cryo	neuro.
12	53	m	10	OU	?	no	no	Yers.
13	33	m	30	OU	no	no	cryo	no
14	29	m	36	OS	?	no	no	no
15	25	m	132	OS	?	no	no	no
16	18	f	5	OU	steroids	yes	no	no

(?=unknown, cryo=retinal cryocoagulation, Tbc=tuberculosis in childhood, cat=cataract extraction, JCA=juvenile chronic arthritis, Yers. = Yersinia enteropathy, neuro.=neurodermitis)

For TNF-α analysis specimens were thawed and allowed to reach room temperature within 1 hour prior to testing. A commercially available ELISA-test was used to measure TNF-α (Human TNF-α ELISA-kit, Endogen Inc., 451 D St., Boston MA 02210, U.S.A., lot no. 312011). The test was performed according to the manufacturer's instructions. The limits of test sensitivity are 5 to 1900 ng/ml. The analysis of CD68 and HLA-DR cell surface molecules was done as previously outlined [11].

RESULTS

The test results are listed in table 2. Out of 16 serum samples only two had small amount of TNF-α (10, 30 pg/ml). However, 5 out of 16 undiluted vitreous specimens showed detectable amounts of TNF-α, although the levels are very small (range 5-35 pg/ml). A large proportion of vitreous inflammatory cells bear cell surface markers characteristic for macrophages/monocytes (CD68) and HLA-DR, respectively.

Table 2
Serum/vitreous TNF-α and cell surface markers on vitreous cells

No.	serum TNF-α [pg/ml]	vitreous TNF-α [pg/ml]	vitreous cells (% of MNC)	
			CD68 (macrophages)	HLA-DR
1	0	0	17	14
2	0	0	23	8
3	0	0	15	74
4	0	0	59	30
5	0	20	49	60
6	0	0	29	30
7	0	0	n.t.	n.t.
8	10	5	38	42
9	0	0	n.t.	n.t.
10	0	25	34	42
11	30	0	25	48
12	0	9	5	27
13	0	35	17	29
14	0	0	20	13
15	0	0	25	32
16	0	0	12	24 n.t. = not tested

DISCUSSION

Experimental studies in rabbits and rats describe TNF-α to be released early during endotoxin induced uveitis [1]. Cytokine studies in human ocular tissue are rarely performed. this may be due to difficulties in obtaining ocular tissues or fluids in such amounts to test various cytokine specificities. Another problem is the time of surgical intervention. Most patients need eye surgery in late stages of the disease and probably then a change in the immunopathogenesis of uveitis could have been happened.

The patients of the present study all had a history of chronic smoldering intermediate uveitis lasting for at least 5 months. Possibly the detection of TNF-α will give higher amounts in active, non-treated subjects.

Ten of 16 specimens did not have detectable levels of TNF-α in serum and/or vitreous, although a proportion of about one third of all mononuclear vitreous cells bears CD68 antigen, characteristic for macrophages/monocytes. In previous studies a large part of those CD68-positive vitreous cells were in addition positive for a cell activation marker HLA-DR. Despite to this only 5 out of 16 vitreous samples and 2 out of 16 sera showed low amounts of TNF-α.

ELISA-tests in general are able to detect biologically active and inactive fragments of cytokines. This could mean an unknown amount of the TNF-α may be biologically inactive. Therefore, the small levels of vitreous TNF-α should be considered with caution in respect to pathogenesis of uveitis. Further studies are requested with various test methods in parallel for each cytokine in clinical acute stages of inflammation.

REFERENCES

1   de Vos AF, Hoekzema R, and Kijlstra A. Curr Eye Res 1992; 11: 581-597.
2   Beutler B and Cerami A. Ann Rev Immunol 1989; 7: 625-655.
3   Fernandez-Botran R. FASEB J. 1991; 5: 2567-2574.
4   Kulkarni PS and Srinivasan BD. Exp Eye Res 1988; 46: 631-633.
5   Rosenbaum JT, Howes ET, Rubin RM, and Samples JR. Am J Pathol 1988; 133: 47-53.
6   Fleisher LN, Ferrell JB, and McGahan MC. Inflammation 1990; 14: 325-335.
7   Fleisher LN, Ferrell JB, and McGahan MC. Invest Ophthalmol Vis Sci 1992; 33: 2120-2127.
8   Hofman FM and Hinton DR. Invest Ophthalmol Vis Sci 1992; 33: 1829-1835.
9   Böke W. In: Böke WRF, Manthey KF, and Nussenblatt RB (eds.). Intermedia te Uveitis. Dev Ophthalmol. Basel: Karger, 1992; 23: 20-27.
10 Eckardt C and Bacskulin A. In: Böke WRF, Manthey KF, and Nussenblatt RB (eds.). Intermediate Uveitis. Dev Ophthalmol. Basel: Karger, 1992; 23: 232-238.
11 Nölle B and Eckardt C. In: Böke WRF, Manthey KF, and Nussenblatt RB (eds.). Intermediate Uveitis. Dev Ophthalmol. Basel: Karger, 1992; 23: 145-149.

© 1994 Elsevier Science B.V. All rights reserved.
Advances in Ocular Immunology
R.B. Nussenblatt, S.M. Whitcup, R.R. Caspi and I. Gery, eds.

Prognostic value of antineutrophil cytoplasmic antibodies in limited ocular Wegener's granulomatosis

W. J. Power, A. Rodriguez, R. A. Neves, L. Lane and C. S. Foster.

Immunology and Uveitis Service, Department of Ophthalmology, Massachusetts Eye and Ear Infirmary, Boston, USA.

INTRODUCTION

Wegener's granulomatosis (WG) was first described as a distinct clinicopathologic entity by Friedrich Wegener in 1939.[1] It is a necrotizing granulomatous vasculitis with a predilection typically for the upper and lower airways and the kidneys. However WG encompasses a wide spectrum of disease,and limited forms have been described.[2] The limited forms of the disease seem to be more common than first reported, probably because of increased awareness of the disease and its earlier diagnosis.[3] The diagnosis of WG is based on typical clinical findings and supporting histologic data (American College of Rheumatology classification).[4] Typical histopathologic features include inflammation of small and, less often, medium-sized vessels, necrosis, and granuloma formation.

Prior to the use of cyclophosphamide most patients with generalized WG experienced a rapidly progressive fatal illness with more than 90% dying within two years.[5,6] In prospective studies, it has been conclusively shown that Wegener's granulomatosis can be effectively treated using daily cyclophosphamide and glucocorticoids.[2,7]

Antineutrophil cytoplasmic antibodies (ANCA) have recently been described as specific markers for a group of closely related vasculitic conditions. At least two distinct classes of ANCA have been described, differentiated by characteristic immunofluorescence patterns using neutrophils as substrate for indirect immunofluorescence assay (IFA). The classic 'cytoplasmic' staining pattern (cANCA) is usually seen in WG and the perinuclear pattern (pANCA) is associated with necrotizing and crescentic glomerulonephritis (renal vasculitis) and with microscopic polyarteritis. The specificity of cANCA for biopsy-proven WG has been shown to be around 90%.[8] The sensitivity depends on the extent and activity of the disease and is about 50% for patients in the initial phase and close to 100% for patients with active generalized disease.[9] It has been suggested that rising titters may predict relapse in patients with generalized disease.[10]

The purpose of the present study was to evaluate the possible prognostic role of serum ANCAs in a group of patients with limited ocular Wegener's granulomatosis.

MATERIALS AND METHODS

Eight patients, none of whom had been diagnosed with WG before referral, were seen at the Immunology Service of the Massachusetts Eye and Ear Infirmary between 1990 and 1993. A complete ocular and systemic medical history was obtained from each patient with particular emphasis on symptoms of previous sinus, respiratory or renal disease. Standard laboratory evaluations included a complete blood count, sedimentation rate, urinalysis, serum blood urea nitrogen, creatinine, rheumatoid factor, VDRL, FTA-ABS, antinuclear antibodies (ANA), circulating immune complexes (C1q binding and Raji cell assay), and soluble interleukin 2 receptor levels. Patients also had chest and sinus x-rays performed.

At initial presentation serum from all eight patients was examined for ANCA at the Massachusetts General Hospital Immunopathology Laboratory. Serum was examined by indirect immunofluorescence staining of ethanol-fixed normal human neutrophils looking for the classic cytoplasmic staining pattern (cANCA) or the perinuclear pattern (pANCA). If positive by immunofluorescence, enzyme linked immunosorbent assay (ELISA) for the presence of specific antibodies to proteinase 3 (PR3) or myeloperoxidase (MPO) was performed. All patients had serial ANCAs performed during the course of their follow-up.

The diagnosis of limited WG was made based on the established criteria of the American College of Rheumatology classification.[6] All patients had a complete ocular examination including ultrasound, fluorescein angiography and imaging studies where appropriate. Tissue for biopsy was obtained for histopathological examination in seven of the eight patients. Tissue was harvested from conjunctiva and/or sclera.

Patients were treated with oral cyclophosphamide with the addition of oral prednisone in some cases. The goal of treatment was to achieve quiescence of active clinical disease and where possible to keep the patients' white blood cell counts (WBC) in the 3-4,000/mm^3 range. Patients were initially treated with cyclophosphamide, 2mg/kg body weight/day. Prednisone was prescribed at a dose of 1mg/kg body weight/day. Drug dosage adjustment was based on clinical response, tolerance, and hematologic parameters.

RESULTS

Eight patients (6 male and 2 female) were studied. The mean age was 52 years (range 22-71 years). The mean follow-up time was 27 months (range 7-57 months). The mean duration between onset of symptoms and referral to the Immunology Service was 9 weeks (range 2-64 weeks). Biopsy of ophthalmic tissue was characteristic of or consistent with Wegener's granulomatosis in seven patients. Four of five scleral biopsies showed features characteristic of the disease. Tissue was not available in one case. All patients achieved clinical disease remission following systemic immunosuppressive chemotherapy.

In five cases the serum ANCA did not return to normal levels during treatment. Of these five patients, three suffered ocular relapse following discontinuation of treatment. All three patients had a minimum of one year clinical disease remission before treatment was withdrawn. One of the five patients developed acute renal failure ten months after treatment was discontinued. The fifth patient, with a follow-up of 10 months has yet to convert to a negative serum ANCA although serial ANCAs have progressively decreased since treatment was instituted. The three cases who reverted to a negative serum ANCA on treatment have all remained in clinical remission to date.

DISCUSSION

ANCA's were first described in 1982 in a group of patients with necrotizing glomerulonephritis but without immune complex deposition in the basement membrane.[11] In a multicenter study reported by van der Woude, serum ANCA was found to be a sensitive marker for WG.[4] The presence and titer of these antibodies was felt to correlate with disease activity and was therefore considered a reliable serological marker for WG.[12] Two major types of ANCA have been described with indirect immunofluorescence microscopy using ethanol-fixed neutrophils as substrate; a diffuse cytoplasmic staining (cANCA) and a perinuclear staining pattern (pANCA). The former has been shown to be specific for a 29 kD serine proteinase, proteinase 3 (PR 3) which is present in neutrophil azurophilic granules.[13] The latter is specific to various lysosomal enzymes such as myeloperoxidase, cathepsin G, elastase and lactoferrin. When produced by antibodies to myeloperoxidase, as demonstrated by ELISA, pANCA is a specific marker of a disease which is characterized by a necrotizing crescentic glomerulonephritis which is often associated with a systemic microscopic polyarteritis.

Although a very sensitive serological marker in the diagnosis of WG, the correlation and prognostic value of ANCA titers with disease activity is currently still under debate. It has been suggested that a rise in serum ANCA titer during remission may in fact represent subclinical illness and justify the re commencement of immunosuppressive therapy.[10] The usefulness of ANCA in monitoring response to therapy and reactivation of disease has not been previously evaluated in patients presenting with limited ophthalmic WG. In the present longitudinal analysis of 8 patients presenting with limited ocular WG we have shown that failure to convert to a negative serum ANCA during treatment may be associated with a poorer subsequent prognosis.

REFERENCES

1.   Wegener F. Über generalisierte septische Gefäberkrankungen. Verh Dtsch Ges Pathol 1936;29:202-209.
2.   Fauci As, Wolff SM. Wegener's granulomatosis: studies in eighteen patients and a review of the literature. Medicine 1973;52:535-561.
3.   Andrews M, Edmunds M, Campbell A et al. Systemic vasculitis in the 1980's- is there an increasing incidence of Wegener's granulomatosis and microscopic polyarteritis? J Royal Coll Physiol 1990;24:284-288.
4.   Leavitt RY, Fauci AS, Block DA. Criteria for the classification of Wegener's granulomatosis. American College of Rheumatology. Arthritis Rheum 1990;33:1101-1106.
5.   Walton EW. Giant cell granuloma of the respiratory tract (Wegener's granulomatosis). Br Med J (Clin Res) 1958;2:265-270.
6.   Hollander D, Manning RT. The use of alkylating agents in the treatment of Wegener's granulomatosis. Ann Intern Med 1967;67:393-398.
7.   Fauci AS, Barton H, Katz P et al. Wegener's granulomatosis: prospective clinical and therapeutic experience with 85 patients for 21 years. Ann Int Med 1983;98:76-85.
8.   van der Woude FJ, Rasmussen N, Lobatto S et al. Autoantibodies against neutrophils and monocytes: tools for diagnosis and marker of disease activity in Wegener's granulomatosis. Lancet 1985;1:425-429.
9.   Cohen Terveart JW, van der Woude FJ, Fauci AS et al. Association between active Wegener's granulomatosis and anticytoplasmic antibodies. Arch Intern Med 1989;49:2461-2465.
10.   Cohen Terveart JW, Huitema MG, Hene RJ et el. Prevention of relapses in Wegener's granulomatosis by treatment based on antineutrophil cytoplasmic titre. Lancet 1990;336:709-711.
11.   Davies DJ, Moran JE, Niall JF et al. Segmental necrotizing glomerulonephritis with antineutrophil antibody: possible arbovirus etiology. Br Med J 1982;2:606.
12.   Lüdermann G, Gross WL. Autoantibodies against cytoplasmic structures of neutrophil granulocytes in Wegener's granulomatosis. Clin Exp Immun 1987;69:350-357.
13.   Niles JL, McCluskey Rt, Ahmad MF, Arnaout MA. Wegener's granulomatosis autoantigen is a novel neutrophil serine protease. Blood 1989;74:1888-1893.

Advances in Ocular Immunology
R.B. Nussenblatt, S.M. Whitcup, R.R. Caspi and I. Gery, eds.

Cytokine Profile in Uveitis : A Point Prevalence Study

A.H.Rahi, *A.Al-Kaff, S.L.Rahi & **J.S.Rahi,
Ministry of Health, Dammam & *KKESH, Riyadh, Saudi Arabia,
and **Institute of Ophthalmology, London.

In spite of major developments in the field of immunology and molecular biology, the precise nature of uveitis remains enigmatic. Although several distinct clinical entities are known, at best these represent a pattern-matching exercise and at worst these are simply terms of convenience which conceal our ignorance. Is uveitis an isolated phenomenon or does it represent a sick eye within a sick body? This is one of the most contentious issues in ophthalmology.

Much of our understanding of intra-ocular inflammation is derived from **experimental models of uveitis and uveo-retinitis**[1,2,3] induced by *foreign proteins* (such as BSA), gram -ve bacterial *endotoxin, ocular antigens* [such as lens protein, crude extracts of retina/choroid, retinal s-antigen, inter-retinal binding protein (IRBP), opsin, phosducin, retinal pigment epithelial protein], *synthetic uveitogenic peptides* and *cross-reacting foreign antigens* such as yeast histone (H3). Intra-ocular injection of *cytokines* such as IL-1, IL-2, IL-6, IL-8, TNF-a and GM-CSF can also produce uveitis[4,5]. It is not surprising, therefore, that the **inflammatory pathways in uveitis** are varied; these exert their influence either singly or in concert with other mediators of inflammation which include *cytokines*, various *neuropeptides* (SP, VIP, CGRP), *prostaglandins, leukotrienes* (LTB4, LTC4), *histamine, platelet activation factor* (PAF) and other *mast cell products, bradykinin*, break-down products of *complement* and various tissue destructive *enzymes* produced by inflammatory cells.

A variety of immunological abnormalities have been described in patients with uveitis which can be conveniently described under 5 headings. Abnormalities of **humoral immunity**;[6,7,8,9,10] these include raised levels of immunoglobulins (eg.IgG, IgM, IgA), circulating immune-complexes and various non-organ and organ-specific antibodies such as ANA, smooth muscle antibody, anti-vascular endothelial antibody, anti-cardiolipin antibody, anti-neutrophil cytoplasmic antibody (ANCA) and auto-antibodies to ocular antigens (eg. anti-sAg, anti-IRBP). Abnormalities of **cellular immunity**[11] include in-vitro blastogenic response of patients lymphocytes against antigens derived from retina, uvea and lens proteins and in-vivo release of cytokines. Qualitative or quantitative abnormalities of **lymphocyte subsets**[11,12,13] have also been observed in patients with uveitides. Thus helper-T cells appear to be low, whereas CD8 +ve suppressor T-cells are increased in patients with VKH, Behcet's disease and sarcoidosis. Helper T-cells are a heterogenous mixture of helper-inducer and suppressor-inducer CD4 +ve T-cells; the latter appear to increase in patients with active VKH. Although the aetiology of Behcet's is unknown, patients may show reduced activity of CD16 & CD56 +ve natural killer (NK) cells. T-cells in the peripheral blood of patients with uveitis also show evidence of in-vivo activation and express HLA-DR and IL-2 receptor (CD25) on their surface. Raised levels of several **cytokines**[14,15,16,17] (eg. IL-1, IL-2, IL-6, IL-8, TNF) have been reported in patients' serum, aqueous humor, vitreous and other ocular tissues and in several instances in situ hybridization technique has demonstrated evidence of IL-2, TNF-ß and IL-4 gene expression in the inflamed eye[18]. Furthermore, soluble IL-2 receptor (sCD25) has been demonstrated in patients' serum indicating over activity of T-cells in uveitis[19,20]. More recently soluble **adhesion molecules** such as intercellular adhesion molecule-1 (sICAM-1) and E-selectin which are derived from vascular endothelium have been found to be raised in patients with recurrent idiopathic uveo-retinitis[10]. Similarly, LFA-1 another adhesion molecule associated with lymphocytes has also been demonstrated in inflamed ocular tissues[21].

Data gathered from experimental models of uveitis and from analyses of humoral and cellular immune responses as well as of levels of cytokines and adhesion molecules in ocular tissues and blood from patient's with intra-ocular inflammation suggest that endogenous uveitis can be classified into 5 aetiopathogenetic groups.

1. **Hetero-immune uveitis**, which could be infective or non-infective.
2. **Auto-immune uveitis** triggered by immune response to lens proteins, various retinal or pigment epithelial antigens or by anti-endothelial, anti-phospholipid, or anti-neutrophil cytoplasmic (ANCA) antibodies.
3. **Uveitis associated with endothelial dysfunction** due to aberrant expression of adhesion molecules in the blood vessels of the retina and the uvea.
4. **Reactive uveitis** similar in pathogenesis to reactive arthritis following gut, genito-urinary or other infections in which endotoxin and other bacterial products supposedly play important role in collaboration with IL-1, IL-6, IL-8 & TNF.
5. **Idiopathic uveitis**; in this miscellaneous group, there is no obvious cellular, humoral or cytokine abnormality. This possibly includes cases which belong to one of the 4 groups mentioned above, but may not be obvious at the initial stages.

Recent studies indicate that antigen presenting cells hand over immunogenic peptides to helper-T cells in association with class II histocompatibility antigens. These cells in turn secrete interleukin-2 and thus recruit other helper T-cells to initiate humoral and cellular immune responses. T-helper 1 (TH1) mediates cellular immunity by secreting IL-2, gamma-IFN and lymphotoxin (TNF-ß) and by activating cytotoxic T-cells, macrophages and NK-cells. T-helper 2 (TH2) on the other hand modulates antibody-mediated responses by secreting IL-4, IL-5, IL-6, IL-10, IL-13. There is also evidence, that TH1 & TH2 can suppress the activity of each other through gamma-interferon and IL-10 respectively. The roles of TH1 & TH2 are well established in rodents, but their significance in human disease has not been well established except in few conditions such as leprosy & leishmaniasis. The pathogenetic role of TH1 in experimental and clinical uveo-retinitis seems to be certain, but the significance of TH2 has not been established. The purpose of this investigation is to examine the relative roles of cytokines derived from TH1 & TH2 in the pathogenesis of uveitis. Serum has been examined in the present study even though the examination of aqueous humor may have been apparently more meaningful, because if the serum shows abnormality, it will mean that uveitis is a localized manifestation of a generalized disease, which may or may not become manifest at the time of presentation or during the course of uveitis.

Method & Material

Forty-five patients with various types of uveitis [Behcet's (20), VKH (5), retinal vasculitis (9) & chronic anterior uveitis (11)] were included in the present study. Serum from these patients and 41 healthy blood donors were tested for interleukin-2, IL-6, gamma-interferon and TNF-a by ELISA using commercial kits (Genzyme, Cambridge, MA). The standard curve was generated by a computer programme, which allowed modification of lower level of detection by extrapolation. The manufacturer's lower level of detection limit based on linear correlation was 100 pg/ml for IL-2 & g-IFN, 18 pg/ml for IL-6 and 10 pg/ml for TNF-a. Except for gamma-interferon (in normal controls and Behcet's disease), other cytokine levels were not normally distributed, therefore non-parametric analyses were carried out using the Mann-Whitney U test and Spearman's rank correlation test to evaluate associations between the cytokines.

Results

The results are summarized in the table below. IL-2 & g-IFN (both products of TH1) were raised in all patients with uveitis, whereas IL-6 (product of TH2) and TNF-a were significantly raised only in patients with retinal vasculitis. A negative correlation was observed between levels of IL-2 & IL-6 ($p < 0.05$) in patients with Behcet's disease and VKH, whereas, there was positive correlation between IL-2, IL-6 & g-IFN in retinal vasculitis ($p < 0.05$)

Table I : Cytokine levels in uveitis

	IL-2 (pg/ml)		G-IFN (pg/ml)		IL-6 (pg/ml)		TNF-a (pg/ml)	
	Median (Range)	p Value	Median (Range)	p Value	Median (Range)	p Value	Median (Range)	p Value
Control (41)	50 (1-260)		48 (7-78)		2.5 (1-6)		2 (1-5)	
Behcet's (20)	646 (76-6142)	<0.001	206 (128-240)	<0.001	3 (1-20)	NS	2 (1-10)	NS
Retinal Vasculitis (9)	288 (76-1700)	<0.001	176 (108-220)	<0.001	18 (8-68)	<0.001	153 (82-504)	<0.001
VKH (5)	740 (294-2670)	<0.001	192 (184-216)	<0.001	2 (1.5-8)	NS	2 (1-4)	NS
Chronic Ant. Uveitis (11)	288 (64-2600)	<0.001	184 (16-220)	<0.001	3 (1-13)	NS	3 (2-15)	<0.05

Discussion

Although the aetiology of endogenous intra-ocular inflammation is unknown, both experimental and clinical studies suggest that interleukins and other cytokines play significant roles in the pathogenesis of uveitis. The present study shows high levels of IL-2 and g-IFN, not only in those cases of uveitis in which there is known systemic involvement (eg. VKH & Behcet's disease), but also in cases of isolated retinal vasculitis and chronic anterior uveitis in which, there were no obvious systemic manifestations. From this, it can be assumed that uveitis is a localized disease resulting from generalized activation of the immune system due to an apparent or inapparent systemic disease. The presence of high levels of IL-6 in retinal vasculitis suggests that in this disease, humoral auto-immune responses may also be significant. It is of relevance in this context that in patients with retinal vasculitis, high levels of anti-endothelial and anti-phospholipid antibodies have been reported[9,10]. To the best of our knowledge, no such study has been carried out before, in which the relative significance of these 4 cytokines in uveitis has been examined. Raised levels of g-IFN have been reported, however, in serum from few cases of VKH[15]. Raised IL-6 in aqueous humor appears to be a feature not only of VKH, but also of heterochromic cyclitis and ocular toxoplasmosis[13,14]. Apart from TH2, ocular tissues, such as retinal pigment epithelium may also contribute to IL-6 levels[22]. Patients with Behcet's disease and retinal vasculitis not only have high levels of IL-2 in their blood (as shown in this study), but they also seem to produce soluble IL-2 receptor[20] possibly as a compensatory protective response. Soluble IL-2 receptor is also raised in serum from patients with retinal vasculitis and heterochromic cyclitis[19]. Raised levels of IL-2, TNF & IL-6 have been demonstrated in vitreous specimens from patients who had suffered from intra-ocular inflammation in the past[16].

In a recent study, levels of IL-6 and TNF-a were examined in patients with intra-ocular inflammation as well as cicatricial pemphigoid[23]. Raised levels of TNF were found only in the latter group. Vitreous from patients with proliferative vitro-retinopathy following retinal detachment also contains high levels of IL-6[16]. In situ hybridization techniques have demonstrated presence of mRNA for IL-2, IL-4 & lymphotoxin in T-lymphocytes infiltrating ocular tissues in experimental auto-immune uveo-retinitis[3,18]. Since IL-2 was raised in all the 4 varieties of uveitis studied, it can be concluded that cyclosporin A could be used for the management of most recalcitrant cases.

Summary & Conclusions

IL-2 & g-IFN were raised in serum from patients with Behcet's disease, VKH, isolated retinal vasculitis and chronic anterior uveitis. This suggests that even if there is no clinically apparent systemic disease, uveitis may result from generalized stimulation of the immune system. Presence of IL-6 & TNF-a in retinal vasculitis suggests additional pathogenetic role of these cytokines either directly or through modulation of humoral immunity. Immuno-suppressive drugs such as cyclosporin A can suppress the IL-2 production, whereas anti-cytokine antibodies can be used to neutralize the activity of other cytokines. Enthusiasm must, however, be tempered with caution since anti-cytokine may act as a double-edged sword: it may sometimes perpetuate uveitis by interfering with the catabolism of the cytokine.

References

1. Nussenblatt R : Invest.Oph.Vis.Sc. 1991; 32 : 3131-3140.
2. Dick A, Cheng Y, Liversidge J & Forrester J : Eye, 1994; 8 : 52-59.
3. Barton K & Lightman S : Eye, 1994; 8 : 60-65.
4. Kulkarni PS & Mancino M : Exp.Eye.Res. 1993; 56 : 275-79.
5. Samples JR, Boney RS, Rosenbaum T : Curr.Eye.Res. 1993; 12 : 649-54.
6. Rahi AHS & Garner A:Immunopath. of the Eye.Oxford,Blackwell Scientific, 1976.
7. Rahi AHS, Holborow E, Perkins E, et al : Trans.Ophth.Soc.UK.1976; 96 : 113-21.
8. Rahi AHS, Kanski J & Fielder A : Trans.Ophth.Soc.UK. 1977; 97 : 217-22.
9. Rahi A, Rahi S & Rahi J:Ocular Immunol Today, Elsevier Sc.Publ. 1990; 317-20.
10. Zaman A, Edelsten C, Stanford M et al : Clin.exp.Immunol. 1994; 95 : 60-65.
11. Hamzaoui K, Ayed K, Slim A et al : Clin.exp.Immunol. 1990; 79 : 28-34.
12. Nussenblatt R, Cevario S, Gery I : Lancet 1980; 2 : 722.
13. Norose K, Yanow A, Wang XC : Invest.Ophth.Vis.Sc. 1994; 35 : 33-39.
14. Murray P, Hoekzema R, VanHaren M, et al : Invest.Oph.Vis.Sc. 1990; 31:917-20.
15. Hirayama M,Kiyosawa K,Nakazaki S et al:Rien.Schin(Clin.Neurol)1990;30:552-59.
16. Franks WA, Limb GA, Stanford MR, et al : Curr.Eye.Res. 1992; 11(5) : 187-91.
17. de Boer JA, Hack CE, Verhoevan AJ, et al : Invest.Ophthal.Vis.Sc. 1993; 34:3376-85.
18. Charteris DG & Lightman SL : Immunology 1993; 78 : 387-92.
19. Murray PI & Young DW : Curr.Eye.Res. 1993; 11(Suppl) : 193-95.
20. Ben Ezra D, Maftzir G, Kalichman I, et al : Amer.J.Ophth. 1993; 115 : 26-30.
21. Whitcup SM, Chan CC, Li Q, et al : Arch.Ophth. 1992; 110 : 662-66.
22. Benson MT, Shepherd L, Rees RC, et al : Curr.Eye.Res. 1992; 11(S) : 173-79.
23. Lee SJ, Li Z, Sherman B, et al : Invest.Oph.Vis.Sc. 1993; 34 : 3522-25.

© 1994 Elsevier Science B.V. All rights reserved.
Advances in Ocular Immunology
R.B. Nussenblatt, S.M. Whitcup, R.R. Caspi and I. Gery, eds.

Ocular prognosis of scleritis and systemic vasculitic diseases

M. Sainz de la Maza[a] and C.S. Foster[b]

[a] Ophthalmology Department, Hospital Clinico, Central University of Barcelona, Urgel 224, Barcelona 08036, Spain

[b] Immunology Service, Massachusetts Eye and Ear Infirmary Hospital, Harvard Medical School, 243 Charles St., Boston, MA 02114, USA

INTRODUCTION

Scleritis may occur isolated or in association with several types of diseases. Immune-mediated diseases, such as the vasculitides, are not only the most frequent but also the most severe systemic conditions which may involve sclera [1]. The vasculitides include the connective tissue diseases and other inflammatory conditions in which vasculitis may occur, and the primary vasculitic diseases. They are characterized by inflammatory vascular lesions in many organs of the body, including the eye. Inflammatory vascular lesions in sclera may be a manifestation of a generalized systemic vasculitis.

The detection of SVD in patients with scleritis is a sign of poor general prognosis because it indicates serious systemic complications [2]. However, it is not clear whether or not the detection of a SVD in patients with scleritis alters significatively the ocular outcome.

The purpose of this study was to evaluate the ocular prognosis of patients with scleritis associated with SVD. Results may have therapeutic implications.

MATERIAL AND METHODS

We reviewed the records of 172 patients (231 eyes) with scleritis seen on the Immunology Service at the Massachusetts Eye and Ear Infirmary during an 11-year period and classified them into those with and without associated systemic vasculitic disease (SVD).

Scleritis was characterized following the classification of Watson and Hayreh as anterior (diffuse, nodular, necrotizing, and scleromalacia perforans) and posterior [3].

Criteria for diagnoses of the different SVD associated with scleritis have been published elsewhere [4]. The diagnostic approach was repeated every six months in cases where scleritis could not be ascribed to any associated disease.

Demographic information, bilaterality of scleritis, and follow-up were recorded. The following conditions were considered as ocular complications: decrease in vision (defined as loss of vision equal or greater to two Snellen lines at the end of the follow-up period or vision equal or worse than 20/80 at presentation), anterior uveitis, peripheral ulcerative keratitis, glaucoma, and cataract.

Comparisons were made between patients with scleritis with and without SVD. Statistical analysis was performed using a multifactorial analysis of variance (statistically significant: $p < 0.05$) for all conditions except age (Mann-Whitney non parametric test).

RESULTS

A total of 82 patients (113 eyes) with scleritis had an associated SVD (47.67%). Patients with scleritis with SVD were compared with patients with scleritis without SVD (90 patients, 118 eyes) (Table 1).

Thirty of the patients with scleritis associated with SVD had diffuse scleritis, 15 patients had nodular scleritis, 29 patients had necrotizing scleritis, 4 patients had scleromalacia perforans, and 4 patients had posterior scleritis. Comparisons of types of scleritis between patients with scleritis with and without SVD showed that diffuse scleritis was significantly more frequent in patients without SVD (p=0.0396) and necrotizing scleritis was significantly more frequent in patients with SVD (p=0.0001). Nodular scleritis did not differ significantly when compared in patients with scleritis with and without SVD.

Patients with scleritis with SVD (mean age: 55.24 years; range 15-81 years) were older than those without SVD (mean age: 48.29 years; range 11-87 years) (p=0.0062). Forty-eight of the patients (58.54%) with scleritis with SVD were female and 34 (41.46%) were male. This female predominance did not differ significantly when patients with scleritis with and without SVD were compared. Scleritis was bilateral in 31 patients (37.80%) with SVD and in 28 patients (31.11%) without SVD. This difference was not statistically significant.

In patients with scleritis with SVD, decrease in vision was detected in 40 (48.78%), anterior uveitis in 39 (47.56%), peripheral ulcerative keratitis in 20 (24.39%), glaucoma in 14 (17.03%), and cataract in 20 (24.39%). Comparisons of these conditions between patients with and without SVD revealed that decrease in vision and peripheral ulcerative keratitis were significantly more frequently found in patients with SVD (p=0.0026 and p=0.0001, respectively), and that anterior uveitis, glaucoma, and cataract were found in a similar proportion of patients in both groups.

Table 1
Comparisons between Scleritis with and without
Systemic Vasculitic Diseases

Condition	Scleritis with SVD (%) (n=82)	Scleritis without SVD (%) (n=90)	
Type of Scleritis			
Diffuse	30 (36.58)	47 (52.22)	p=0.0396
Nodular	15 (18.29)	24 (26.67)	NS
Necrotizing	29 (35.37)	10 (11.11)	p=0.0001
Scleromalacia*	4 (4.88)	2 (2.22)	
Posterior*	4 (4.88)	7 (7.78)	
Sex: Female/Male	48 / 34	57 / 33	NS
Bilaterality	31 (37.80)	28 (31.11)	NS
Decrease in Vision	40 (48.78)	24 (26.67)	p=0.0026
Anterior Uveitis	39 (47.56)	34 (37.78)	NS
PUK	20 (24.39)	4 (4.44)	p=0.0001
Glaucoma	14 (17.03)	8 (8.89)	NS
Cataract	20 (24.39)	9 (10)	NS

SVD: systemic vasculitic disease; PUK: peripheral ulcerative keratitis; NS: non significant (p>0.05); * not included in the multifactorial analysis of variance due to small number of patients

DISCUSSION

Scleritis may occur alone or as a manifestation of a variety of non immune-mediated or immune-mediated disorders. Within the immune-mediated disorders, SVD are the most frequent conditions associated with scleritis [1]. The histopathologic and immunofluorescence detection of immune complex inflammatory microangiopathy in affected scleral biopsy specimens [5], the absence of vascular perfusion in severe types of scleritis on anterior segment fluorescein angiography [6], and the favorable response of scleritis to immunosuppressive drugs [7], suggest that scleritis associated with SVD shares the same pathogenetic process of the underlying disease, including vessel damage and tissue destruction, as well as cell-mediated immune reactions [5]. As the results of this study show, SVD are the most severe and destructive conditions which may involve sclera; the detection of SVD in a patient with scleritis carries a poor ocular prognosis since patients with scleritis with SVD more commonly have necrotizing scleritis, decrease in vision, and peripheral ulcerative keratitis than do patients with scleritis without SVD.

Since the presence of scleritis may indicate an underlying potentially lethal systemic vasculitis, it is essential to detect the ocular and the systemic condition as early as possible, so that vigorous treatment can favorably alter the ocular and systemic prognosis of these patients. We conclude from this study that the detection of a SVD in a patient with scleritis provides valuable ocular prognostic information since patients with scleritis with SVD have a worse ocular prognosis than do patients with scleritis without SVD.

REFERENCES

1   Sainz de la Maza M, Jabbur NS, Foster CS. Severity of scleritis and episcleritis. Ophthalmology 1994; 101:389-96.
2   Foster CS, Forstot SL, Wilson LA. Mortality rate in rheumatoid arthritis patients developing necrotizing scleritis or peripheral ulcerative keratitis. Ophthalmology 1984; 91:1253-63.
3   Watson PG, Hayreh SS. Scleritis and episcleritis. Br J Ophthalmol 1976; 60:163-91.
4   Foster CS, Sainz de la Maza M. The Sclera. New York: Springer-Verlag, 1994; chapter 6.
5   Fong LP, Sainz de la Maza M, Rice BA, Foster CS. Immunopathology of scleritis. Ophthalmology 1991; 98:472-79.
6   Hakin KN, Watson PG. Systemic associations of scleritis. Int Ophthalmol Clin 1991; 31(3):111-29.
7   Sainz de la Maza M, Jabbur NS, Foster CS. An analysis of therapeutic decision for scleritis. Ophthalmology 1993; 100:1372-6.

Advances in Ocular Immunology
R.B. Nussenblatt, S.M. Whitcup, R.R. Caspi and I. Gery, eds.

THYGESON'S SUPERFICIAL PUNCTATE KERATITIS: MANAGEMENT USING
IMMUNOMODULATORS. Mark D. Sherman, Douglas S. Holsclaw, and Ira G.
Wong. The Francis I. Proctor Foundation, Southern California Permanente Medical
Group, Northern California Permanente Medical Group, and University of California,
San Francisco. San Francisco, California USA 94143

INTRODUCTION

Thygeson's superficial punctate keratitis (TSPK) is a chronic recurrent inflammatory disorder affecting the cornea. The condition is characterized by repeated episodes of photophobia, tearing and foreign body sensation. Exacerbations may last 2 to 4 weeks, followed by remissions lasting 4 to 6 weeks. The cycle of exacerbations and remissions may occur over 30 years. On examination, the eye displays multiple coarse, punctate, elevated corneal epithelial lesions. Under high magnification, these lesions appear as a conglomeration of smaller white or grey dots that stain with fluorescein when the disease is active. The surrounding corneal tissue is clear and the bulbar conjunctiva is usually quiet. When the disease is inactive, the classic lesions generally disappear and the patient is asymptomatic. Subepithelial lesions are rare and have been associated with previous use of antiviral medications. Bilateral lesions are found in over 90% of the cases. TSPK has been described in individuals from 2 1/2 to 85 years of age. There is no sexual predilection. An etiologic agent has not been consistently identified, although a viral etiology has been proposed.

In 1950, Thygeson described 26 patients with superficial punctate keratitis that he had been studying for 20 years. Although he could not successfully culture a viral agent from these epithelial lesions, he noted the striking clinical resemblance to other known viral infections affecting the corneal epithelium. Braley (1953) described a case of superficial punctate keratitis in which a viral agent was grown in embryo mouse brain tissue culture and caused corneal lesions in a rabbit model. His experiments have never been successfully repeated. Braley noted that topical steroids caused the epithelial lesions to resolve. Lemp (1974) reported the isolation of varicella-zoster virus from the epithelial surface of a 10 year old boy with TSPK. The child had contracted varicella six years earlier. Further efforts to isolate a microbial agent from patients with TSPK have been unsuccessful. Ostler (1993) has suggested that the condition is caused by a slow virus, which would explain its long course of exacerbations and remissions and the difficulty in obtaining culture and serologic evidence of infection. In 1981, Darrell reported an association of TSPK with HLA-DR3, further supporting the idea that immune mechanisms modulate the expression of this condition.

Management of TSPK has included patching, contact lenses, epithelial debridement, topical antivirals and topical steroids. The effective use of topical cyclosporin A has recently been described (Holsclaw et al, 1994). The purpose of this study was to review our treatment of 24 recent cases of TSPK.

Materials and Methods

We retrospectively reviewed the records of 24 consecutive patients with TSPK referred to our Cornea/External Disease Service during the past three years. Each patient underwent a detailed history and complete eye examination. The diagnosis of TSPK was based on standard clinical criteria outlined by Thygeson (1966). During the initial examination, patients were offered a variety of therapeutic options, including patching, contact lenses, topical NSAIDs (ketorolac, flurbiprofen) and topical steroids (fluorometholone alcohol 0.1%, prednisolone acetate 0.12%, prednisolone acetate 1.0%). The choice of initial therapy was determined by each patient's previous treatment history and the severity of their symptoms, as well as the patient's own preference following a discussion of the potential side effects of each treatment modality. All topical medications were prescribed for a QID regimen. Treatment success was defined as symptomatic improvement and reduction of the number of epithelial lesions after one week of medications. Treatment failure was defined as persistence of symptoms following one week of QID treatment for topical medications. In the case of treatment failure, patients were offered the option to increase the potency of their medications in a step-wise fashion (e.g. topical NSAID, FML, Pred mild, Pred forte, cyclosporin A). Patients were examined at weekly intervals while their disease was active.

Results

Our collection of 24 patients with TSPK included 12 males and 12 females. The average age was 34 years. The age range was 14 to 70 years. Thirteen patients received a topical NSAID eyedrop. Two of these patients demonstrated a positive response (NSAID = 2/13). Five out of 17 patients showed a positive response to fluorometholone alcohol 0.1% (FML = 5/17). Three out of 5 patients showed a positive response to prednisolone acetate 1/8% (Pred mild = 3/5). Eight out of 12 patients showed a positive response to prednisolone acetate 1.0% (Pred forte = 8/12). Two patients that showed a favorable response to Pred forte had a significant rise in intraocular pressure (IOP). The Pred forte was discontinued and they were started on topical cyclosporin A 2%. Their IOP returned to normal and they showed a positive response to cyclosporin. A total of 7 patients were given Cyclosporin A 2%. All 7 showed a positive response (CycA = 7/7).

Discussion

TSPK is a recurrent inflammatory eye condition that can cause incapacitating symptoms. Several features of the disease suggest a viral etiology, although an etiologic agent has never been consistently isolated. The exquisite sensitivity to topical steroids and topical cyclosporin A demonstrated in this review supports the idea of immunologic mechanisms modulating the expression of this condition.

As a referral center, most of our patients had already failed more conservative treatments by their own ophthalmologists. However, some patients may initially respond to patching, artificial tears, contact lenses, or other approaches. Forstot et al (1979) reported the effective use of soft contact lenses for TSPK. They noted this therapy avoids the potential complications of long-term steroid use, such as cataracts, glaucoma, and supra-infections. Goldberg et al (1980) found patching to be another effective form of therapy. Nesburn (1984) has reported success using 1% trifluridine. However, others have not had similar success with antiviral medications. Idoxuridine has been associated with the development of subepithelial opacities (Tabbara, 1981). The potential for corneal scarring (even without the use of antivirals) in prolonged disease has also been described by Abbott et al (1979).

Our review of 24 recent cases of TSPK supports the use of topical steroids as the mainstay in the treatment of this condition. An effort to start patients on the lowest dose of steroids should be made prior to using stronger agents. Patients that are placed on topical steroids must be carefully followed, as the risk of "self-medication" is high in this chronic/recurrent condition and a rise in IOP may occur. Cyclosporin A appears to be an excellent alternative to steroids for recalcitrant cases of TSPK. The long term effects of topical cyclosporin A requires further investigation.

References

Abbott, R.L., Forster, R.K.: Superficial punctate keratitis of Thygeson associated with scarring and Salzmann's nodular degeneration. Am. J. Ophthalmol., 87: 296, 1979.

Braley, A.E., Alexander, R.C.: Superficial punctate keratitis. Isolation of a virus. Arch. Ophthalmol., 50: 147, 1953.

Darrell, R.W., Suiciu-Foca, N.: HLA DR3 in Thygeson's superficial punctate keratitis. Tissue Antigens, 18: 203, 1981.

Forstot, S.L., Binder, P.S.: Treatment of Thygeson's superficial punctate keratopathy with soft contact lenses. Am. J. Ophthalmol., 88: 186, 1979.

Goldberg, D.B., Schanzlin, D.J., Brown, S.I.: Management of Thygeson's superficial punctate keratitis. Am. J. Ophthalmol., 89: 22, 1980.

Holsclaw, D.S., Wong, I.G., Sherman, M.D.: Masked trial of topical cyclosporine A in the treatment of refractory Thygeson's superficial punctate keratitis. Invest. Ophthalmol (supp.) 35: 1302, 1994.

Lemp, M.A., Chambers, R.W., Lurdy, J.: Viral isolation in superficial punctate keratitis. Arch. Ophthalmol. 91: 8, 1974.

380

Nesburn, A.B., Lowe, G.H., Lepoff, N.J., Maguen, E.: Effect of topical trifluridine on Thygeson's superficial punctate keratitis. Ophthalmology 91: 1188, 1984.

Ostler, H.B.: Diseases of the external eye and adnexa. Baltimore: Williams and Wilkins, 1993.

Tabbara, K.F., Ostler, H.B., Dawson, C., Oh, J.: Thygeson's superficial punctate keratitis. Ophthalmology, 88: 75, 1981.

Thygeson, P.: Superficial punctate keratitis. JAMA, 144: 1544, 1950.

Thygeson, P.: Further observations on superficial punctate keratitis. Arch. Ophthalmol., 66: 34, 1961.

Thygeson, P.: Clinical and laboratory observations on superficial punctate keratitis. Am. J. Ophthalmol. 61: 1344, 1966.

Advances in Ocular Immunology
R.B. Nussenblatt, S.M. Whitcup, R.R. Caspi and I. Gery, eds.

Serology in the ophthalmic oncology - findings and outlook for the future

S. Suchkov[a], A. Gabibov[b], G. Gololobov[b], T. Loginova[a], N. Yurovskaya[a], and A. Brovkina[a]

[a]Helmholtz Eye Research Institute, 14/19 Sadovaya Chernogryazskaya Street, P.O. Box 103064, Moscow, Russia

[b]Engelhardt Institute of Molecular Biology, 32 Vavilov Street, Moscow, Russia

INTRODUCTION

Sera of patients with intraocular tumors apart from having the primary antigen, contained, in some cases, the corresponding autoantibodies (Suchkov et al., 1993). The latter finding is especially interesting in that some of those autoantibodies could represent some of the features of the primary antigen, including the catalytic activity pertaining to the antigen.

The nature of those autoantibodies (abzymes) is now a subject of intensive studies; so is the mechanism of their catalytic function. In similar but earlier studies, it was shown that sera of patients with systemic autoimmunity conditions, e.g. lupus (SLE), rheumatoid arthritis, mixed connective tissue diseases, and *myasthenia gravis* contained autoantibodies and anti-idiotypic antibodies to DNA, DNA-binding proteins, and topoisomerase I. The latter finding is especially interesting in that anti-idiotypic autoantibodies to topoisomerase I reveal a high affinity to DNA, a specific substrate for the primary autoantigen (Gabibov et al., 1992). Autoantibodies catalyzing the cleavage of peptide bonds have been also found in sera of patients with systemic autoimmunity. The same was established to be partly true for local (ophthalmic) autoimmune conditions, e.g. autoimmune uveitis and sympathetic ophthalmia (Suchkov et al., 1992, 1993). Little is known about the distribution profile of those autoantibodies in patients harboring different types of the intraocular tumors. The main purpose of this study is to assess properly possible diagnostic and prognostic values of the identified parallels within a group of the intraocular tumors.

PATIENTS, MATERIALS AND METHODS

We investigated topoisomerase I immunoreactivity as well as the occurrence of the anti-topoisomerase I autoantibodies of the 1st and 2nd orders (including DNA-binding and DNA-cleavage activity of the latter) in sera and tears of 47 patients with intraocular tumors (including 37 well-differentiated retinoblastomas and 10 uveal melanomas) using topoisomerase I and the corresponding autoantibodies as probes. Control samples were taken from healthy volunteers and the patients with breast carcinomas as well.

From a cohort of patients harboring retinoblastomas, 17 were with the bilateral tumor and 20 - with the unilateral one, aged from 3 to 42.

Screening of sera was done both for the presence of topoisomeraseI-specific autoantibodies and the appropriate anti-idiotypic autoantibodies by ELISA, and for the presence of and level of the catalytic activity of DNA-specific autoantibodies by agarose gel electrophoresis. ELISA and immunoblotting were used as reported (Gololobov et al., 1989). Tears from patients with intraocular tumors conditions were screened only for the presence of topoisomerase I-specific autoantibodies and the appropriate anti-idiotypic autoantibodies by ELISA as mentioned above.

Isolation of the catalytic autoantibodies (abzymes) from the serum of a patient with a full-blown picture of SLE was done by a combination of different column chromatography techniques, including affinity chromatography on Protein A-Sepharose and DNA-cellulose. The purification was completed by using of HPLC (TSK 3000 SW) and ion-exchange chromatography (Mono Q column).

RESULTS

In total, 69 serum and 37 tears samples were examined (Table 1).

Table 1.
Samples analyzed for topoisomerase I immunoreactivity.

Subjects	Fluid	Number
Normal	serum	13
	tears	7
Malignant melanoma	serum	10
	tears	7
Retinoblastoma	serum	37
	tears	20

- bilateral	serum	17
	tears	10
- unilateral	serum	20
	tears	10
Breast carcinoma	serum	9
	tears	3

No anti-topoisomerase I immunoreactivity was detected in normal (healthy volunteers) serum and tears samples. There was an evidence of both topoisomerase I and anti-topoisomerase I immunoreactivity in sera of 100% and in tears of 69% of breast carcinomas. Serum anti-topoisomerase I was also found in 37% retinoblastomas and in 30% uveal melanomas. In tears, the distribution of the anti-topoisomerase I appeared to be as 32% in retinoblastoma and as 27% - in uveal melanoma. Statistically significant titres of anti-topoisomerase I autoantibodies were found in bilateral retinoblastomas both in tears and serum samples. Irrespective of type of the tumor, the frequency of the second-order autoantibodies was lower than 18-20% as compared that for the first order ones. However, in bilateral retinoblastomas high titres of those autoantibodies were persistent in serum and tears samples in 68% of cases.

It is interesting that in patients with retinoblastoma aged between 3 and 10, serum titres of anti-topoisomerase I autoantibodies and corresponding abzymes were statistically higher than in adult patients with the same type of malignancy. No correlation was found in tears samples between those groups. No differences in anti-topoisomerase I immunoreactivity were also found within a group of patients with intraocular malignant melanoma.

DISCUSSION

Our results further substantiate the specific humoral immune mechanisms involvement into the intraocular tumor pathogenesis, and stress the clinical significance of further studies of the role of the non-specific (broad-range) tissue antigens and the autoantibodies network in those patients.

It appears to be of particular importance to have the differences found in the anti-topoisomerase I immunoreactivity between two cohorts of patients - with retinoblastoma and intraocular malignant melanomas. The problem is that intraocular malignant melanoma is usually typical for all ages, but retinoblastoma is the commonest malignancy of infancy.

The latter may be also bilateral or unilateral. Correct diagnosis and proper prediction, without recourse, is vital, since it is undiserable both to enucleate an eye for binign condition and to miss a fatal, though potentially curable, malignant tumor. If doubt about the diagnosis still exists after tests, such as a CT, scan have been performed, methods such as the biochemical assay of aqueous humour enzymes or non-specific immunotests have been advocated. However, very similar interpretation of the above-mentioned tests might be made for other conditions, such as ophthalmic autoimmunity conditions or Coats's disease. As we have established, retinoblastoma is associated with increased levels of anti-topoisomerase I autoantibodies and the corresponding abzymes. While serum criteria proposed may be of a diagnostic and prognostic help for an ophthalmic surgeon, there might be occasions when the similar tears' indices are valuable for diagnosis as well. However, further studies need to be performed on a larger population to assess the full potential of this approach.

REFERENCES

1   Suchkov S, Yurovskaya N Oftalmologiya (in Russian) 1982; 8: 21-26.

2   Suchkov S, Yurovskaya N Vestnik Oftalmologii (in Russian) 1983; 3: 70-72.

3   Suchkov S, Trebukhina E, Yurovskaya N, Sukhanov V . In: Abelev G, eds.18th Meeting of the International Society for Oncodevelopmental Biology and Medicine. Moscow: 1990; 85.

4   Gabibov A, Gololobov G, Kvashuk O, Shuster A Science 1992; 4: 679-686.

Advances in Ocular Immunology
R.B. Nussenblatt, S.M. Whitcup, R.R. Caspi and I. Gery, eds.

Flow cytometric analysis of surface markers of cerebrospinal fluid cells and peripheral blood lymphocytes from VKH disease

M. SUGITA[a], S. NAKAMURA[a], S. TANAKA[b], F. ISODA[c], K. OKUDA[c] and S. OHNO[a]

[a]Department of Ophthalmology, [b]Department of 3rd Internal medicine and [c]Department of Bacteriology,Yokohama City University School of Medicine, 3-9 Fuku-ura, Knazawa-ku, Yokohama 236, Japan

INTRODUCTON

Vogt-Koyanagi-Harada's disease (VKH disease) is believed to be an autoimmune disease affecting melanocytes[1]. Pleocytosis in cerebrospinal fluid (CSF) usually occurs during the acute phase of the disease. It was reported that CD4 positive cells were higher in CSF than in peripheral blood (PB) from VKH patients[2]. Recently, two new T cell subsets have been identified by CD45RA and CD45RO monoclonal antibodies. These are probably involved in the regulation of immunological memory. CD45RA positive cells are called virgin or naive cells and CD45RO positive cells are called memory cells[3]. There are no reports about these surface markers of VKH disease. To investigate the immunological mechanisms of VKH disease, we analysed CD45RA and CD45RO of the CSF cells and PB lymphocytes (PBL) from VKH patients before and after the treatment with flow cytometry in this study.

MATERIAL AND METHODS

We studied 11 patients with VKH disease (7 males and 4 females). The mean age was 38 years, ranging from 22 to 66. CSF cells and PBL were collected before and 4 weeks after the systemic treatment. Seven were treated with systemic corticosteroids and 4 were treated with new immunosuppressant, FK506.

Cell Preparation

Immediately after sterile lumbar puncture, CSF cells were collected from 2 to 5 ml of CSF by centrifugation for 10 minutes at 1700 rpm, and were suspended by PBS contained 0.3% BSA and 0.1% NaN_3.

On the same day, PBL were obtained from the heparinized venous blood. Both CSF cells and PBL were stained by mAbs as described below.

Monoclonal antibodies

Fluorescine-conjugated mAbs, anti-CD4 (Anti-Leu 3a), CD8 (Leu 2a), CD25 (Anti-IL 2R) and CD45RA (Leu 18) and phycoerytrin-conjugated mAbs, anti-CD3 (Anti-Leu 4a), CD4 (Leu 3a), CD19 (Leu 12) and CD45RO (Leu 45RO) (Becton & Dickinson) were used.

Flow cytometry

Two color analysis was carried out on EPICS ELITE Flow Cytometer (Coulter) equipped with a dual laser for green (FITC) and red (PE) fluorescence. All results were expressed as percentages of each subset to total lymphocytes. Each subset of CSF cells was compared with that of PBL. Furthermore, each subset of CSF cells and PBL was compared between before and after the treatment. The Student's t test and Mann-Whitney test were used for statistical comparisons.

RESULTS

Before systemic treatment, CD3$^+$, CD4$^+$, CD4$^+$CD45RO$^+$ cells were significantly higher in CSF cells than in PBL, whereas CD8$^+$, CD4$^+$CD45RA$^+$ cells were significantly lower in CSF cells than in PBL. Therefore CD4$^+$/CD8$^+$ ratio and CD45RO$^+$/CD45RA$^+$ ratio in CSF were higher than in PBL (p<0.01). CD19$^+$ and CD4$^+$CD25$^+$ cells in CSF were similar to those in PBL. As the rate of CD4$^+$ and CD8$^+$ in CSF became similar to those in PB, CD4$^+$/CD8$^+$ ratio in CSF was not high after the treatment. On the other hand, CD45RO$^+$/CD45RA$^+$ ratio remained in high level after the treatment as CD4$^+$CD45RO$^+$ cells did not reduce after the treatment (Figure 1, 2). The rate of CD19$^+$ and CD8$^+$ in CSF were increased after the treatment (Table 1). There was no significant difference in each subset between corticosteroid treated group and FK506 treated group.

Table 1. Mean percentage of T and B cell subsets in the CSF and PB of before and after thetreatment.

		CSF			PB			p
CD3$^+$	before	89.4	±	6.3^a	73.7	±	7.8	0.01
	after	81.7	±	9.3^a	69.7	±	10.0	0.05
CD19$^+$	before	3.0	±	1.5^b	9.2	±	5.3	0.01
	after	12.6	±	6.7^b	15.3	±	6.5	N.S.
CD4$^+$	before	68.8	±	7.8^c	46.4	±	9.9	0.01
	after	53.4	±	14.2^c	45.6	±	6.2	N.S.
CD8$^+$	before	20.2	±	5.6^d	31.3	±	11.3	0.01
	after	26.9	±	8.7^d	30.4	±	7.5	N.S.
CD4$^+$ CD25$^+$	before	11.2	±	2.9^e	12.1	±	13.5	N.S.
	after	5.1	±	2.9^e	13.8	±	11.7	N.S.
CD4$^+$ CD45RA$^+$	before	3.71	±	3.1^f	19.2	±	12.2	0.01
	after	1.42	±	1.6^f	20.2	±	13.6	0.01
CD4$^+$ CD45RO$^+$	before	60.7	±	11.1	32.2	±	17.1	0.01
	after	50.4	±	13.6	22.2	±	5.8	0.01

[b,c,e,f]: p<0.01   [a,d,g]: p<0.05

before treatment   4 weeks after treatment

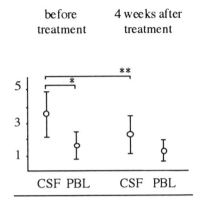

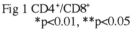

CSF PBL   CSF PBL

Fig 1 CD4⁺/CD8⁺
*p<0.01, **p<0.05

before treatment   4weeks after treatment

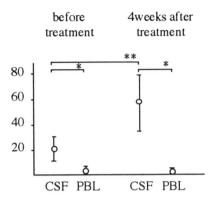

CSF PBL   CSF PBL

Fig 2 CD4⁺CD45RO⁺/CD4⁺CD45RA⁺
*p<0.01, **p<0.05

DISCUSSION

In VKH disease, pleocytosis in cerebrospinal fluid usually occurs from a reaction against melanocytes of meningen. Analysis of surface markers of CSF cells might be useful to investigate the immunological response in VKH disease. Similar to the previous reports[3,4], the most of the CSF cells were CD3 positive (T cells) and CD4 positive cells (T helper cells) and were higher in CSF than in PB in our results. Furthermore, CD4⁺CD45RO⁺ cells were significantly higher and CD4⁺CD45RA⁺ cells were lower in CSF than in PB. Then CD4/CD8 ratio and CD45RO⁺/CD45RA⁺ ratio in CSF were higher than in PBL ($p<0.01$).

T helper cells are subdivided by monoclonal antibodies to isoforms of CD45 (CD45RA and CD45RO). In human CD45RO cells respond to recall antigens by proliferation or the generation of virus-specific effector cells[2]. There are important difference between CD45RA cells (virgin or naive cell) and CD45RO (memory cells) cells. CD45RO cells express higher levels of several adherent molecules such as LFA-1, LFA-3 and ICAM-1 and also express low levels of several molecules (CD25, major histocompatibility complex class II), and secret several cytokines (IL-1 alpha, IL-2, IL-4, IL-5, IFN-gamma). On the other hand, CD45RA cells express no adherent molocules and secret IL-1alpha, and IL-2 only[5]. It has been reported that CD45RO⁺ cells are dominant in the site of inflammation because of these functions.

In CSF with multiple sclerosis, an inflammatory disease which involves the white matter of the CNS and shows pleocytosis, a reduction of CD4⁺CD45RA⁺ cells and an increase of CD4⁺CD45RO⁺ cells were reported [6,7]. In this study, after systemic corticosteroids or immunosuprressive treatment, the rate of CD4⁺CD45RO⁺ was remained higher in CSF than in PB from VKH patiants. Therefore, this subset may play an important role in immunopathogenesis in VKH disease.

REFFERENCES

1)S Sugiura: Vogt-Koyanagi-Harada disease. Jpn J Ophthalmol. 22: 9-35, 1978.
2)K Norose, A Yano, F Aosai and K Segawa: Immunologic Analysis of Cerebrospinal Fluid Lymphocytes in Vogt-Koyanagi-Harada Disease. Invest Ophthalmol Vis Sci. 31:1210-1216, 1990.
3)M Kogiso, Y Tanouti, S Miki and Y Miura: Characterizition of T-cell subsets, soluble Interleukin-2 receptors and Interleukin-6 in Vogt-Koyanagi-Harada disease. Jpn J

Ophthalmol. 36: 37-43, 1992.

4)LT Clement: Isoforms of the CD45 Common Leukocyte Antigen Family: Markers for Human T-Cell Differentiation. J Clin Immunol. 12:1-10, 1992.

5)K Kristensson, CAK Borrebaeck and R Carlsson: Human CD4⁺T cells expressing CD45RA acquire the lymphokine gene expression of CD45RO⁺T-helper cells after activation *in vitro*. Immunol. 76:103-109, 1992.

6) M Zaffaroni, L Gallo, A Ghezzi and CL Cazzullo: CD4⁺ lymphocyte subsets in the cerebrospinal fluid of multiple sclerosis and non-inflammatory neutological diseases. J Neurol. 238: 209-211, 1991.

7) M Matsui, K J Mori and T Saida: Cellular Immunoregulatory Mechanisms in the Central Nervous System: Characterization of Noninfammatory and Inflammatory Cerebrofpinal Fluid Lymphocytes. Ann Neurol. 27: 647-651, 1990.

Advances in Ocular Immunology
R.B. Nussenblatt, S.M. Whitcup, R.R. Caspi and I. Gery, eds.

THE ROLE OF CHLAMYDIA TRACHOMATIS IN RECURRENT ACUTE ANTERIOR UVEITIS HLA B-27 POSITIVE AND HLA B-27 NEGATIVE: A BACKGROUND INVESTIGATION DURING THE NON-INFLAMMATORY PHASE OF THE DISEASE.

M.S. Tognon, R. Cusinato*, B. Turrini, L. Tollot, G. Bombi*, G. Meloni* and A.G. Secchi

Department of Physiopathological Optics and Microbiology*, Padua University. Padova, ITALY.

INTRODUCTION

Acute Anterior Uveitis (AAU) is the most common form of intraocular inflammation. In the majority of cases its etiology remains unknown, but a strong association with the HLA B27 phenotype has been confirmed by a large number of investigators (1, 2).

In HLA B27 related diseases other than AAU, enteric and\or urogenital infections with Gram negative bacteria and Chlamydia trachomatis have been thought to play an important role (3, 4), although the elucidation of the role played by HLA B27 molecule and its interactions with microbial antigens in producing disease remains to be clarified.

In the past a possible role of Chlamydia trachomatis infection in the development of AAU has been investigated, but no definitive data are available in the literature.

Significant antibody titers to Chlamydia trachomatis have been found in AAU patients (5) and, furthermore an increased linphocyte tranformation response to chlamydial antigens in HLA B27 positive AAU patients when compared to HLA B27 negative patients and controls, has been demonstrated (6).

Recently a high incidence of asymptomatic infection of the urethra and/or cervix with Chlamydia trachomatis has been detected in AAU patients (7).

The present study was designed in order to investigate the prevalence of antibody titers to Chlamydia trachomatis, and the prevalence of urogenital and conjunctival infection with Chlamydia trachomatis in our AAU patients, both HLA B27 positive and negative.

MATERIALS AND METHODS

We have performed a retrospective study among our patients affected by idiopathic AAU not previously tested for HLA B27. Ninty-six patients have been enrolled in the study.

Each patient has been investigated for the presence of the HLA B27 phenotype.

In each patient a previous contact with Chlamydia trachomatis has been investigated by the search of serum antibodies against the microorganism. The sera, previously stored at -80°C, were tested for specific antibodies by complement fixation test (CFT) using a group specific antigen (PLT) (Virion Roche).

Furthermore, the prevalence of symptomatic or asymptomatic urogenital and conjunctival infection with Chlamydia trachomatis has been investigated by Polymerase Chain Reaction (PCR) detection of specific genomic sequences in conjunctival scraping and endocervical, vaginal and/or urethral swabs in each patient (8). The swabs and the conjunctival scrapings were immediately placed in 1 ml of Phosphate-buffered saline solution (PBS) pH 7,4 and stored at -80°C.

To prepare the DNA, after thawing, 1 ml of PBS washing of specimen was treated with a digestion solution. DNA was estacted and precipitated with a phenol-chlorophorm-isoamyl-alcohol solution and ethanol method. Dried and resuspended in sterile water the specimen was then ready for DNA amplification.

The oligonucleotide primers, derived from highly conserved regions of the published DNA sequences for the MOMPS (Major Outer Membrane Proteins) of Chlamydia trachomatis, were sintetized with a Beckman DNA-SM automated DNA synthetizer. The primer pair used yielded and amplified a fragment of 530 bp.

For DNA amplification, PCR was performed on 10 μl of resuspended DNA extract in sterile water. The final reaction mixture (total volume of 100 ul) contained 1 μM of each primer, 200 μM each of d-ATP, d-CTP, d-GPT and d-TTP, 50 mM of KCl, 10 mM of TRIS pH 8.3, 1.5 mM MgCl2, 2.5 U Amplitaq DNA polymerase (Perkin Elmer Cetus Norwalk CT). It was overlayed with mineral oil. Samples were subjected to 30-40 cycles of amplification in a DNA termal Cycler, Perkin Elmer Cetus. An amplification cycle consisted of denaturation for 30 sec at 95°C, primer annealing to template at 55°C for 30 sec and primer extension at 72°C for 45 sec. For each experiment a positive and a negative control were added.

The reaction products were examined by electrophoresis on 2.5% agarose gel stained with ethidium bromide and photographed under ultraviolet illumination for the detection of the amplified product.

RESULTS

HLA B27 TYPING:

Thirty-nine out of 96 patients (41%) resulted positive for HLA B27 phenotype. No differences were noted as far as the age of onset of the disease, and the number of recurrences were concerned between HLA B27 positive and negative patients.

On the contrary as far as gender was concernd, in the HLA B27 positive group 76% of patients were males and 24% were females, while in the HLA B27 negative group 28% of patients were males and 72% were females.

CHLAMYDIA TRACHOMATIS INFECTIONS:
Only one patient, in the HLA B27 negative group, resulted
positive for serum antibidies against Chlamydia Trachomatis
among our patients. In the same patients the vaginal swab was
also positive for Chlamydia trachomatis DNA sequences.
In all of the other patients PCR resulted negative both in
conjunctival scraping and urogenital swab and the serology for
Chlamydia trachomatis was negative.

DISCUSSION AND CONCLUSIONS

In HLA B27 related diseases other than AAU, Reiter
syndrome and ankylosing spondilitis above all, a pathogenetic
role of Gram negative bacteria and/or Chlamydia trachomatis
has been suggested. Such a pathogenentisc role, either
directly or through a molecular mimicry, has been supposed
also in AAU (9. 10).
The aim of the present study was to evaluate a possible
role of Chlamydia Trachomatis in the development of AAU in HLA
B27 positive and/or negative patients.
The first step of our investigation was to evaluate the
prevalence of HLA B27 phenotype among our patients affected by
AAU. The results of our study show that the prevalence of HLA
B27 phenotype among our patients is similar to other previous
reports.
While no differences were noted between our HLA B27 positive
and negative patients as far as the age of onset of the
disease and the number of recurrences were concerned, our
study also confirmed the high prevalence of males among HLA
B27 AAU patients.
The second step of our study was to investigate in our AAU
patients a previous contact with Chlamydia trachomatis. In
only one case of AAU it has been possible to demonstrate serum
antibodies against Chlamydia trachomatis and specific DNA
sequences in the urogenital swab. This patient, moreover, was
HLA B27 negative.
In conclusion the results of our study did not support the
possibility that Chlamidia trachomatis plays a role in the
occurrence of acute anterior uveitis. All of our HLA B27
positive AAU patients, and all but one of our HLA B27 negative
AAU patients, in fact, did not show any previous contact with
the microorganism. It is possible to maintain from our
findings that Chlamydia trachomatis should not be considered
as a causative agent for AAU both HLA B27 positive and HLA B27
negative.

TABLE: HLA B27+ vs HLA B27-: CLINICAL CARACTERISTICS, RESULTS		
	HLA B27+	HLA B27-
Age of onset	38+/-17	34+/-17
Number of recurrences	3.8+/-3.9	4.5+/-4.3
Gender (males)	**30/39**	**17/57**
Antibodies against C. t.	0/39	1/57
Urogenital swab + for C. t.	0/39	1/57
Conjunctival scraping + for C. t.	0/39	0/57

C. t. = Chlamydia trachomatis

REFERENCES
1. T.E.W. Feltkamp - Current Eye Research 9:213-218, 1990
2. A. Linssen, A. Rothova, H.A. Valkenburg, A.J. Dekker-Saeys, L. Luyendijk, A. Kijlstra, and T.E.W. Feltkamp - Invest. Ophthalmol. Vis. Sci. 32(9):2568-2578, 1991
3. C.J. Eastmond, M. Calguner, R. Shinebaum, E.M. Cooke - Ann. Rheum. Dis. 41:15-25, 1982
4. A.E. Good - Ann. Rheum. Dis. 38:119-122, 1979
5. J.M. Aguettaz, E. Vadot, M. Mouillon, J.L. Bonnet - J. Fr. Ophtalmol., 10,11:679, 1987
6. D. Wakefield, R. Penny - Clin. Exp. Immunol. 51:191, 1983
7. W. Graninger, E. Arocker-Mettinger, H. Kiener, A. Benke, J. Szots-Sotz, R. Knobler, J. Smolen -Documenta Ophthlmologica 82:217, 1992
8. J. Sambrook, E.S. Fritsch, T Maniatis - Molecular cloning.A laboratory manual. Second Edition, CSH
9. D. Wakefield, T.H. Stahlberg, A. Toivanen, K. Granfors, C. Tennant - Arch. Ophthalmol. 108:219-221, 1990
10.L.White, R. McCoy, B. Tait, R. Ebringer - Br.J.Ophthalmol. 68:750-755, 1984

© 1994 Elsevier Science B.V. All rights reserved.
Advances in Ocular Immunology
R.B. Nussenblatt, S.M. Whitcup, R.R. Caspi and I. Gery, eds.

LOCAL IgG ANTIBODY PRODUCTION IN THE AQUEOUS HUMOR OF PATIENTS WITH UVEITIS OF VARIOUS ORIGIN.

C. Trichet[a] S. Koscielny[b], P. Thulliez[c], P. Lambin[d] and E. Bloch-Michel[a].

[a]Department of Ophthalmology CHU Bicêtre, Fac Med Paris Sud, France

[b]Department of Statistic, Instiut Gustave Roussy, Villejuif, France

[c]Institut de Puériculture, Laboratoire de la Toxoplasmose, Paris

[d]Institut National de Transfusion Sanguine, Paris

We previously reported an increased level of antibody to measles in the Aqueous humor (A.H) of patients with multiple sclerosis related uveitis (1). We also found a significant association between MRI lesions and high A.H and blood level of measles antibody (2). More recently we showed that the presence of such white matter MRI lesions could be linked to an increased level of IgG in A.H as judged by the elevation of the ratio R = R2/R1 (3). The purpose of this paper is to determine in which other type of uveitis the ratio R2/R1 may be also modified to study the variations of this according to the type of uveitis.

PATIENTS AND METHODS

903 patients with uveitis of all kinds were tested in this study, including 223 cases of uveitis of known etiology and 680 with negative work up.

Those uveitis of known origin included 16 Behcet, 23 Birshot, 43 Fuchs H.C., 57 herpes, 14 Posner-Schlossmann, 14 presumed measles-linked uveitis, 12 sarcoidosis, 11 MS, 33 toxoplasmosis. In all cases the ACP had been performed before the real etiology was definitively found.

Quotient R = R2/R1. In this quotient R2 represents the ratio IgG/Albumin in A.H while R1 represents the ratio IgG/Albumin in serum (4).

METHODS

Aqueous and seric IgG and Albumin were estimated with laser nephelometry. Comparison between mean values of R according to the groups of patients was performed with the Wilcoxon Test. For each etiology the mean value of R1, R2 and R and also of albumin and IgG was compared with the mean value of the ten other groups. (Each group was made up with the sum of all 903 cases minus those of the considered etiology).

RESULTS

R1 (IgG/Alb in serum) :
> - There was no difference between any of the 9 groups. This finding allowed us to exclusively consider values of R2.

R2 : (IgG/Alb in AH) :
> - In FUCHS HC. a significant elevation of R2 was observed : $P < 0,001$ while level of IgG was not different from control groups
> - In MS associated uveitis a significant increase of R2 was also present : $P < 0,003$
> - On the other hand, R2 was significantly decreased in Behcet's disease : $P < 0,02$

Separate Values :
> - In F.H.C. the level of albumin was significantly decreased in the aqueous humor : $P < 0,01$
>   while IgG level did not differ with control $P = 0,39$
> - In MS associated uveitis the level of IgG was increased and nearly but not completely significant : $P = 0,06$
> - In Behcet's disease the level of albumin in aqueous was significantly increased : $P < 0,02$.

DISCUSSION

Local production of non specific antibodies has been considered so far in different types of uveitis by several authors using apparently different but very similar methods. Dernouchamps (5) using the RCR (Relative Concentration of Ratio) was the first to demonstrate the significant relative elevation of IgG in patients with Fuchs H.C. Later on, Quentin and Reiber identified an IgG production in 5 out of 6 patients with MS associated uveitis. This finding is of great importance. It would indicate that the same phenomena may be found in aqueous A.H as well as in the spinal fluid (6).

However data obtained in such studies were evaluated by the comparison with presumed normal subjects and also were made on a limited number of cases. The purpose of our study was to make a comparison between 10 groups of patients without having recourse to "normal" values whose interpretation was debatable since aqueous sampling were obtained from cataract patients. The extensive aspect of this study with 903 patients with uveitis should also be considered. The elevation of R results confirmed the previous findings of Dernouchamps on F.H.C. as well as those by Quentin and Reiber on MS associated uveitis.

In F.H.C. elevation of R seemed to be due not to a relative excess of IgG (difference with control was not significant) but to an unexpected but significant decrease of albumin in A.H. This finding which is visible in Murray's article (7) would require further investigation.

In MS associated uveitis the discrete ($P = 0,06$) lack of significant production of IgG in aqueous is presumably linked to the limited number of cases (11 as compared to 43 F.H.C. for instance) of the disease. If this finding was confirmed it would supply an additional argument to the similarity of immunologic findings in both A.H and final fluid in MS

The significant decrease of R2 in Behcet's disease on the other hand was imputable to an abnormal elevation of albumin in the aqueous.It could be related to both very acute inflammatory process with excessive permeability of the barrier that are suggested by the usual clinical course of this disease.

REFERENCES

1 Bloch-Michel E. Helleboid L. Hill C. Koscielny S. Dussaix E. Measles virus antibody in aqueous humour of patients with uveitis associated with multiple sclerosis. The Lancet 1992; 339: 750-751.

2 Bloch-Michel E. Iba-Zizen MT Koscielny S.Trichet C. Delvalle A. Doyon D. Dussaix E. and Cabanis EA. MRJ and idiopathic uveitis. In Dernouchamps JP. and al. Eds Recent advances in Uveitis Amsterdam N-York 1993; 459-460

3 Koscielny S. Thulliez P. Cabanis EA Iba-Zizen Trichet C. Helleboid L. Dussaix E. and Bloch- Michel E. Local IgG production in brain MRI(+) and MRI(-) uveitis patients (submitted).

4 - Grabner G. Zehetbauer G. Bettelheim H. Hönigesmann C. and Dorda W. The blood-aqueous barrier and its permeability for proteins of different molecular weight. Albrecht V. Graefes Arch klin exp Ophthal:1978; 207:137-142.

5 Dernouchamps JP. Herremans JF Molecular sieve effect of the blood-aqueous barrier. Exp. Eye. Res. 1975;21:288-297.

6 Waksman BH. Multiple sclerosis. Curr. Opin. Immunol 1989;1: 733-739.

7 Murray PJ. Hoekzema R. Luyendijlk L. Koning S. and Kijlstra A. Analysis of aqueous humor immunoglobulin G in uveitis by Enzyme-Linked immuno absorbent assay, Isoelectric Focusing, and immuno blotting. Invest. Ophthalmol Vis. Sci. 1990; 31: 2129-2135.

Advances in Ocular Immunology
R.B. Nussenblatt, S.M. Whitcup, R.R. Caspi and I. Gery, eds.

IgE-RAST and clinical features in ocular disease complicating atopic dermatitis

E. Uchio[a], Z. Ikezawa[b], and S. Ohno[a]

Departments of [a]Ophthalmology and [b]Dermatology, Yokohama City University, 3-9 Fuku-ura, Kanazawa-ku, Yokohama 236, Japan.

Abstract

We examined clinical factors and data from recent cases of Atopic dermatitis (AD) (with or without ocular complications) and non-AD to evaluate the mechanism of ocular complications. IgE-RAST (CAP system; Kabi Pharmacia Diagnostics, Uppsala, Sweden) for several allergens including rice, egg and mite were measured in 166 patients with AD (47 ocular type, 119 non-ocular type) and 59 non-AD individuals. Serum IgE was also analyzed. The positive rates of IgE-RAST for rice and wheat were significantly higher in ocular type AD as compared with those in non-ocular type AD. IgE-RAST of almost all allergens in non-AD individuals showed significant lower positive rate than that in AD patients. Dermatologically severer cases were more common in patients with ocular complications than in non-ocular disease complicating patients. These results suggest that ocular type AD belongs to the severest part of AD, and that some kind of cereals might contribute to the pathological role in atopic ocular complications.

Introduction

Atopic dermatitis (AD) is a recurrent, itching, eczematous skin disease which may arise from a disordered regulation of IgE- and T-cell-mediated hypersensitivity reactions and vascular responses [1]. However, it has still not been demonstrated what mechanisms underlie the development or exacerbation of AD and its ocular complications. Inhalants such as mites, pollens and molds and many kinds of foods have been suggested as etiological agents in AD, since IgE antibodies to these antigens are present in the sera of AD patients [2-3]. Recently, the severe type of AD, which is not well controlled by local steroid treatment, has been noted to be increasing in Japan [3]. The probable involvement of rice allergy in many severe cases of AD is suggested from a statistical analysis of the correlation between rice-RAST score and dermatological severity in AD patients [3]. Although the characteristics of ocular complications of AD have been reported [4], to our knowledge, the pathophysiological features of ocular complications of AD have not been described. In this paper we compared the clinical and immunological features of the ocular and non-ocular types of AD patients and examined what kinds of allergens may be related specifically to the development of atopic ocular complications.

Materials and methods

One hundred sixty-six patients with typical and atypical lesions of AD were included in this study. Typical eczematous eruptions on flexural areas were considered typical lesions of AD, as described by Hanifin et al. [5]. Definite AD was diagnosed by presence of four items: 1) itching, 2) chronic course of more than one year, 3) atopic history, and 4) typical lesions of AD. All the clinically diagnosed definite AD patients were referred to ophthalmologists and examined for signs of ocular disease. Ocular complicated AD patients consisted of 47 patients (group 1). Non-ocular AD group was divided into 3 groups according to the other complications outer the eye as follows. The first series of patients were AD without any complications (group 2, pure AD group), the second series of patients had bronchial asthma (group 3, AD+BA group), and the third series of patients had allergic rhinitis (group 4, AD+AR group). Serum samples from 59 healthy individuals were also examined (group 5, Controls). The clinical severity of the AD lesions was graded as of mild, moderate, or severe type, according to expansion of the lesions, response to therapy, frequency of relapse and the clinical course [3]. Serum IgE antibodies specific to inhalant and food antigens were determined with the CAP system (Pharmacia CAP System RAST FEIA, Kabi Pharmacia Diagnostics, Uppsala, Sweden). The concentration of the patient samples was read from a standard curve. The results were expressed in kU_A/l and classified with RAST scoring system (score 0: < 0.35 kU_A/l, score 1: 0.35 ~ 0.69, score 2: 0.7 ~ 3.4, score 3: 3.5 ~ 17.4, and score 4: $\geqq$ 17.5 kU_A/l). A result exceeding 0.69 kU_A/l (score $\geqq$ 2) was considered positive. Serum total IgE level was also measured. Significant differences of percentage positivity of IgE RAST between groups were calculated by χ^2 - test. Mann-Whitney test was used to identify differences of serum total IgE levels between groups.

Results

Table 1 compares the dermatological severity between two patient groups in AD; patients who had ocular complications (group 1) and patients who showed no ocular complications (group 2-4). Severe cases of AD were observed in 22/47 (47%) of group 1 and 37/119 (31%) of group 2-4. This difference was significant (p < 0.01), indicating that the dermatological severity of AD was related to the presence of ocular complications.

Table 1.
Relation between dermatological severity and prevalence of ocular complications in patients with AD

	n	Dermatological severity		
		mild	moderate	severe
AD with ocular complications (group 1)	47	3	22	22
AD without ocular complications (group 2-4)	119	34	48	37

p < 0.001 between group 1 and group 2-4 (χ^2-goodness test).

The results of RAST scores for all patient groups are presented in Table 2. IgE-RAST of almost all allergens in non-AD individuals (group 5) showed significantly lower positive rate than that in AD patients (groups 1-4). The RAST values for wheat were positive in 25 of 47 patients (53.2%) with AD having ocular complications, whereas values were positive in only 27 of 81 patients (33.3%) and 3 of 19 patients (15.8%) with pure AD (group 2) and with AD+AR (group 4), respectively.   These difference were significant (p < 0.05).   The RAST values for rice were also significantly elevated in patients with AD and ocular complications (group 1) (33/47 (70.2%)) compared to those with pure AD (group 2) (27/81 (33.3%)) and those with AD+AR (group 4) (4/19 (21.1%)).

Table 2.
Comparison of IgE RAST reactions to inhalant and food allergens among patient groups

	n	RAST positive patients (%)						
		Antigen						
		DF	Candida	Milk	Egg white	Soybean	Wheat	Rice
AD + OD (group 1)	47	76.6*	42.6*	4.3	23.4[§]	36.2*	53.2[¶]	70.2*
pure AD (group 2)	81	74.1*	50.6*	17.3[§]	17.3	28.4*	33.3[¶]	33.3[¶]
AD+BA (group 3)	19	94.7*	47.4[¶]	26.3[†]	36.8[¶]	21.1[§]	36.8[¶]	36.8[¶]
AD+AR (group 4)	19	78.9[¶]	52.6*	0	0	15.8	15.8	21.1[§]
Controls (group 5)	59	35.6	10.2	3.4	5.1	1.7	1.7	3.4

Abbreviations: OD, ocular diseases; DF, *Dermatophagoides farinae*, mite antigen; Candida, *Candida albicans*.   Significance between patient group and controls is indicated by symbols: p < 0.001, * ; p < 0.005, [¶] ; p < 0.01, [†]; p < 0.05, [§].   Significance among patient groups is as follows.   Milk: p < 0.05 between group 1 and group 2, and group 1 and group 3.   Egg white: p < 0.005 between group 3 and group 4.   Wheat: p < 0.05 between group 1 and group 2, and group1 and group 4.   Rice: p < 0.005 between group 1 and group 2, and group 1 and group 4.   p < 0.05 between group 1 and group 3.

We compared serum IgE levels in patients with AD and ocular complications in three dermatological severity groups. As shown in Figure 1 the serum IgE values were significantly elevated in patients with severe type compared to those in patients with moderate type (p < 0.05).   The levels of serum IgE in patients with mild skin disease were lower than those in patients with severe skin disease, although the difference did not reach significance.

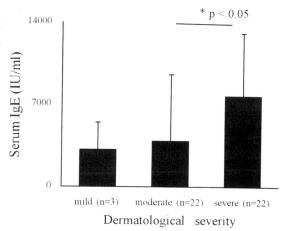

Figure 1.   Serum IgE levels in mild, moderate, and severe types of AD patients. Each bar represents the mean and standard deviation of serum IgE levels.

Discussion

Positive RAST reactions to *Dermatophagoides farinae* (DF; mite antigen) have been reported in 73% of Japanese patients [6].   Although the DF-RAST positivity was the highest in the AD+BA group (94.7%), controls also showed a comparatively high positive rate (35.6%) probably due to the wet and hot climate and housing style using mats in Japan.   As shown in Table 2, among food antigens the positive RAST rate of rice and wheat were significantly higher in patients with ocular-complicated AD than those in patients with AD of other types.   The positive RAST rate to rice and wheat antigens are reported to be 38 - 49.7% and 21 - 32%, respectively, in Japan [3,6].   In contrast, a positive reaction against rice and wheat are obtained in 0 - 7% and 13 - 19%, respectively, in the USA [7-8].   The reason of these different RAST reactions to cereal antigens between Japan and western countries has not yet been clearly explained.   It is reported that epitopes of rice, wheat and soy bean antigens which are related to exacerbations of AD may fall into two groups [3].   One group is composed of hapten-like epitopes, which react with IgE-antibodies, and the other consists of carrier-like epitopes which induce the production of IgE-antibodies, probably by the induction of helper T (Th_2) cells.   The Th (Th_1) cells induced by the carrier-like epitopes may also induce delayed hypersensitivity reactions, which are believed to join a major part of the inflammatory reaction in AD [3]. Therefore, carrier epitopes of rice antigens inducing the production of IgE-antibodies to not only rice but also to other cereal antigens may play an important role in the development of severe AD in Japan and south east Asia, where rice foods are the most popular cereals. However, it has still not been elucidated how oral tolerance to cereal antigens, which is believed to exist normally might be broken down in the severe type of AD.   One possibility is that these patients are inherently susceptible to the breakdown of oral tolerance, perhaps mediated through some kinds of allergens such as mites or bacteria which act as immunomodulators.   Our data confirm the observation that the incidence of type 1 allergy to foods has an important role in the development of severe AD and its ocular complications.   However, there remains controversy whether the severity of AD can be explained only by the extent of type 1 allergy.   It is reported that type 4 allergy may also play a critical role in the pathogenesis of AD [9].   In conclusion, although further studies are needed for more distinct immunological mechanism of severe AD with ocular complications, our data indicate a clear correlation between presence of ocular complications and high serum IgE levels or positive rate of RAST scores to cereals.

References

1. Hanifin JM.   J Allergy Clin Immunol 1984;73:211-226.
2. Okudaira H, Hongo O, Ogita T, Haida M, et al.   Ann Allergy 1983;50:51-54.
3. Ikezawa Z, Miyakawa K, Komatsu H, Suga C, et al. Acta Derm Venereol Suppl (Stockh) 1992;176:103-107.
4. Garrity JA, Liseseang TJ. Can J Ophthalmol 1984;19:21-24.
5. Hanifin JH, Rajka G.   Acta Derm Venereol Suppl (Stockh) 1980,92:44-47.
6. Miyakawa K. Arerugi 1991;40:1500-1510
7. Sampson HA, McCaskill CC.   J Pediatr 1985;107:669-675.
8. Sampson HA. J Allergy Clin Immunol 1983;71:473-480.
9. Wierenga EA, Snoek M, de Groot C, Cheretien I, et al. J Immunol 1990;144:4651-4656

Advances in Ocular Immunology
R.B. Nussenblatt, S.M. Whitcup, R.R. Caspi and I. Gery, eds.

S-ANTIGEN SPECIFIC T CELL CLONES FROM A PATIENT WITH BEHÇET'S DISEASE

J.H.YAMAMOTO [a,b], Y.FUJINO [b], C.LIN [c], M.NIEDA [c], T.JUJI [c] and K.MASUDA [b]

[a] Division of Ophthalmology and Laboratory of Transplant Immunology-Heart Institute, School of Medicine, University of São Paulo, Av. Dr. Éneas Carvalho Aguiar, 500 3º and., São Paulo 05403-000, Brazil

[b] Department of Ophthalmology, School of Medicine, University of Tokyo, 7-3-1 Hongo, Bunkyo-ku, Tokyo 113, Japan

[c] Department of Transfusion Medicine and Immunohematology, School of Medicine, University of Tokyo, 7-3-1 Hongo, Bunkyo-ku, Tokyo 113, Japan

INTRODUCTION

T cell clones or lines specific to retinal antigens are valuable tools to further understanding the mechanisms of retinal autoimmunity in uveitis in humans. Peripheral blood lymphocytes from patients with Behçet's disease (BD) are reported to be sensitized to S-antigen (S-Ag) [1]. So far, very little has been reported about isolation of T cell clones or lines specific to retinal antigens from patients with uveitis [2]. In the present study, we report on the isolation and establishment of T cell clones specific toward S-Ag from a patient with BD.

SUBJECTS, MATERIALS AND METHODS

Patient. Peripheral blood was obtained from a 38 year-old male patient with the complete form of BD (diagnostic criteria proposed by Behçet's Disease Research Committee of Japan-1974), in whom cellular immune responses of peripheral blood lymphocytes at proliferative assays to S-Ag, peptides M and G were previously detected. The patient's HLA was A2, Bw46, Bw62, Bw6, Cw9, DR9, DR8.1, DRw52, DQw1, DQw3. This study was conducted with the approval of the Ethics Committee of the University of Tokyo under the patient's informed consent.

Establishment of T cell clones. Peripheral blood mononuclear cells (PBMCs) were separated by gradient centrifugation (Ficoll-Paque, Pharmacia, Uppsala, Sweden). 3×10^5 cells/well were cultured with bovine S-Ag ($0.05\mu M$ and $0.2\mu M$), purified by the method of Dorey et al [3], in RPMI 1640 medium with HEPES (GIBCO, Grand Island, NY) supplemented with antibiotics, glutamine (2mM) and 10% heat-inactivated human AB serum (lot nº 29309048, Flow Laboratories, Inc., McLean, VA) (complete medium) in flat-bottom, 96-well microculture plate (Costar, Cambridge, MA). After 5 days of incubation, blast cells were harvested and seeded by limiting dilution method at 0.3 cells/well, 1 cell/well and 3 cells/well in a 96-V C microcloning plate (Biotec, Tokyo, Japan), along with 5 x 10^4 irradiated (2000 R) autologous PBMCs per well, 0.05µM of bovine S-Ag and 500 U/ml of human recombinant interleukine 2 (r-IL2, S-6920, Shionogi Pharmaceutical Industry, Osaka, Japan) in AIM-V medium (GIBCO) with 10% human AB serum. After 7 to 14 days, the growing cells of positive wells were transferred and expanded in 96-well flat-bottom microculture plate (Costar). Following 7 to 14 days of expansion, clones were transferred to a 24-well culture plate (Linbro, Flow Laboratories, Inc., McLean, VA). Every 2 weeks, the cells were restimulated with 0.05µM of S-Ag, irradiated (2000R) PBMCs and 500U/ml of r-IL2. PBMCs from normal volunteers with the same DR antigens as the patient (DR8.1 and DR9) were irradiated (2000 R) and used as pooled antigen-presenting cells (APCs). In the intervals between the restimulation, clones were expanded in the presence of 500U/ml of r-IL2. This cycle was repeated to maintain the cell clones.

Surface phenotyping. The following monoclonal antibodies (mAbs), labelled with fluorescein isothiocyanate (FITC), were used: anti-human CD3 (Leu-4), CD4 (Leu-3a), CD8 (Leu-2a), TCR αβ (TCR-1αβ) and TCRγδ (TCR-γδ-1) (Becton-Dickinson, Immunocytometry systems, San Jose, CA). Goat anti-mouse IgG-FITC (Becton-Dickinson) was used for the indirect immunofluorescence analysis. Mouse IgG$_1$ conjugated to FITC (G1CL, Becton-Dickinson) was used as control. After a resting period of at least 10 days after the stimulation cycle, T cell clones (10^5 cells per mAb) were directly or indirectly stained with FITC-conjugated mouse mAbs with specificity toward human CD3, CD4, CD8, TCRαβ and TCRγδ. Anti-TCR antibody was used in combination with goat anti-mouse IgG-FITC for indirect immunofluorescence analysis. Cell suspensions were incubated with the antibodies for 30 minutes at 4°C, washed and analyzed on a Ortho Spectrum III (Ortho Diagnostic Systems Inc., Laser Flow Cytometry System, Westwood, MA). A commercial control FITC-conjugated mouse IgG$_1$ was used as a negative background control.

Proliferative studies. 2 x 10^4 resting T cells were cultured, in triplicate, in 96-well round-bottomed microplates (Costar) for 72 hr with or without bovine S-Ag (0.05µM and 0.2µM) in the presence of 10^5 irradiated (2000 R) autologous PBMCs in complete medium. Responses to the S-Ag-derived peptides, peptide M and peptide G, were similarly assayed. Peptides M and G, derived from the sequence of human S-Ag [4], were synthesized by Bio Science Lab., Fujiya Co. Ltd., Kanagawa, Japan according to the t-BOC method using a peptide synthesizer 430A (Applied Biosystems, Foster City, CA, USA). Peptide M corresponds to positions 306 to 323 (DTNLASSTIIKEGIDRTV) [5] while peptide G corresponds to positions 343 to 362 (GELTSSEVATEVPFRLMHPQ) [6] of the human S-Ag. For the analysis of *the HLA restriction pattern,* murine anti-HLA-DR (Becton-Dickinson), anti-HLA-DQ (Leu-10, Becton-Dickinson) and anti-HLA-class I (Sera-lab, Crawley Down, Sussex) mAbs were added to culture plates at 0.1µg/ml final concentration. Microcultures were pulsed with 0.5µCi of tritiated thymidine (^{3}H-TdR, New England, Boston, MA, USA; 2Ci/mmol) per microwell 16 hr prior to harvesting. Cell proliferation was evaluated by incorporated radioactivity counted by a liquid scintillation counter. The results were expressed as disintegration per minute (DPM) or stimulation index (S.I.=DPM in culture wells with antigen/DPM in culture wells without antigen). The inhibitory effect of anti-HLA mAb on the antigen-induced proliferative responses was calculated with the following equation:

$$\% \text{ response} = \frac{\text{(DPM in culture wells with antigen and mAb)-(DPM in culture wells without antigen or mAb)}}{\text{(DPM in culture wells with antigen)-(DPM in culture wells without antigen or mAb)}} \times 100$$

Cytotoxicity assays. Autologous EBV-transformed B cells, allogeneic DR9 EBV-transformed B cells, K562 and Daudi cells, used as target cells, were labelled with 100μCi chromium-51 (CJS 11, Amersham Life Science, Tokyo, Japan) and subsequently washed 3 times with RPMI 1640 medium containing 10% fetal bovine serum (FBS). Target cells were then incubated in RPMI 1640 medium plus 10% FBS only or added with bovine S-Ag (1 mg/ml) for 1 hr at 37°C. Effector cells (T cell clones) were incubated in triplicate with 1 x 10^4 ^{51}Cr-labelled S-Ag-preincubated or not preincubated target cells, at effector to target ratios of 1:1 and 20:1 in 96-well round-bottomed microwells for 4 hr at 37°C. Supernatants were then harvested and measured for radioactivity in a gamma counter. Chromium release of the labelled target cells is given as experimental release. Maximum release and spontaneous release of chromium were measured in wells containing target cells in the presence of detergent or medium alone, respectively. The percentage of specific release was calculated according to the following equation:

$$\% \text{ specific lysis} = \frac{\text{experimental release - spontaneous release}}{\text{maximum release - spontaneous release}} \times 100$$

RESULTS AND DISCUSSION

Four long-term (12 weeks) T cell clones were established from the peripheral blood of a patient with BD. Their characteristics are represented in Table 1.

Table 1
Characteristics of the T cell clones

Clone	Phenotype	S.I.[a] to S-Ag	Cytotoxicity[b] Daudi cells	K562
Clone 2	CD3$^+$CD4$^+$TCRαβ$^+$	6.8	0%	0%
Clone 10	CD3$^+$CD8$^+$TCRαβ$^+$	4.4	0%	0%
Clone 30	CD3$^+$CD4$^-$CD8$^-$TCRαβ$^+$	1.5	10%	10%
Clone 6	CD3$^+$CD4$^-$CD8$^-$TCRγδ$^+$	1.0	72%	46%

[a] S.I.=stimulation index; [b] cytotoxicity represented as percent of specific lysis.

The *clones CD4$^+$ (clone 2) and CD8$^+$(clone 10)* proliferated specifically to bovine S-Ag, but their responses to the S-Ag-derived synthetic peptides M and G were weak (S.I. ranging from 1.7 to 2.4), suggesting that sites of human T cell recognition of S-Ag may be different from those established in experimental models [5,6]. Anti-DR mAb reduced proliferation by approximately 40%, even for the CD8$^+$clone, whilst the anti-class I mAb had no effect on either clone. The inhibition of a CD8$^+$ T cell clone response to S-Ag with anti-class II mAb was rather unusual, since CD8$^+$ T cells are usually restricted by class I. However, a few exceptions to this association of CD8 with MHC antigens have been reported [7]. The S-Ag specific T cell clones were stained with mAbs to Vβ5.1, Vβ5.2, Vβ5.3, Vβ6.7, Vβ8, Vβ12 and Vα2 TCR variable region genes (Diversi-Tm αβTCR Screening Panel 1A; T Cell Sciences Inc., Cambridge, MA), but they were negative, pointing out to another Vβ and Vα variable region.

Clones 2 and 10 did not show any specific killing activity against the autologous EBV-transformed B cells, nor to any of the other lines tested. Since there are various types of cells that function as antigen-presenting cells with varying capacity of processing and presenting antigens, an antigen-specific killing function cannot be totally disregarded. Moreover, a hypothetical dominant peptide-specific killing activity could also have been undetected in our assay using whole S-Ag.

The *CD3⁺CD4⁻CD8⁻(DN) T cell clones, clones 30 and 6*, were not specific to S-Ag. Clone 30 (CD3⁺ DN/ αβTCR⁺) was devoid of cytotoxic activity towards all target cells tested, contrary to the described cytotoxic function for DN, αβTCR⁺ T cells [8]. Clone 6 (CD3⁺ DN/ γδTCR⁺) lysed K562 and Daudi target cell lines independent on the presence of S-Ag. γδ⁺ T cells are thought to represent a separate lineage with a capacity of antigen-independent killing. Reports of increased peripheral blood γδ⁺ T cells in patients with BD [9] suggest that these cells may play a role in the physiopathogenesis of this disease.

Additional human T cell lines and clones specific to retinal antigens will provide the framework necessary to examine the events that lead to ocular inflammation.

ACKNOWLEDGMENTS

The author, J.H. Yamamoto, was a grantee of a scholarship from the Japanese Ministry of Education, Health and Sciences. This study was sponsored by the research grant No 05771389 from the Ministry of Education and Culture, Japan.

REFERENCES

1. Yamamoto JH, Minami M, Goro I, Masuda K, Mochizuki M. Cellular autoimmunity to retinal specific antigens in patients with Behçet's disease. *Br J Ophthalmol.*1993;77:584-9.
2. Nussenblatt RB, Palestine AG, El-Saied M. Long-term antigens specific and non-specific T-cell lines and clones in uveitis. *Curr Eye Res.* 1984;3:299-305.
3. Dorey C, Cozette J, Faure JP. A simple and rapid method for isolation of retinal S-antigen. *Ophthalmic Res.* 1982;14:249-55.
4. Yamaki K, Tsuda M, Shinohara T. The sequence of human retinal S-antigen reveals similarities with α-transducin. *FEBS Lett.* 1988;234:39-43.
5. Donoso LA, Yamaki K, Merrymand CF, Shinohara T, Yue S, Sery TW. Human S-antigen: characterization of uveitopathogenic sites. *Curr Eye Res.* 1988; 7:1077-85.
6. Gregerson DS, Merryman CM, Obritsch WF, Donoso LA. Identification of a potent new pathogenic site in human retinal S-antigen which induces experimental autoimmune uveoretinitis in LEW rats. *Cell Immunol.* 1990;128:209-19.
7. Sprent J, Schaefer M. Antigen-presenting cells for unprimed T cell. *Immunol Today.* 1989;10:17-22.
8. Matsumoto M, Yasukawa M, Inatsuki A, Kobayashi Y. Human double-negative(CD4⁻CD8⁻) T cells bearing alpha beta T cell receptor possess both helper and cytotoxic activities. *Clin Exp Immunol.* 1991;858:525-30.
9. Suzuki Y, Hoshi K, Matsuda T, Mizushima Y. Increased peripheral blood γδ⁺T cells and natural killer cells in Behçet's disease. *J Rheumatol.* 1992;19:588-92.

© 1994 Elsevier Science B.V. All rights reserved.
Advances in Ocular Immunology
R.B. Nussenblatt, S.M. Whitcup, R.R. Caspi and I. Gery, eds.

Tear immunoglobulins and secretory component of humoral immunological disorders

J.-C. Zhao and L. Bielory

Immuno-Ophthalmology Service, Departments of Ophthalmology and Medicine, University of Medicine and Dentistry of New Jersey, Newark, NJ, 07103-2499, USA.

INTRODUCTION

Immunodeficiency (ID) and hypergammaglobulinemia (HG) are two common immune dysfunctional disorders. Humoral immunodeficiency disorders (HID) include a diverse spectrum of disorders from the complete absence of mature recirculating B cells, plasma cells and immunoglobulin (Ig) to the selective absence of only certain Ig classes or subclasses. Selective IgA immunodeficiency (IgAID) is the most common form of HID with a reported prevalence between 1/500-1/700 in studies of asymptomatic individuals and blood donors [1]. Common variable immunodeficiency (CVID) is a broad diagnostic category that refers to a heterogeneous group of disorders that are associated with late-onset ID, poor antibody response following antigenic challenge, and increase incidence of infections. HG is defined as an increase in serum Ig which includes a diverse spectrum of disorders. AIDS patients often have elevated IgG, IgA and normal IgM levels [2], as well as other autoimmune diseases such as chronic granulomatous diseases, sarcoid, rheumatoid arthritis, lupus erythematosus and liver diseases [3-7]. In order to further discern that whether the immune dysfunctional disorders have any effect on tear fluid (TF) immunological contents, TF immunoglobulins (Igs) and secretory component (SC) were analyzed in the HID, HG and control groups.

MATERIALS AND METHODS

Subjects: Twenty patients with humoral dysfunctional diseases (HID group: n=8, male=2, female=6; IgAID=2, CVID=6; 28-70 yrs., mean=41.9 yrs. HG group: n=12; including HG-HIV-positive: n=6, male=1, female=5; 33-49 yrs., mean=39.7 yrs.; and HG-HIV-negative: n=6, male=4, female=2; 34-66 yrs., mean=50.2 yrs.) and eight controls (male=4, female=4; 27-66 yrs., mean=42.2 yrs.) without clinical signs of ocular disease were recruited. None of the individuals were taking any medication that could interfere with tear production. Informed consent was obtained from all subjects prior to entry into this study.

Tears collection: Tears were collected with a P-20 pipetteman utilizing a soft tipped gel loading pipette tip (Bio-Rad Laboratories, Inc., CA) from the inferior conjunctival sac. Care was taken not to touch or irritate the eye directly. TF samples were stored at -70 °C until analyzed.

Tear electrophoresis and Western blot: One ul TF samples (1:10 dilution in nonreducing denaturing sample buffer) were run on 10-15% gradient sodium dodecyl sulphate polyacrylamide gel electrophoresis (SDS-PAGE) using an automated electrophoresis system (PhastSystem, Pharmacia, LKB Biotechnology, Piscataway, NJ). After electrophoresis, one gel was developed and silver stained while the other gel was transferred to nitrocellulose membrane using a PhastTransfer (PhastSystem, Pharmacia, LKB Biotechnology, Piscataway, NJ). After transfer, proteins on the nitrocellulose membrane were identified for IgA, IgG, IgM and SC with different immunologic probes by standard immunohistochemistry described before [8]. Commercial antiserum conjugated with alkaline phosphate were used as follows: antihuman IgA (a chain), antihuman IgM (u chain), and IgA, G, M (H&L). For SC, sheep antihuman SC (IgG) was used as the primary antibody and biotin conjugated donkey antisheep IgG (H&L) as secondary antibody (The Binding Site Inc., CA).

Igs and free SC quantity: TF IgA, IgG and free SC were quantified with radial immunodiffusion (RID) plate (Turbo UL IgA, IgG and SC RID, The Binding Site Inc., CA). Student's t-test was used for statistical analyses.

RESULTS

Electrophoresis of TF from control, ID and HG patients in SDS-PAGE revealed similar binding profiles ($\geq$ 12 bands ranging from 10-$\geq$200 kD). TF from HID patients (n=8) contained the major tear proteins similar to those found in the controls, but in the region over 200 kD one staining pattern was lacking in 6 HID samples.

Immunoblotting with immunological probes: Immunoblots revealed that all samples from controls contained one wide band of IgA (>200 kD), three-four bands of SC (50->200 kD), two-three bands of IgG (160->200 kD). Traces of IgM (>200 kD) were detected in three (3/8) control TF. In the HID group, there was no staining in the IgA region in 6 TF samples. IgM was clearly found in 7 of 8 TF samples including the one with no serum IgM and another IgAID individual who had markedly increased TF IgM with no IgA in TF.

Quantity of Igs and free SC: See table 1.

Table 1
TF Igs and free SC in humoral immunological disorders (mg/l) *

Mean value		IgA	IgG	SC
Control	(n=8)	331.13	33.14	37.41
HID	(n=8)	4.55 ($\leq$.01)	64.66 ($\leq$.05)	108.49 ($\leq$.05)
HG:HIV+	(n=6)	15.68 ($\leq$.05)	168.50 ($\leq$.05)	141.98 ($\leq$.05)
HIV-	(n=6)	521.50 (NS)#	110.87 ($\leq$.05)	13.36 ($\leq$.01)

* TF IgA, IgG and SC in humoral immunodeficiency disorders (HID) and HIV+ or HIV- hypergammaglobulinemia (HG: HIV+ or HIV-) are compared to those in control group respectively. #NS=No statistical difference.

DISCUSSION

Tears which constantly bathe the ocular surface contain various immunologically active proteins including Igs, lysozyme, prealbumin and lactoferrin [9] and therefore, reflect the immunologic environment of ocular surface. The evaluation of tear components in different diseases can provide a unique opportunity to assess the immunologic state of the eye and their correlations.

The significant higher TF IgG in HID group than the control group and the presence of TF IgM in 7 of 8 HID cases , who were deficient in IgA (one case contained TF IgA with no IgM in TF) suggest that elevated TF IgG and IgM may indicate increased production to compensate for the ocular defense of HID group in the absence or low level of TF IgA.

It is interesting to note that one HID patient in this study contained IgM in TF, though he had no IgM in serum. This is similar to the study of Kuizenga et al [10] who reported secretory IgM in TF of IgAID patients. The presence of TF IgM when IgM is absence in the peripheral circulation suggests local synthesis of IgM at the mucosal surface. Brandtzaeg et al [11] have shown that there is local synthesis of IgM at colonic glands of mucosal surfaces in IgAID patients.

In the external secretion, especially for IgA, SC required by dimeric IgA as it is transported through the epithelial cells is a 70 kD polypeptide produced by epithelial cells of mucous membrane and found in ocular tissue, salivary gland, gastrointestinal, respiratory and the genitourinary tracts. SC acts as a receptor for dimeric IgA and appears to function as a mechanism for transport of Igs across the mucosal surface into secretory fluid and it was thought to be a regulator for the secretory Igs [12, 13]. But in the present study, we found TF free SC in HID group was significantly higher than the control group which may indicate that SC production is independent of the secretion of TF IgA.

Using immunoblotting, we found TF IgM in 7 of 8 HID cases. Moreover, the IgM was associated with/bound to SC. Theoretically, not only dimeric IgA but any other class Ig that has an attached J chain can bind to the SC. The presence of the J chain protein in IgM structure allow its molecule to fit the receptor on secretory cells where it is transported across epithelial linings to the external secretion. Therefore, pentameric IgM can also be transported into TF by those mechanism for dimeric IgA. The presence of the SC appears to protect secretory Ig such as IgA, IgM rending them less susceptible to the proteolytic enzymes present in the TF. Thus IgM appearing in TF is a true secretory Ig, like IgA. In addition, IgM may be more effective than that of IgG in the defense of ocular surface, especially in the absence of IgA in HID individuals. IgM is more efficient than IgG at activation complement, neutralizing virus and bacteria.

In HG group, the significantly higher TF IgG level than control may indicate the correlation between local concentration and serum production. The levels of TF IgA and free SC may also indicate that TF free SC is produced independently of TF IgA. The differences of TF IgA level between HIV+ and HIV- groups suggest that there may be different pathological mechanism of IgA production/secretion and further study remains.

REFERENCES

1   Clark JA, Callicoat PA, Bradley CA, et al. Am J Clin Pathol 1983;80:210-213.
2   Skokanova V, Kaminkova J, Vacek Z, et al. Casopis Lekaru Ceskych 1993; 132(12):369-372.
3   Hay EM, Freemont AJ, Kay RA, et al. Ann Rheum Dis 1990;49:373-377.
4   Lam S, Tessler HH. Am J Ophthalmol 1990;110(4):440-441.
5   Ehrenstein MR, Isenberg DA. Ann Rheum Dis 1992;51:1185-1187.
6   Spronic PE, v.d. Gun BT, Limburg PC, et al. Clin Exp Immunol 1993;93(1):39-44.
7   Kawamoto H, Sakaguchi K, Takaki A, et al. Acta Medica Okayama 1993;47(5): 305-310.
8   Coyle PK, Sibony PA, Johnson C. Invest Ophthalmol Vis Sci 1989;30:1872-1878.
9   Kuizenga A, van Haeringen NJ, Kijlstrat A. Invest Ophthalmol Vis Sci 1991;32:3277-3284.
10   Kuizenga A, Stolwijk TR, van Agtmaal EJ, et al. Curr Eye Res 1990;9(10):997-1005.
11   Brandtzaeg P, Fjellanger I, Gjeruldsen ST. Science 1968;160:789-791.
12   Solari R, Kraehenbuhl JP. Immunol Today 1985;6:17-20.
13   Franklin RM. Curr Eye Res 1989;8(6):599-606.

1. Inflammatory Disease
b. Therapeutic Approaches

Advances in Ocular Immunology
R.B. Nussenblatt, S.M. Whitcup, R.R. Caspi and I. Gery, eds.

411

EFFICACY AND SAFETY OF 1% RIMEXOLONE OPHTHALMIC SUSPENSION VS. 1% PREDNISOLONE ACETATE (PRED FORTE®) FOR TREATMENT OF UVEITIS

C.S.Foster*, M.Drake^, F.D.Turner^, J.L.Crabb~, C.I.Santos**, and The Rimexolone Uveitis Study Group

* Massachusetts Eye & Ear Infirmary, Harvard Medical School, Boston, MA., 02114 (USA)

^ Alcon Laboratories, Inc., 6201 South West Freeway, Fort Worth, TX., 76134 (USA)

~ 5405 Knight Arnold, Memphis, TN., 38115 (USA)

** 269 Pinero Ave., Rio Piedras, Puerto Rico, 00927

INTRODUCTION

Uveitis is an ocular inflammatory process affecting the iris, ciliary body and/or choroid. While the inflammation is usually limited to anterior regions (1), it can affect the posterior segment or as panuveitis it can involve both regions simultaneously. Uveitis occurs acutely, recurrently or chronically and can lead to cataract formation, glaucoma, hypotony, neovascularization and vitreal opacification (2) if not treated successfully.

Noninfectious anterior segment uveitis responds to treatment with corticosteroids, immunosuppressive drugs, and/or non-steroidal anti-inflammatory agents. Currently, topical corticosteroids are the most commonly prescribed drugs for patients with this potentially blinding disease (3). However, steroids have undesirable side-effects, the most dangerous being their tendency to raise the intraocular pressure (IOP) of some patients (4,5).

A new topical corticosteriod, Rimexolone 1% Ophthalmic Suspension, has been shown to be an effective anti-inflammatory with a reduced tendency to raise IOP levels. The clinical study reported here was conducted to evaluate the efficacy and safety of Rimexolone 1% compared to a commonly prescribed corticosteroid, 1% prednisolone acetate (Pred Forte®), in patients with uveitis for whom a topical steroid was indicated.

MATERIALS & METHODS

The study reported here was a 28-day double-masked study in which 160 patients with uveitis were evaluated for both safety and efficacy after being randomized to treatment with either Rimexolone 1% or 1% Prednisolone Acetate. A demographic analysis of patient age, sex, iris color, area of inflammation and specific diagnosis indicated that the study group was representative of similar populations reported in the literature (1). Analysis also showed that the two treatment groups were uniformly composed. Acute uveitis was seen in 57.5% of the study patients, while 21.5% were diagnosed with recurrent uveitis and 21% with chronic uveitis.

412

This 4-week study included five examinations (on Days 3-4, 7-10, 14, 21 and 28) during which visual acuity and IOP levels were measured, and both slit lamp and external ophthalmic evaluations were made. At each examination, six clinical parameters of the disease were evaluated: anterior chamber cells; anterior chamber flare; ciliary flush; keratic precipitates; photophobia; discomfort. Patients in both the Rimexolone 1% treatment group (N=77) and the 1% Prednisolone Acetate treatment group (N=83) were medicated as described below:

Day 1 to 7:   1-2 drops in affected eye(s) <u>every hour</u> (while awake)
Day 8 to 14:   1-2 drops in affected eye(s) <u>every 2 hours</u>
Day 15 to 21: 1-2 drops in affected eye(s) <u>every 3 hours</u>
Day 22 to 25: 1-2 drops in affected eye(s) <u>every 12 hours</u>
Day 26 to 28: 1-2 drops in affected eye(s) <u>every 24 hours</u>
Day 28: study terminated, with a follow-up examination at 36-48 hours

RESULTS

The presence of cells in the anterior chamber is a semi-quantitative measurement of the severity of uveitis. The 77 Rimexolone-treated patients and the 83 Prednisolone Acetate-treated patients were evaluated at all five of the examinations for the presence of these anterior chamber cells. No clinically or statistically significant differences between the Rimexolone-treated and Prednisolone Acetate-treated groups were seen at any point, as shown in FIGURE 1.

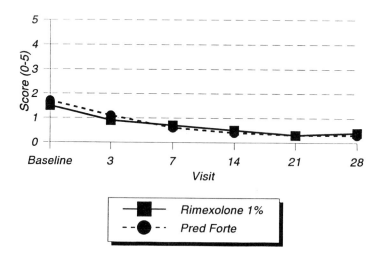

<u>FIGURE 1</u>: A comparison of mean scores of anterior chamber cells for patients in both groups at each examination. A grading scale of 0-5 was used, with 0 = <5 cells, 2 = moderate (11-20 cells) and 5 = hypopyon.

A second measurable sign of the severity of uveitis is the presence of anterior chamber flare. The 77 Rimexolone-treated patients and the 83 Prednisolone Acetate-treated patients were evaluated during each study examination for the presence of this clinical sign. Once again, no clinically or statistically significant differences were seen between the two treatment groups at any point, as shown in FIGURE 2.

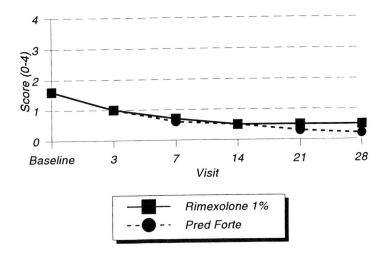

FIGURE 2: A comparison of mean scores of anterior chamber flare for patients in both treatment groups at each examination. A grading scale of 0-4 was used, with 0 = none to trace, 2 = moderate without plastic aqueous and 4 = severe with heavy fibrin deposits and clots.

In addition to anterior chamber cells and flare, other parameters of disease severity such as ciliary flush, keratic precipitates, photophobia and discomfort were evaluated in both treatment groups. No clinically significant differences between the treatment groups were seen at Day 28 for any of these four clinical signs of uveitis (data not shown).

As described above, the evaluation of six clinical parameters of uveitis indicated that Rimexolone 1% and 1% Prednisolone Acetate are equally effective for treating patients with uveitis. In order to compare the tendency of these two topical corticosteroids to raise IOP levels, the Rimexolone-treated and Prednisolone Acetate-treated patients in this study were evaluated at each examination with Goldmann applanation tonometry. Any increase from a patient's baseline IOP levels of 10 mm Hg or more was defined as clinically significant. Our results indicated that patients treated with Rimexolone 1% were significantly less likely to develop such IOP increases than were Prednisolone Acetate-treated patients. Whereas by Day 28 only 6.8% of Rimexolone-treated patients developed one or more clinically significant IOP increases, 11.8% of the 1% Prednisolone Acetate-treated patients developed this treatment complication (p = 0.0302 using Fisher's Exact Test). The relative frequency of clinically significant IOP increases in the two groups is shown in FIGURE 3.

414

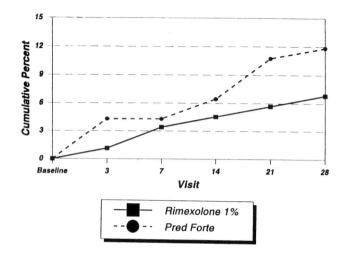

FIGURE 3: The cumulative percentage of patients in both treatment groups exhibiting a clinically significant IOP increase (ie. 10 mm Hg or more over baseline) is plotted over time.

In addition to a significantly decreased tendency to raise IOP levels in the uveitis patients studied here (FIGURE 3), our results suggest that Rimexolone 1% Ophthalmic Formulation is safe and well-tolerated by these patients. Adverse reactions to Rimexolone 1% were generally mild, nonserious, usually resolved without treatment and did not result in sequelae. No serious events related to Rimexolone 1% were reported, and no patient discontinued from the study due to a treatment-related event. The most common adverse reactions to this medication were ocular discomfort (3.4%) and ocular discharge (3.4%). No post-treatment rebound effect was observed in the patients using Rimexolone 1% for four weeks. When adverse reactions in the Rimexolone-treated and Prednisoloe Acetate-treated groups were compared demographically, no clinically significant differences were seen.

CONCLUSIONS

Uveitis is a potentially blinding inflammatory disease. Currently, topical steroid treatment is indicated for many uveitis patients. In this study a new topical steroid, Rimexolone 1% Ophthalmic Suspension, was compared with the commonly prescribed 1% prednisolone acetate (Pred Forte®) in patients with acute as well as recurrent and chronic uveitis. Results indicate that Rimexolone 1% was as effective as 1% Prednisolone Acetate for treating patients with uveitis. In addition to being as effective as 1% Prednisolone Acetate, Rimexolone 1% was also shown to be safe and well-tolerated by the patients in this study. Our results also show that Rimexolone 1% was significantly less likely than 1% Prednisolone Acetate to cause potentially dangerous increases (10 mm Hg or more) in the IOP levels of patients with uveitis for whom topical steroid treatment was indicated.

PARTICIPATING MEMBERS OF THE UVEITIS STUDY GROUP

Kerry K. Assil, M.D.   (Bethesda Eye Institute, St. Louis, MO.)
Robert Caine, M.D.   (Cambridge St., Fredricksburg, VA.)
James L. Crabb, M.D.   (Eye-Tech, Memphis, TN.)
C. Stephen Foster, M.D.   (Massachusetts Eye & Ear Infirmary, Boston, MA.)
Kenneth Fox, M.D.   (Cambridge St., Fredricksburg, VA.)
Rudolph M. Franklin, M.D.   (Genois St., New Orleans, LA, & Bob Hope Eye
                                             Research Center, Houston, TX.)
Henry J. Kaplan, M.D.   (Euclid Ave., St. Louis, MO.)
Martin J. Kreshon, M.D.   (Charlotte Eye, Ear, Nose Assoc., Charlotte, NC.)
James P. McCulley, M.D.   (Dept. Ophthalmol, Dallas, TX.)
Kenneth W. Olander, M.D.   (Eye Physician Assoc., Milwaukee, Wi.)
Alan Gary Palestine, M.D.   (19th St., Washington, D.C.)
F. Temple Reikhof, M.D.   (E. St., Salt Lake City, UT.)
Carmen I. Santos, M.D.   (Rio Piedras, P.R.)
Stephen V. Scoper, M.D.   (Univ of VA HSC, Charlottesville, VA.)
Daniel H. Spitzberg, M.D.   (Capital Ave., Indianopolis, IN.)
Joseph Tauber, M.D.   (Eye Found. of K.C., Kansas City, MO.)
Howard H. Tessler, M.D.   (W. Taylor, Chicago, IL.)
Paul L. Zimmerman, M.D.   (Rocky Mountain Eye Cntr., Salt Lake City, UT.)

REFERENCES

1 Darrell RW, Kurland L, Wagenerti P. Arch Ophthalmol 1962; 68: 4.
2 Foster CS. In: Boke WRF, Manthey KF, Nussenblatt RB, eds. Intermediate
      Ophthalmology. Dev Ophthalmol. Basel: Karger, 1992; 23: 156.
3 Ellis PP. Int Ophthalmol Clinics 1966; 6: 799.
4 Becker B. Investig Ophthalmol Vis Sci 1965; 4: 198.
5 Armaly MF. Investig Ophthalmol Vis Sci 1965; 4: 187.

Advances in Ocular Immunology
R.B. Nussenblatt, S.M. Whitcup, R.R. Caspi and I. Gery, eds.

TOPICAL CYCLOSPORIN A REDUCES EOSINOPHIL ACTIVATION IN VERNAL KERATOCONJUNCTIVITIS.

A. Leonardi[a], F. Borghesan[b], M. Salmaso[a], M. Plebani[b], and A. G. Secchi[a].

[a]Institute of Clinical Ophthalmology, Department of Physiological Optics

[b]Department of Laboratory Medicine; University of Padua, Padua, Italy

INTRODUCTION

Vernal keratoconjunctivitis (VKC) is an ocular allergic disease predominantly observed in children and young adults living in warm, southern climates. Topical treatment with Cyclosporine A 2% has proven effective in the management of severe VKC cases [1] in which topical steroids and/or mast cell stabilizers are not sufficient therapy or are contraindicated.

Eosinophils play a major role in the development of allergic diseases, releasing upon activation, granule-stored, pharmacologically specific mediators. Eosinophil cationic protein (ECP) comprises 30% of the eosinophil granule matrix [2]. Its toxic effect on human corneal epithelial cells has recently been demonstrated in vitro [3]. ECP levels in biological fluids correlate with the severity of some allergic diseases and its presence in biological fluids and tissues is now considered a marker for eosinophil activation.

In this study, tear ECP levels were measured in normal subjects and in patients with active VKC treated with various topical, ocular drug therapies as a means of evaluating drug efficacy.

MATERIALS AND METHODS

Using a capillary micro-pipette, tear samples from 9 eyes of 7 normal volunteers (mean age: 16 ± 2.1 years; 3 males, 4 females) were collected. A 5 ml aliquot was used for tear cytology, with the remainder stored at -20° for subsequent determination of ECP.

23 patients affected by bilateral active (VKC) (mean age: 13 ± 5.0 years; 16 males, 7 females) were enrolled in the study. After clinical evaluation of ocular signs and symptoms, tear samples were collected, as above, for tear cytology and ECP determination. Of the 23 VKC patients, 9 were treated bilaterally four times daily with cyclosporine A 2% (CsA) in castor oil, 5 with dexamethasone 0.1% (Dex), 3 with disodium cromoglycate 4% (DSCG) and 6 with Lodoxamide 0.1% (Lod). Clinical evaluation and tear collection (for tear cytology and ECP

measurement) were repeated 5-7 days after commencement of steroid therapy and 2 weeks after DSCG and CsA. From the 46 VKC eyes, 42 baseline and 40 post-therapy tear samples were available.

A clinical score (0-4) was determined at each visit and for each eye for the four major symptoms: itching, tearing, photophobia, and foreign body sensation, and for the five major signs: conjunctival erythema, eye swelling, discharge, papillae/follicles and epithelial disease (corneal involvement).

Tear cytology was evaluated using pre-colored slides (Testsimplet,® Boehringer, Mannheim, Germany), counting the eosinophils present in 5 microscopic fields of 0.15 mm^2 each.

ECP was measured using a commercially available radioimmunoassay technique (Kabi Pharmacia, Uppsala, Sweden). The results were expressed as micrograms per liter (mg/L).

Statistical analyses were performed using the Student's t test, the Mann-Whitney U-test or the Wilcoxon Signed-Rank test, where appropriate. Results are listed as the mean ± standard error of the mean (SEM). Correlation coefficents were obtained by the use of linear correlation analysis. For statistical significance, the assigned p value was ≤ 0.05.

RESULTS

The mean ECP level measured in the 9 tear samples from 7 normal volunteers was 7.1 ± 0.6 mg/L (range: 5 to 10 mg/L). No subject had any signs or symptoms of external eye disease. Tear cytology demonstrated no eosinophils. In the 42 tear samples from untreated VKC patients at baseline, mean ECP levels were 847.3 ± 111.8 mg/L (range 24 to 2530 mg/L). After miscellaneous drug therapies, (40 samples available), mean ECP levels were significantly decreased (p <0.01) to 383.8 ± 83.2 mg/L (6 to 2387 mg/L). Both levels were significantly increased compared to controls (p<0.01).

The individual drug effects on ECP levels in VKC patients are listed in Table 1. Only Cyclosporin A and dexamethasone significantly decreased ECP levels, however, lodoxamide showed a very strong trend towards significance (p = 0.06).

The clinical scores of both signs and symptoms decreased significantly after treatment with CsA, Dex and Lod (Figures 1 and 2). In patients with severe VKC treated with only DSCG, the mean clinical score was increased after treatment, with a worsening of corneal involvement and conjunctival inflammation. The number of eosinophils in tears was significantly reduced only in patients treated with topical CsA (p<0.01).

ECP levels and number of eosinophils in tears were significantly correlated (r = 0.55, p < 0.01). Significant correlations were also observed between ECP levels in all samples (independent of therapy) and 1) signs (r = 0.466, p < 0.001); 2) symptoms (r = 0.551, p <0.001) and 3) corneal involvement (r = 0.836, p<0.0001).

Table 1
ECP levels in tears (mg/L) before and after topical treatments

	Cs A	Dex	DSCG	Lod
Before	932.5 ± 143 (186-2075) (N=17)	1291.7 ± 314.3 (24-2530) (N=9)	734.5 ± 213.6 (260-1690) (N=6)	476.1 ± 196.3 (25-2010) (N=10)
After	166 ± 44.8 (6-612) (N=15)	628.5 ± 173.4 (9-1300) (N=9)	1426.4 ± 410.3 (255-2387) (N=5)	130.7 ± 61.2 (7-696) (N=11)
P value	0.0004	0.002	n.s.	n.s. (0.06)

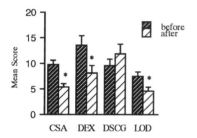

Figure 1 Ocular signs before and after therapies (*=p<0.001).

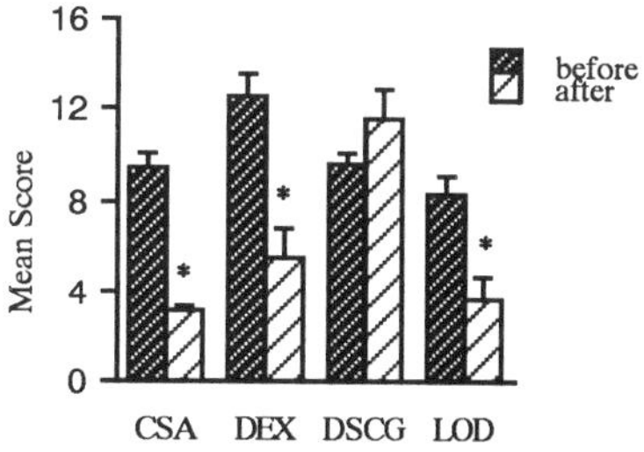

Figure 2. Ocular symptoms before and after therapies (*=p<0.001).

DISCUSSION

The typical histological features of VKC are the conjunctival infiltration of eosinophils and basophils, a constant, increased number of mast cells and an increased deposition of collagen [4]. An accumulation of Th2-like helper T cells, producing interleukins 3, 4 and 5, has also been shown to occur in VKC, accounting for the frequent occurrence of high levels of tear immunoglobulin E, mast cell proliferation, and the abundant presence of eosinophils [5]. Activated eosinophils are known to release toxic factors such as the presently studied ECP, in addition to EMBP, eosinophil peroxidase, eosinophil-derived neurotoxin, and eosinophil protein-X. Eosinophil major basic protein (EMBP) has already been shown to play a role in the pathogenesis of epithelial erosions observed in VKC, indicating the importance of eosinophil activation in severe forms of this disease

420

[6]. Conjunctival eosinophil activation and degranulation, accompanied by high levels of tear ECP, was also previously reported in 7 VKC patients [7].

In this study, ECP was easily detectable and measurable in tears with a high degree of sensitivity. The wide variations of ECP levels found in baseline tears of VKC patients (24 to 2530 mg/L) may reflect a varying range of activation of eosinophils. The significant correlation between ECP levels and corneal involvement, in addition to the known toxic effect of ECP on corneal epithelium, suggests a relationship between this mediator and VKC-related corneal damage. Tear ECP was dramatically reduced by CsA 2% and dexamethasone, suggesting a down-regulating activity of these drugs on eosinophil activation. CsA seemed to be the most effective therapy for severe VKC, also reducing the number of tear eosinophils. The effect of CsA on eosinophil chemotaxis and activation is probably secondary to its effect on T-helper lymphocytes rather than a direct effect on the eosinophil cell membrane. Lodoxamide reduced tear ECP, but not significantly, while DSCG did not have any effect on ECP in severe VKC patients. Clinical signs and symptoms were significantly reduced by treatment with CsA, dexamethasone and lodoxamide.

ECP levels were found to highly correlate with both signs and symptoms, in addition to corneal involvement. Thus, the measurement of ECP is useful not only in the monitoring of ocular allergic diseases, but also in the evaluation of new therapies, for which an objective parameter is needed to complement clinical assessments.

REFERENCES

1   Secchi AG, Tognon MS, Leonardi A. Am J Ophthalmol 1990; 110: 137-142.
2   Olsson I, Venge P. Blood 1974; 44: 235-46.
3   Hallberg CK, Brysk MM, Tyring SK, Gleich GJ, Trocme SD. Invest Ophthalmol Visual Sci 1994; 35 (4) (Suppl.): 1943 (Abstract).
4   Leonardi A, Albanese C, Abatangelo G, Secchi AG. Invest Ophthalmol Visual Sci 1993; 34 (4) (Suppl.): 700 (Abstract).
5   Maggi E, Biswas P, Del Prete G, et al. J Immunol 1991; 146: 1169-74.
6   Trocme SD, Kephart GM, Burne WM, Buckley RJ, Gleich GJ. Am J Ophthalmol 1993; 115: 640-43.
7   Saiga T, Ueno N, Shimizu Y. Invest Ophthalmol Visual Sci 1991; 32 (4) (Suppl.): 682 (Abstract).

© 1994 Elsevier Science B.V. All rights reserved.
Advances in Ocular Immunology
R.B. Nussenblatt, S.M. Whitcup, R.R. Caspi and I. Gery, eds.

INCREASED RISK OF MALIGNANCY IN PATIENTS WITH UVEITIS TREATED WITH SYSTEMIC IMMUNOSUPPRESIVE THERAPY

N. L. Murray, P. J. McCluskey and D. Wakefield
Laboratory of Ocular Immunology, School of Pathology, University of N.S.W. Sydney, NSW. Australia

INTRODUCTION

Systemic therapy with immunosuppressive drugs is a sight saving treatment in selected patients with severe uveitis. Despite the lack of clear data regarding the risk of developing a malignancy, the use of cytotoxic drugs for the treatment of uveitis is a major concern. Results from studies of patients treated with systemic immunosuppression for transplantation and diseases such as rheumatoid arthritis, Sjogren's syndrome, systemic lupus erythematosus (SLE) and Crohn's disease clearly show an increased risk of malignancy.[1] However, even without immunosuppressive therapy, an increased risk of malignancy is observed in patients with such autoimmune diseases [1].

To evaluate this problem, we performed a retrospective analysis of patients with uveitis who had received systemic immunosuppressive therapy to ascertain the incidence and risk of malignancy. These subjects were compared with patients with uveitis who were treated with systemic corticosteroids alone, a well accepted agent for control of severe uveitis with no known increased risk of malignancy. [2]

METHODS

Patients with severe uveitis requiring prolonged systemic immunosuppressive therapy and attending the Ocular Immunology Clinic at St Vincent's Hospital, Sydney, Australia between 1980 and February 1992 were reviewed. Forty six patients who had received systemic immunosuppressive therapy and had regular follow up for at least twelve months were studied. Follow up involved detailed ophthalmic and systemic review. A detailed history was obtained, complete ophthalmic and physical examinations were performed on all subjects, and all previous records reviewed. Appropriate investigations were performed to assess current disease status. Ocular inflammation was graded according to a previously published uveitis scoring system.[11] Patients with uveitis who received immunosuppressive therapy, but with incomplete follow up data, were excluded. All patients with an associated systemic disease with a known increased risk of malignancy, including patients with rheumatoid arthritis, Sjogren's syndrome, SLE, and Crohn's disease, were excluded. The frequency of neoplasms in the patients with uveitis were compared with the reported frequency of these tumours in the Australian population as obtained from the State Cancer Council of New South Wales.

RESULTS

Forty six patients received systemic immunosuppressive (cytotoxic) treatment for control of their uveitis. There were 28 females and 13 males with a mean age of 42 years (range 13-71 years). Forty one patients were treated with corticosteroids alone. There were 29 females in this group; the mean age was 42 years with a range of 14-72 years. Duration of uveitis ranged from 4 to 60 months for the corticosteroid treated group, and 3 to 70 months for the cytotoxic treatment patients. Pre treatment uveitis scores were 7 (range 3-11) for the corticosteroid treatment group and 7 (range 3-12) for the group treated with cytotoxic drugs. There were no differences between the corticosteroid treated and cytotoxic treated uveitis patient groups (p > 0.05 for age, sex, duration and uveitis score).

Thirty five of the corticosteroid treated group of patients had idiopathic disease, four had sarcoidosis and two Behcet's syndrome. Thirty four of the cytotoxic treatment group had idiopathic disease, six sarcoidosis, 3 Behcet's syndrome, 2 sympathetic ophthalmia and one patient had VKH.

Table 1
Observed and expected number of malignancies in patients with uveitis treated with immunosuppressive drugs

Malignancy	Observed (N=46)	Expected	Relative risk
Non Hodgkins Lymphoma	1	4.3/1000	5.2
Cervical cancer	3	7.7/1000	9.0
Squamous cell cancer	1	1.7/1000	13.1
Basal cell cancer	2	6.6/1000	6.8
Prostate cancer	1	4.9/1000	4.5

Two patients treated with systemic corticosteroids only developed malignancies during the course of this study. One man with idiopathic uveitis developed a biopsy proven basal cell carcinoma of the arm, whilst a woman with idiopathic uveitis was diagnosed as having carcinoma of the cervix (CIN 2). Both neoplasms were surgically treated without evidence of recurrence at follow up. Nine malignancies were detected in seven patients treated with immunosuppressive drugs. Three patients developed skin cancers and three subjects were diagnosed as having cervical carcinoma. One patient developed an adenocarcinoma of the prostate whilst another manifested non-Hodgkin's lymphoma. The incidence of malignancy was higher in the patients treated with cytotoxic drugs than in those treated with corticosteroids only. The only association with a particular immunosuppressive agent and malignancy was that observed with chlorambucil. Four of the six patients treated with chlorambucil developed malignancies during the course of this study (p<0.05). Multiple models containing potential risk factors for the development of malignancy were tested using logistic regression analysis. Age, sex, nature and duration of uveitis and smoking history were not related to an increased risk of malignancy.

DISCUSSION
Although the number of patients with uveitis in this study is small, we observed an increased risk of malignancy in patients treated with cytotoxic drugs. Furthermore, patients treated with corticosteroids alone do not exhibit the same increase in systemic malignancy. The malignancies observed in patients with uveitis who received combination immunosuppressive therapy (corticosteroids and Cytotoxics) are similar to those observed in other immunosuppressed patient groups. Non Hodgkin's lymphoma (NHL), skin and cervical cancer in particular, have been noted in earlier studies. The development of malignancy appears to be related to the degree and duration of immunosuppressive therapy[1], rather than to a specific drug or clinical situation.

We present what we believe to be the first report of an increased prevalence of cervical malignancy in patients with uveitis treated with cytotoxic drugs. This result is in keeping with observations made on immunosuppressed transplant patients. There is a need for ongoing careful surveillance and preventative measures in patients with uveitis treated with cytotoxic and immunosuppressive drugs. Currently we regularly perform haematological, biochemical and urine analysis. All patients are instructed with regard to ultraviolet light protection and all suspicious skin lesions are biopsied and treated as indicated. We advise regular colposcopy - cervical smears alone are now accepted as inadequate screening in high risk groups. We believe appropriate preventative screening can minimise the significant oncogenic risks to uveitis patients treated with cytotoxic drugs.

Alkylating agents are, in our experience, the most effective agents in inducing a disease remission in severe refractory cases of uveitis. We initially used chlorambucil in the early 1980's, as did others. More recently we have used cyclophosphamide in both oral and pulsed intravenous form. The side effect profile of alkylating agents is significant, in particular sterility, alopecia and malignancy[2]. "Safe" quantities of both chlorambucil (total dose < 1g) and cyclophosphamide (total dose < 50g), or treatment with either for less than six months has been proposed[2,4]. Interestingly, chlorambucil was used in six of our patients, two with doses exceeding 1g (1.8g, 2.1g). Both these patients developed skin carcinoma (BCC). Cyclophosphamide was used in nine patients, four having doses exceeding 50g, no tumours have developed in any of these subjects. However, one patient who received (6g total dose) cyclophosphamide subsequently developed a SCC of the skin. Currently we use cyclophosphamide (2-3 mg/kg/day PO) for six months then review its role in the immunosuppression of the patient, cognisant that if disease control is not achieved alternate treatment is indicated and the possibility of malignancy may be increased if treatment is continued beyond this period. Idiopathic uveitis treated with systemic corticosteroids does not appear to be associated with an increased risk of malignancy. Malignancies occur in immunosuppressed uveitis patients as in other patients with autoimmune disease treated with Cytotoxics.

REFERENCES:
1. Penn I. Tumours of the immunocompromised patient. *Ann Rev Med* 1988; 63-73.
2. Hemady R, Tauber J, Foster C.S. Immunosuppresive drugs in immune and inflammatory ocular disease. *Surv Ophthal* 1991; 35: 369-385.
3. Nussenblatt R.B, Palestine A.G, Chan C.C. Cyclosporin A therapy in the treatment of intraocular inflammatory disease resistant to systemic corticosteroids and cytotoxic agents. *Am J Ophthalmol* 1983; 96: 275-282.
4. Baker G.L, Kahl Le Zee B.C. et al Malignancy following treatment of rheumatoid arthritis with cyclophosphamide. *Am J Med* 1987; 83: 1-9.
5. Porreco R, Penn I. Proegemueller W. et al. Gynaecological malignancies in immunosuppressed organ homograft recipients. *Obstet Gynaecol* 1975; 45: 359-364.
6. Walder B.K, Charlesworth J.A, McDonald G.J. et al. The skin and immunosuppression. *Aust J Derm* 1970; 17: 94-97.
7. Mc Cleod A.M, Catto G.R. Cancer after transplantation. *Br Med J* 1988; 297: 4-5.
8. Ben Ezra D, Forrester J.V, Nussenblatt R.B. et al. Uveitis scoring system Springer Verlage, Berlin 1991.
9. Hogan M.D, Kimura S.J, Thygeson P. Signs and symptoms of uveitis, I. Anterior uveitis. *Am J Ophthalmol* 1959 (47 supp): 155-170.
10. Kimura S.J, Thygeson P, Hogan M.D. Signs and symptoms of uveitis II Classifications of the posterior manifestations of uveitis. *Am J Ophthalmol* 1959 (47 supp): 171-180.
11. Nussenblatt R.B, Palestine A.G, Chan C.C. et al. Standard of vitreal inflammatory activity in intermediate and posterior uveitis. *Ophthalmol* 1985; 92: 467-471.
12. Wakefield D, McCluskey P. Intravenous pulse methylprednisolone therapy in severe inflammatory eye disease. *Arch Ophthalmol* 1986; 104: 847-851.

© 1994 Elsevier Science B.V. All rights reserved.
Advances in Ocular Immunology
R.B. Nussenblatt, S.M. Whitcup, R.R. Caspi and I. Gery, eds.   425

IMMUNOSUPPRESSIVE THERAPY FOR COGAN'S SYNDROME

P. Pivetti-Pezzi, M. Accorinti, M. La Cava, R.A.M. Colabelli Gisoldi

Institute of Ophthalmology, Ocular Immunovirology Service, University "La Sapienza", Rome - Italy

INTRODUCTION

Cogan's syndrome is an uncommon disease of young adults characterized by episodes of acute non-syphilitic interstitial keratitis associated with vestibuloauditory dysfunction resembling Meniere's disease (1). The outlook for vision is generally good, while deafness is often profound and is the main handicap.
Ocular symptoms may also include conjunctivitis, episcleritis, iritis, orbital pseudotumor, papillitis, posterior scleritis, retinal haemorrhages and maculopathy with severe vision impairment (2,3,4). Furthermore in about 50% of the patients it is possible to find systemic manifestations, such as vasculitis, aortitis and aortic valvular disease, renal involvement, gastrointestinal haemorrhage, arthralgias, lymphoadenopathy and muscoloskeletal disease (2-4).
The aetiology of Cogan's syndrome is unclear but there is some evidence of autoimmune reactivity to both corneal and inner-ear antigens as well as the possibility of a cell-mediated immunity suggested by the presence of lymphocytes in ocular and vestibulo-auditory tissues (5). Therefore Cogan's syndrome is probably a manifestation of a systemic vasculitis (3,4,6,).The audiovestibular symptoms may partially respond to oral prednisone therapy as well as the milder forms of eye inflammation. Nevertheless the possible serious outcome of this syndrome and the suspected autoimmune pathogenesis may suggest a stronger therapeutic appoach with immunosuppressive agents.
We report our experience with Cyclosporine - A treatment in two cases of Cogan's syndrome in which the therapy stopped the progression of both corneal and audiovestibular lesions with no recurrences after a mean time of 23 months from the withdrawal of therapy.

CASE N°1

In July 1989 a 23-year-old woman developed an acute progressive bilateral hearing deficiency with nystagmus and vertigo. Neurological examination, as well as a computerized tomography of the brain were normal while the audiometry revealed a deep sensorineural hearing loss.
Two weeks later the patient also complained of bilateral eye redness, pain and photofobia because of a decreased tear secretion. A "sicca syndrome with corneal oedema" was suspected and lacrimal substitutes administered.

Despite a steroid treatment (0.5 mg/Kg/day of pednisone) in the following 10 months, recurrences of the eye symptoms and the appearance of arthralgias, myalgias and lower limb paresthesia were noted, while no improvement in the hearing loss was noted. We examined the patients for the first time in April 1990 and we observed deep-seated infiltrates in the cornea of both eyes (peripheral the in left eye; peripheral and central in the right eye). Anterior segment, intraocular pressure and fundus oculi were normal. The best-corrected visual acuity was 10/10 in both eyes, Schirmer's test and retinal fluorescein angiography was also normal.

At laboratory evaluation she presented an increased ESR, while the following exams resulted normal : complete blood count, chemistries, VDRL, TPHA, FTA-ABS, complement and immunoglobulin levels, protein electrphoresis, auto-antibodies, rheumatoid factor, circulating immunocomplexes, chest X-ray, electrocardiogram and echocardiogram, serology for Lyme disease, computerized tomography.

Both otorhinolaryngological and physical examinations revealed a complete bilateral sensorineural hearing loss, no nystagmus, positive capillaroscopy, the persistence of arthralgias, myalgias and lower limb paresthesia. A diagnosis of Cogan's syndrome was made and Cyclosporine - A (5 mg/Kg/day) administered for 14 months in combination with a short course of topical steroids (4 times daily for 1 week then slowly tapered). During the first 6 months of therapy we observed two mild relapses of interstitial keratitis that completely disappeared after a 7-day course of topical steroids, the disappearence of arthralgias, myalgias and paresthesia of the lower limbs, normal laboratory values, persisting bilateral deefness, no other organ involvement and no drug-related side-effects. Cyclosporine - A therapy was discontinued after 14 months and the patient has received no treatment now for 34 months without any symptoms of the disease.

CASE N° 2

In September 1991 a 27-year-old woman complained of bilateral high - frequency hearing loss (greater on the right), tinnitus, vertigo and nausea together with pain and redness in both eyes.

A diagnosis of bilateral iridocyclitis was made and steroid therapy (prednisone: 0.5 mg/Kg/day), bethametasone and mydriatic eye drops administered. After two months in which no improvement of the hearing deficiency was obtained the patient was admitted to our Institute.

We found a visual acuity of 8/10 in RE and 10/10 in LE, bilateral central deep-seated white corneal infiltrates and corneal oedema, no reaction in the anterior and vitreous chamber, and a cotton-wool like spot along the supero-temporal vascular arcade in right eye.

The audiogram revealed a sensoryneural defect for high-frequencies. An increased ESR and a mild leukocytosis were present while all the other following exams were normal: complete blood count, chemistries, VDRL, TPHA, FTA-ABS, complement and immunoglobulin levels, protein electrophoresis, auto-antibodies, rheumatoid factor, circulating immunocomplexes, chest X-ray, electrocardiogram and echocardiogram, serology for Lyme disease.

Both neurological and physical examinations were normal, as was the NMR.

A diagnosis of Cogan's syndrome was made and the patient was administered Cyclosporine-A (5 mg/Kg/day) and prednisone 1 mg/Kg/day for 5 days which was then gradually reduced in 45 days and bethametasone eye drops were also prescribed for 20 days.

Ocular symptoms subsided in 15 days while a partial recovery of the high frequency hearing loss was obtained. Cyclosporine - A therapy was administered for 12 months, than tapered in 4 months and then stopped.

During the follow-up we observed no recurrences of neither interstitial keratitis nor audiovestibulary symptoms. Furthermore no other organ involvement nor drug-related side-effects appeared and the patients has been out of therapy from 12 months.

RESULTS

At the time of observation both patients showed a typical interstitial keratitis, with a probable concomitant onset of the audiovestibular symptoms. One of them also displayed arthralgias, myalgias, paresthesia and complete deafness in spite of the previously administered steroid therapy.

After a complete ophthalmologic, otholaryngologic, neurologic and systemic evaluation a treatment with Cyclosporine-A was started (initial dose : 5 mg/Kg/day) and prolonged for 14 and 16 months in order to avoid further progression of the ocular/audiovestibular symptoms and the onset of other systemic manifestations.

Two mild ocular relapses of interstitial keratitis occurred after two and three months of therapy in case n° 1 but promptly subsided after a brief steroid eye drop treatment.

Now at the end of follow-up (50 and 31 months from our first examination, respectively) we have obtained a complete control of ocular inflammation, a partial improvement in hearing in case n° 2, no audiometric changes in patient n°1 because of a previously diagnosed complete deafness but a total resolution of vestibular troubles, and the absence of any other possible systemic manifestations.

No drug-related side-effects appeared and now the patients are in a therapy-free period from 34 and 12 months respectively.

COMMENT

Cogan's syndrome is a rare disease mainly characterized by interstitial keratitis and audiovestibular symptoms. Ocular involvement is usually mild and it may be resolved without therapy (1) or with the use of topical corticosteroids and cycloplegis; on the contrary deafness is usually irreversible (4,7), even if a prompt steroid treatment may limit its progression (2,6,8,10). Furthermore in patients affected by Cogan's syndrome a severe sight-threatening ocular inflammation has been described as well as systemic involvement, mainly constituted by large-vessel vasculitis (2,3,4).

A successful treatment of all these complications may be achieved with systemic steroids, while other immunosuppressive agents (cyclophosphamide, cyclosporine-A, FK 506) have proved useful in more severe cases (9,11,12).

Cyclosporine-A has been used since 1982 for the treatment of some ocular autoimmune disease and, at the maximum dosage of 5 mg/kg/day, seems not to have any toxic effects. With this in mind and the possibility of a progression towards deafness in one patient, of the possible more severe ocular involvement (one patient presented signs of retinal vasculopathy), of the possible onset of systemic manifestations, we administered Cyclosporine-A in two patients with Cogan's syndrome. While still on treatment with Cyclosporine-A in both our patients we obtained a good control of the disease without any onset of audiovestibular symptoms and of systemic manifestations. One of the patients during this period experienced only two episodes of mild interstitial keratitis which resolved after a short period of topical steroids. The rarity of the disease does not allow the execution of prospective trials to investigate the efficacy of different therapies. The absence of drug-related side-effects and the good control of ocular and systemic conditions achieved in our patients and mantained for 34 and 12 months from the end of Cyclosporine-A therapy, may suggest a prompt immunosuppressive approach, particularly with Cyclosporine-A, for the treatment of Cogan's syndrome in order to prevent an irreversible hearing loss, a vision threatning inflammatory eye disease and a systemic vasculitis.

REFERENCES

1) Cogan DG.: Arch. Ophthalmol. 1945; 33: 144-49.

2) Anonimus: The Lancet 1991; 337:1011-1012.

3) Vollertsenn RS.: Rheum. Dis. Clin. N. Am. 1990; 16: 433-39.

4) Haynes B.F., Kaiser-Kupfer M.I., Mason P., Fauci A.S.: Medicine (Baltimore) 1980; 59: 426-41.

5) Majoor M.H., Albers F.W., Gmelig-Meyling F., Van Der Gaag R., Huizing E.H.: Ann. Otol. Rhinol. Laryngol. 1992; 101: 679-684.

6) Cheson B.D., Bluming A.Z., Alroy J.: Am. J. Med. 1976; 60: 549-55.

7) Wilder-Smith E., Roelcke U.: J. Clin. Neuro-Ophthalmol. 1990; 10: 261-63.

8) Bachynski B., Wise J.: Can. J. Ophthalmol. 1984; 19: 145-47.

9) Haynes B.F., Pikus A., Kaiser-Kupfer M., Fauci A.S.: Arthritis Rheum. 1981; 24: 501-03.

10) Hebbar M., Gosset D., Savinel P., Hatron P. Y., Devulder B.: La Presse Medicale 1989; 18, n°3: 129.

11) Roat M.I., Thoft R.A., Thompson A.W., Jain A., Fung J.J., Starzl T.E.: Trans. Proc. 1991; 23: 3347.

12) Allen N.B., Cox C.C., Cobo M., Kisslo J., Jacobs M.r., McCallum R.M., Haynes B.F.: Am. J. Med. 1990; 88: 296-301.

Advances in Ocular Immunology
R.B. Nussenblatt, S.M. Whitcup, R.R. Caspi and I. Gery, eds.

Immunosuppression in Behcet's disease: visual outcome

K. F. Tabbara and P. S. Chavis

Department of Ophthalmology, College of Medicine, King Saud University and King Khaled Eye Specialist Hospital, P.O. Box 55307, Riyadh 11534, Saudi Arabia.

INTRODUCTION

Behcet's disease is a chronic multisystem disorder characterized by an underlying vasculitis and recurrent episodes of uveitis, genital ulcers, oral ulceration, and skin lesions [1-15]. The most striking ocular manifestation of the disease is the anterior and posterior uveitis. The eye lesions are the most serious of the major criteria of Behcet's disease and may eventuate in blindness. Cataract formation, anterior and posterior synechiae and glaucoma are common complications of anterior uveitis in patients with Behcet's disease. Glaucoma may be due to peripheral anterior synechiae, neovascular glaucoma, or steroid-induced glaucoma [15]. Posterior manifestations of Behcet's disease include microvascular retinal abnormalities, retinal vasculitis, which may be phlebitis and occasionally an arteritis. The vasculitis may lead to vascular occlusion and retinal hemorrhages. Neovascular formation is seen as a part of the vascular occlusive process. Focal areas of retinitis are frequently seen and cystoid macular edema may occur.

Late complications of Behcet's disease in the posterior segment include optic atrophy and degenerative changes in the macular area.

Treatment with immunomodulating agents may induce remissions and control the inflammation. It is not clear whether these modalities influence the final outcome. Since the disease is variable in its manifestations and runs in remissions and exacerbations the final outcome may or may not be modified by the therapy.

We decided to study retrospectively the long term visual outcome of therapy, given to 63 patients with Behcet's disease.

PATIENTS AND METHODS

A total of 63 consecutive patients with complete Behcet's disease were included. All patients had aphthous ulcers, genital ulcers, skin lesions and retinal vasculitis, and uveitis. The records of patients were reviewed retrospectively. All patients were followed-up for a period ranging from 20 to 124 months, with a mean follow-up period of 61 months. Patients were seen by an ophthalmologist and a rheumatologist. Each patient had a complete ophthalmological examination including visual acuity testing, tonometry, biomicroscopy and ophthalmoscopy. Patients were given one of the following therapeutic regimens:(a) cyclosporine 1 to 5 mg/kg/day, (b) conventional immunosuppressive therapy consisting of either chlorambucil 0.1 mg/kg/day orally, or azathioprine 1 to 2 mg/kg/day orally.

During each follow-up visit, patients underwent complete ophthalmological examination including biomicroscopy and ophthalmoscopy. Laboratory testing included blood cyclosporine trough level for group (a), blood urea nitrogen creatinine, complete blood count, differential count, and platelet count whenever indicated.

RESULTS

There were 60 male (95%) and 3 (5%) female patients. Thirty-five patients received cyclosporine therapy, and 28 patients received conventional therapy. Table 1 shows the bilateral and unilateral blindness among patients with Behcet's disease before and after therapy. The final visual outcome among the two groups; cyclosporine and conventional immunosuppressive therapy is shown in Table 2. Three patients underwent enucleation for a blind painful eye, three patients developed phthisis bulbi and seven patients eventuated in no light perception in both eyes. Table 3 shows the visual loss among 63 patients with Behcet's disease before and after therapy. Thirty-four (54%) had significant visual loss before therapy and 46 (73%) had significant visual loss at the conclusion of therapy.

Tables

Table 1
Blindness among patients with Behcet's disease

	Before Therapy		After Therapy	
Bilateral Blindness	19	(30%)	18	(28%)
Unilateral Blindness	33	(52%)	30	(48%)
Total	52	(82%)	48	(76%)

Table 2
Visual Outcome among 63 cases with Behcet's disease

Treatment Group	Visual Acuity 20/50 or better**		
	18 months*	30 months*	60 months*
Cyclosporine	18/35 (51%)	4/35 (40%)	8/35 (23%)
Conventional Immunosuppressive therapy	12/28 (43%)	15/28 (54%)	7/28 (25%)

* Mean follow-up period
** Best corrected vision

Table 3
Visual loss among 63 patients with Behcet's disease before and after therapy

	Before Therapy	After Therapy
Visual impairment (< 20/50)	15	27
Blindness (< 20/200)	19	19
Visual Loss	34 (54%)	46 (73%)

DISCUSSION

Behcet's disease is characterized by remissions and exacerbations and objectives of therapy should be closely evaluated in each patient and the risk benefit ratio should be well defined [11-13].

Immunosuppressive therapy has been used in patients with uveitis associated with Behcet's disease. Several cytotoxic agents have been used in Behcet's disease including chlorambucil, cyclophosphamide and azathioprine [12]. Some cases may eventuate in blindness despite all therapy [11].

Short term clinical trials have shown that cyclosporine and FK 506 are effective in the treatment of uveitis in Behcet's disease [14]. Despite recent advances in immunology and molecular biology, Behcet's disease remains to be a disorder of unknown etiology, has no diagnostic test, and no known cure. It is believed that the cause of Behcet's disease is multifactorial, the same was true about Lyme disease and syphilis before spirochetes were identified as the etiologic agents. *Streptococcus sanguis* may play a role in the pathogenesis of Behcet's disease [4-7].

Patient's with Behcet's disease have a higher incidence of buccal mucosal colonization with *Streptococcus sanguis* [4-6]. Cross reactivity between the 65 kDa heat shock protein and *Streptococcus sanguis* has been demonstrated [7].

The therapeutic regimen for the treatment of autoimmune disorders affecting the posterior segment of the eye have evolved over the past two decades. The major drugs used for the treatment of ocular Behcet's include: corticosteroids, alkylating agents (cyclophosphamide and chlorambucil), antimetabolites (azathioprine and methotrexate), and immunomodulators (cyclosporine, FK 506). The pillars for future therapy of autoimmune disorders rest on understanding the pathogenesis of the disease and on immunologic intervention. We shall be moving from the age of nonspecific immunologic suppression and cytotoxic therapy to an era of selective immunologic modulation.

The past decade of research has been a progressive discovery of our ignorance in Behcet's disease. It is a distinct obligation of medical researchers in the field of Behcet's disease to reassess our current therapeutic modalities. We do hope to replace speculations with facts, to identify the etiologic factor and to provide a rational, safe and effective long term therapy and better visual outcome in Behcet's disease.

REFERENCES

1   Charteris DG, Champ C, Rosenthal AR, Lightman SL. Behcet's disease: activated T lymphocytes in retinal perivasculitis. British J Ophthalmol 1992;76:499-501.
2   Mizushima Y. Behcet's disease. Curr Opinion Rheumatol 1991;3:32-35.
3   Michelson JB, Chisari FV. Behcet's disease. Surv Ophthalmol 1982;26:190-203.
4   Hamza M, Mizushima Y. Behcet's disease and dental treatment. J Rheumatol 1989;16:1612-1613.
5   The Behcet's Disease and Research Committee of Japan: Skin hypersensitivity to streptococcal antigens and induction of systemic symptoms by the antigens in Behcet's disease: a multicenter study. J Rheumatol 1989;16:506-511.
6   Isogai E, Ohno S, Kotake S, Isogai H, Tsurumizu T, Fuji N, Yokota K, Syuto B, Yamaguchi M, Matsuda H, Oguma K. Chemiluminescence of neutrophils from patients with Behcet's disease and its correlation with an increased proportion of uncommon serotypes of *Streptococcus sanguis* in the oral flora. Arch Oral Biol 1990;35:43-48.
7   Lehner T, Lavery E, Smith R, Van Embden J, Mizushima Y. Cross reactivity between the 65 kDa heat shock protein, *Streptococcus sanguis* and the corresponding antibodies in Behcet's disease. Infect Immun 1990.
8   International Study Group for Behcet's Disease. Criteria for diagnosis of Behcet's disease. Lancet, i:1078-1080.
9   Anonymous: Behcet's disease. Lancet 1989;i:761-762.
10   O'Duffy JD. Behcet's syndrome. N Engl J Med 1990;322:326-328.
11   Tabbara KF. Chlorambucil in Behcet's disease: A reappraisal. Ophthalmology 1993;90:906-908.
12   Yazici H, et al. A controlled trial of azathioprine in Behcet's syndrome. New Engl J Med 1990;332:281-285.
13   Tabbara KF. Azathioprine in Behcet's syndrome. N Engl J Med 1990;323:195.
14   Chavis PS, Antonios SR, Tabbara KF. Cyclosporine effects on optic nerve and retinal vasculitis in Behcet's Disease. Documenta Ophthalmologica 1992;80:133-142.
15   Tabbara KF, Al Balla S. Ocular Manifestations of Behcet's Disease. Asia-Pacific Journal of Ophthalmology 1991;3:8-11.

Advances in Ocular Immunology
R.B. Nussenblatt, S.M. Whitcup, R.R. Caspi and I. Gery, eds.

433

INTRAVENOUS PULSE CYCLOPHOSPHAMIDE THERAPY FOR SEVERE INFLAMMATORY EYE DISEASE.

Denis Wakefield, Yadu N. Singh and Peter J. McCluskey#
Laboratory of Ocular Immunology, School of Pathology, UNSW, Kensington, NSW.
Dept. of Immunology, Prince Henry Hospital, Sydney, NSW and #Dept of Ophthalmology, St. Vincent's Hospital, Sydney, NSW

INTRODUCTION

Severe uveitis and scleritis remain common and difficult clinical management problems. Untreated, they often lead to severe visual impairment. Although cytotoxic drugs are useful in such situations, their use is complicated by adverse effects due to systemic immunosuppression, frequent side effects, treatment failures and disease relapse.[1] Cyclosporin-A is increasingly used in such situations, but is associated with the disadvantage of relapse of disease after stopping therapy.[2-4] Recently, monthly intravenous cyclophosphamide 'pulse' therapy has been found to be effective in systemic inflammatory and autoimmune diseases[5-6] with the advantage of less frequent and less severe adverse effects than daily oral therapy. It has also been used in severe scleritis with encouraging results.[6]

'Pulse' cyclophosphamide therapy has previously been shown to be effective in a multi centre study in patients with inflammatory eye diseases, including a small number of patients with uveitis and scleritis[6]. This earlier study did not use a consistent treatment protocol, used combination therapy (with pulse steroids) and did not utilise a reproducible uveitis or scleritis scoring system to evaluate patient's response to treatment.

In order to further evaluate the safety and efficacy of pulse cyclophosphamide therapy in patients with severe uveitis and scleritis we treated a series of patients using a standardised therapeutic regimen and quantitative assessment systems.

PATIENTS AND METHODS

Eleven patients with severe treatment refractory posterior uveitis and 11 subjects with severe scleritis were studied. Patients were recruited from the eye clinics of Sydney Eye Hospital and St Vincent's Hospital, Sydney, Australia.

There were five males and 6 females with ages ranging from 23 to 73 yrs in the uveitis group. All patients had idiopathic uveitis, except one patient with sarcoidosis. Patients with uveitis had active disease for 8 to 96 months before entry into this study. All had previously received oral prednisolone. Six patients with uveitis had previously been treated with 'pulse' intravenous methylprednisolone. In addition, two each had been treated with azathioprine or Cyclosporin-A, and 4 had received oral cyclophosphamide. While four patients had partial improvement, seven had no improvement with therapy. Adverse drug effects were common in this patient group.

Eleven patients (M:F = 3:8) with scleritis were treated as part of this study with ages ranging from 19-74 years. Eight patients had idiopathic scleritis and 3 had secondary scleritis (1 each with rheumatoid arthritis, post surgical and relapsing polychondritis). The duration of disease prior to treatment ranged from 8 to 120 months. All patients with scleritis had received steroids orally and/or parentally. Three patients had also received cytotoxic drugs (2 Cyclosporine-A and 1 each azathioprine and oral cyclophosphamide). The therapies were either not effective or were only partially effective. There were significant adverse effects to these earlier therapies. After appropriate investigations to define the etiology and exclude infectious diseases, patients were administered intravenous cyclophosphamide at monthly intervals, following a standard protocol. Briefly, cyclophosphamide (dose 750 mg/m2 if glomerular filtration (GFR) rate was >1/3 of normal and 500 mg/m2 if GFR < 1/3 of normal) was given intravenously in 1 litre normal saline over 2 hours following pre hydration with 3 litres of normal saline. Four doses of Mercaptoethane Sulphonate (MESNA, 40% w/w of cyclophosphamide) was used to minimise urinary bladder toxicity. MESNA was given orally or intravenously. Anti emetics were used routinely, and consisted of Lorazepam 1mg, Thiethylperazine 6.5mg and Diphenhydramine 25mg given orally 1 hour before the cyclophosphamide infusion and then 6 hourly for 24 hours. Ondansetron was used if these anti emetics were ineffective in controlling nausea and vomiting. The subsequent monthly dose of cyclophosphamide depended on the nadir of the white cell count. A full blood count was performed on 7th, 10th, 14th day after the infusion and 2 days before the next infusion. If the nadir was less than 1.5×10^9L, the cyclophosphamide dose was reduced by 25 mg/m^2. If nadir was more than 4×10^9/l, the dose was increased by 25 mg/m^2. Urine was checked routinely to detect hematuria.

Prednisolone therapy was continued at the pre infusion dosage for the first month of cyclophosphamide therapy. Subsequently, the dose was slowly reduced depending upon response to treatment.

Each patient was reviewed at monthly intervals prior to the next cyclophosphamide infusion. A detailed evaluation of response, adverse effects, visual acuity and ocular inflammatory activity was made during these visits. A standardised scleritis scoring system was used to access response to therapy and to allow quantitation of disease activity over time.

RESULTS

The number of cyclophosphamide 'pulses' for patients with uveitis ranged from 3 to 9, and the monthly dose varied from 1000 mg to 1900 mg/month. The follow-up period after completion of therapy ranged from 7 to 28 months. Eight patients (16 eyes) showed marked improvement in ocular inflammatory activity and vision. Three patients (4 eyes) had only mild improvement.

Nausea was the commonest adverse effect experienced by 8 patients. Two patients developed significant alopecia which reversed on stopping therapy. One patient developed a urinary tract infection. None of these adverse effects necessitated withdrawal from the study. There was no instance of hemorrhagic cystitis or severe bone marrow suppression. Six patients were able to stop prednisolone, 4 had their corticosteroid therapy significantly reduced. One patient continued to require high dose prednisolone therapy to control ocular inflammation.

Patients with scleritis received 2 - 6 'pulses' of cyclophosphamide with adequate pre and post treatment hydration. The cyclophosphamide dose ranged from 800-2100 mg and follow-up after completion of the treatment ranged from 6 - 12 months. All patients had significant improvement and 6 patients were able to stop all other treatment. The remaining 5 patients were able to significantly reduce the dose of oral steroids.

DISCUSSION

Corticosteroids remain the mainstay of therapy for patients with severe inflammatory eye disease. Cyclosporine-A and other immunosuppressive drugs are usually reserved for severe disease refractory to systemic corticosteroid therapy [1-4]. In recent times intravenous 'pulse' therapy has been used with beneficial effects in the treatment of these patients.[6,7]

Cyclophosphamide has been used with good effect in rheumatoid arthritis. Systemic Lupus Erythematosis Wegener's granulomatosis orbital vasculitis and scleritis.[5,6] Similarly, intravenous cyclophosphamide 'pulse' therapy with both corticosteroids and cytotoxic drugs has been found to be useful in many immunological diseases. In lupus nephritis for example, it was found to be superior to prednisolone, and prednisolone plus azathioprine.[5] With intermittent intravenous therapy, the adverse effects of cyclophosphamide seems to be less frequent than continuous daily oral therapy[5].

Although cyclophosphamide has been reported to improve scleritis[6] and uveitis associated with Behcet's disease, to our knowledge there has been no previous report of the use of 'pulse' cyclophosphamide in the treatment of sight threatening idiopathic posterior uveitis. All patients in this study showed improvement or stabilisation of visual acuity and reduction in ocular inflammatory activity after treatment with pulse cyclophosphamide.

Nausea and vomiting which were common adverse events, were controlled by anti emetics including Ondansetron. No serious adverse event requiring withdrawal from the study was encountered.

Since cyclophosphamide is known to produce a number of significant side effects including: ovarian failure, sterility, pulmonary fibrosis, hemolytic anemia, chromosomal damage, teratogenesis, malignancy, alopecia, haemorrhagic cystitis and bone marrow suppression, the decision to commence this therapy should be taken only after careful consideration of the risks and potential benefits in the individual patient.[5] In addition long term follow-up is important to ensure that patients do not subsequently develop a malignancy.[5]

The results of our study indicate that intravenous 'pulse' cyclophosphamide is effective in the management of patients with severe uveitis and also patients with scleritis who have failed to respond to systemic corticosteroids and other immunosuppressive drugs. Intravenous cyclophosphamide therapy has a number of advantages. It decreases the ocular inflammatory response allowing systemic corticosteroids to be decreased or stopped, it is effective in situations in which other immunosuppressive drugs have failed, it is usually effective after a relatively short period of time and it may produce a long lasting disease remission that may be sustained after the drug is stopped.[5] As in a recent study of patients with Wegener's granulomatosis, intravenous 'pulse' cyclophosphamide produces less side effects, although it is equally effective when compared with oral cyclophosphamide. The disadvantages of intravenous pulse cyclophosphamide therapy include potentially life threatening side effects as a result of severe immunosuppression, or bone marrow depression as well as the potential of this drug to predispose to the development of malignancy. Pulse cyclophosphamide therapy also requires admission to a medical facility and there is a need for good vascular access and careful follow-up. There is a need to conduct a larger randomised comparative trial to validate the findings of this small, open, uncontrolled study of the efficacy of pulse cyclophosphamide therapy in the treatment of severe inflammatory eye disease.

REFERENCES

1.   Hemady R, Tauber J, Foster CS.   Immunosuppresive drugs in immune and inflammatory ocular disease. Surv. Ophthalmol. 1991; 35: 369-85.
2.   Wakefield D, McCluskey P.   Cyclosporine-A therapy in inflammatory eye diseases. J. Ocular Pharmacol. 1991;7:221-26.
3.   Wakefield D, McCluskey P. Cyclosporine therapy for severe scleritis.   Br. J. Ophthalmol. 1989;73: 743-46.
4.   Nussenblatt RB, Palestine AG, Chan CC.   Cyclosporin A therapy in the treatment of intraocular inflammatory disease resistant to systemic corticosteroids and cytotoxic agents. Am. J. Ophthalmol. 1983; 96: 275-82.
5.   Austin HA III, Klippel JH etal.   Therapy of lupus nephritis. Controlled trial of Prednisolone and cytotoxic drugs. N. Engl. J. Med. 1986; 314: 614-19
6.   Meyer PAR, Watson PG, Franks W, Dubord P.   'Pulse' immunosuppressive therapy in the treatment of immunologically induced corneal and scleral disease.   Eye 1987; 1: 487-95.
7.   Wakefield D, McCluskey P, Penny R.   Intravenous pulse methylprednisolone therapy in severe inflammatory eye disease. Arch Ophthalmol. 1986; 104: 847-51.
8.   Williams HJ, Reading JC, Ward JR, O'Brien WM: Comparison of high and low dose cyclophosphamide therapy in rheumatoid arthritis.   Arthritis Rheum. 1980, 23: 521-7.

2. Infectious Diseases: Mechanisms, Manifestations, Diagnosis and Therapeutic Approaches

Advances in Ocular Immunology
R.B. Nussenblatt, S.M. Whitcup, R.R. Caspi and I. Gery, eds.

MULTIPLE OCULAR INFECTIONS IN AIDS PATIENTS.

M.N. Burnier Jr., R. Lewandowski, A. Cabrera, D. Goldstein and J. Deschênes, McGill Ocular Immunopathology Unit; Departments of Ophthalmology and Pathology, McGill University, Montreal, Canada.

INTRODUCTION

AIDS is caused by the human immunodeficiency virus (HIV) which results in profound depression of patients' cellular immunity and subsequent development of multiple opportunistic infections, Kaposi's sarcoma, and other malignancies such as B-cell lymphomas.

HIV is a retrovirus that, by definition, contains only RNA (no DNA) in its genome. It can infect many types of human cells, but much of its pathologic action is secondary to infection of the helper/inducer T cell (CD4+). Because this cell is crucial for the development of cell-mediated immune responses, infection and subsequent death of the CD4+ T cells results in severe immunosuppression. HIV binds to the helper T cell and once in the cell, its RNA is translated into DNA by an enzyme called reverse viral transcriptase. The DNA enters the nucleus and is incorporated into the cell genome. Viral DNA is then capable of directing protein synthesis of new viral proteins using the infected cell's apparatus. These viral particles are then shed from the cell, and the infected cell eventually dies.

The range of manifestations of HIV infections (the spectrum of the disease) may include asymptomatic HIV-positive patients, non-specific signs and symptoms of illness, autoimmune and neurologic disorders, opportunistic infections, and various types of neoplasia.

The ocular manifestations in AIDS patients may be divided into four disease categories: 1) noninfectious retinopathy, 2) opportunistic infections, 3) neoplasms, and 4) neuro-ophthalmic disorders.[1]

PURPOSE

Ocular opportunistic diseases in AIDS may be grouped according to the general category of the offending organism: virus, parasite, fungus, and bacteria.

A strong correlation exists between the level of immunosuppression (CD4 count) and the appearance of particular opportunistic infections.[2]

Table 1

Helper T-cell count	Infection
1000 cells/mm3	none (normal)
200-400 cells/mm3	Candida skin infection, thrush, shingles
< 200 cells/mm3	P. carinii, toxoplasmosis, Cryptococcus
< 100 cells/mm3	Cytomegalovirus, Mycobacterium avium.

The diagnosis of intraocular infection in AIDS patients may be complicated by the presence of more than one infectious agent, although the incidence of this occurrence is not known.

METHODS

42 eyes of 30 AIDS patients with a clinical diagnosis of CMV retinitis were obtained postmortem. Twenty-five sections of each eye were stained with H&E, PAS, and GMS.

RESULTS

All 42 globes had typical CMV lesions of the retina, as well 19 eyes had CMV cells in choroidal vessels. Eight of these CMV infected eyes (19%) contained more than one infectious agent. Three eyes revealed CMV and Pneumocystis carinii, two had CMV and toxoplasmosis, two had evidence of CMV and MAI, and one eye demonstrated concurrent infection with CMV, Pneumocystis carinii and MAI.

DISCUSSION

Cytomegalovirus (CMV) Retinitis

CMV retinitis is the most common ocular infection in AIDS occurring in 20-30% of patients in most clinical series. Immunosuppression associated with organ transplantation (particularly renal transplant) and chemotherapy were the most common causes of CMV retinitis prior to the AIDS epidemic.

CMV is a herpes class virus and contains double-stranded DNA. The majority of patients with AIDS become CMV viremic once their CD4 count drops below 100 (usually less than 50). CMV infection probably reaches the eye through the blood stream, although the possibility of reactivation of latent virus has not been ruled out. CMV retinitis begins as a small white retinal infiltrate that, if seen early, may resemble a large cotton-wool spot. There is usually only minimal vitreous inflammation associated with the disease. The necrotizing retinitis is relentlessly progressive and leaves in its wake atrophic, avascular retina. CMV spreads by direct extension into healthy retina. Newly infected retina may take one to two weeks to "declare" itself. Lesions that occur in the posterior pole are usually associated with significant intraretinal hemorrhage.

Less frequently, patients may present with severe vascular sheathing or "frosted branch angiitis" as their initial manifestation of CMV retinitis.

Histopathologic features include areas of retinal necrosis and characteristic enlarged cells with eosinophilic cytoplasm showing intranuclear "owl's eye" viral inclusions. These cells, CMV-cells, are typically found within the sensory retina, RPE, optic nerve and choroidal blood vessels. Intra-cytoplasmic inclusions may be identified by PAS and GMS stains.[3]

Pneumocystis carinii choroidopathy

P. Carinii is the most common infection in patients with AIDS, causing pneumonia in over 80% of the cases. Pneumocystis carinii pneumonia is the initial manifestation of AIDS in 60% of cases. P. carinii is a protozoan first described by Chagas (1909) and a year later by Canini. It is considered by some investigators to be a fungus. The microorganism exists exclusively in the extracellular spaces.[4]

Ocular Pneumocystis carinii is almost exclusively a choroidal disease that occurs most commonly in the setting of inhaled pentamidine therapy. Clinical presentation my include a single, pale, oval, choroidal lesion with minimal evidence of inflammation. Multiple yellowish, slightly elevated choroidal lesions with no vitritis have also been described. These lesions frequently measure 0.5 - 2 disc diameters. The overlying retinal function is usually preserved. The presence of P. carinii in the choroid may be a marker for disseminated disease. CT scan may demonstrate microcalcifications in other organs such as the kidney or pancreas.[5]

Histopathologically, there is a characteristic choroidal infiltrate that is eosinophilic, acellular, vacuolated, and frothy. These infiltrates are commonly present within the choroidal vessels and choriocapillaries. Gomori's methenamine silver stain (GMS) demonstrates cystic organisms and trophozoites with minimal inflammatory response.

Mycobacterium infection

Mycobacterium avium-intracellulare may occur in the late stages of disease. Clinical data is limited but small, white, evanescent choroidal lesions with no overlying vitreal inflammation has been described. Co-infection with other opportunistic infections is probably more common than clinically realized.

Histopathologically, the inflammatory reaction is much less intense than the tissue response that one should expect for a non-immunosuppressed patient. Frequently the granuloma, in patients with AIDS, is not surrounded by the characteristic lymphocytic halo.

CONCLUSION

While CMV retinitis is the most common intraocular infection in AIDS patients, the diagnosis may be complicated by the presence of a second infectious agent. In this series, 19% of eyes harboured at least one agent in addition to CMV. This should be borne in mind in the presence of CMV retinitis which appears refractory to treatment.

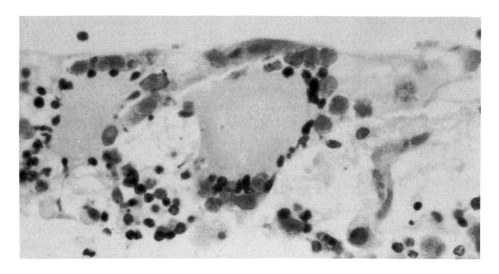

Figure 1. CMV retinitis.
Multinucleated giant cells containing intranuclear and intracytoplasmic viral inclusions (H & E, 200x).

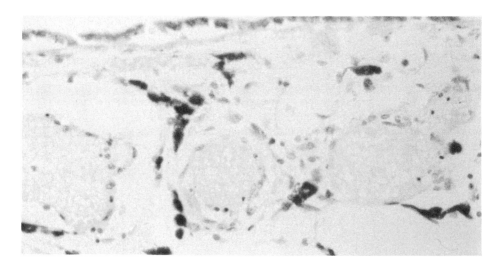

Figure 2. Pneumocystis carinii choroiditis.
Eosinophilic choroidal masses containing pneumocystis carinii organisms.

REFERENCES

1. Holland GN, Pepose JS, Petit TH, et al: Acquired immune deficiency syndrome: ocular manifestations. Ophtalmol 90: 857-73, 1983.

2. Phillips AN, Lee CA, Elford J, et al: Serial CD4 lymphocytes counts and development of AIDS. Lancet 337: 389-92, 1991.

3. Burnier Jr. MN, Chan CC, McLean IW, eta al: The use of various immunohistopathologic techniques in the diagnosis of CMV retinitis in AIDS patients. Inv Ophthalm Vis Sc 32: 764, 1991.

4. Foster RE, Lowder CY, Meisler DM, et al. Presumed Pneumocystis carinii choroiditis: Unifocal presentation, regression with intravenous pentamidine, and choroiditis recurrence. Ophthalmology 98: 1360-5, 1991.

5. Freeman WR, Gross JG, Labelle J, et al: Pneumocystis carinii choroidopathy: a new clinical entity. Arch Ophthalmol 107: 863-7, 1989.

Advances in Ocular Immunology
R.B. Nussenblatt, S.M. Whitcup, R.R. Caspi and I. Gery, eds.

Polymerase Chain Reaction for the Detection of the Mycobacterium tuberculosis in Ocular Tuberculosis

Satoshi Kotake, M.D.[a], Koichi Kimura, M.D.[b], Koji Yoshikawa, M.D.[a], Yoichi Sasamoto, M.D.[a], Akira Matsuda, M.D.[a], Nobuhiro Fujii, Ph.D.[b] and Hidehiko Matsuda, M.D[a]

[a]Departments of Ophthalmology Hokkaido University School of Medicine; Kita-15, Nishi-7, Kita-ku, Sapporo 060, Japan

[b]Department of Microbiology, Sapporo Medical College, Minami-1, Nishi-17, Chuo-ku, Sapporo 060, Japan

INTRODUCTION

The incidence of ocular tuberculosis has had a parallel decline with the systemic disease since the 1940s. The diagnosis of ocular tuberculosis is extremely difficult because we cannot get enough samples. Recently, several attempts have been made to specifically diagnose *Mycobacterium tuberculosis* infection through biological or molecular biological techniques. Among them, special attention has been paid to newly introduced DNA amplification method, PCR. As we recently encountered two representative cases of ocular tuberculosis, we tried to detect *Mycobacterium tuberculosis* by this method.

PATIENTS AND METHODS

Case 1, a 20-year-old man, had a 2-week history of visual loss in his both eyes. Visual acuity was R.E.: 20/200 and L.E.: 20/50. Slit-lamp findings were iridocyclitis in both eyes, mutton-fat keratic precipitates and nodules on trabecular meshwork in a left eye. Ophthalmoscopy revealed florid retinal vasculitis and vitreous hemorrhage in both eyes.

Chest X-ray showed apical consolidation but tubercle bacilli were not cultured from sputum. A surgical biopsy of the cervical lymph nodes was carried-out and pathologically a final diagnosis of tuberculosis was made.

Case 2, a 53-year-old woman, had a history of chorioretinitis of unknown cause with macular scarring of left eye. She was first seen by us in April 1992 because of retinal vasculitis in the right eye. On examination, she had a visual acuity of R.E.:20/30 and L.E.:20/400. Ophthalmoscopy disclosed inactive, chorioretinal scars in both eyes and new, active retinal vasculitis in her right eye. Diagnostic evaluation disclosed a positive tuberculin skin test (17x12mm), but normal results of a chest roentgenogram. In follow-up she was noted to have marked retinal vasculitis and hemorrhage also in her right eye. A presumptive diagnosis of ocular tuberculosis was made.

Approximately 0.1 ml of aqueous humor was obtained by anterior chamber paracentesis by using a 27-gauge needle. Samples were also collected at cataract surgery as controls. In our polymerase chain reaction test for Mycobacterium tuberculosis , we used a sequence which is specific for Mycobacterium tuberculosis coding for the MPB64 protein [1]. In the step of sample preparation and amplifying DNA, we followed the protocol of Narita et al.[2]. A 240 base pair region (nt 460-700) was amplified with the synthetic oligonucleotide primers. When the first step amplification was negative, the second step amplification was carried out. In the second step, we constructed an inner primer pair just within the previous one, to amplify 200 base pair (nt 480-680).

RESULTS

In Figure, both samples from patient 1 and 2 showed positive results in the second step. Samples collected at cataract surgery were negative.

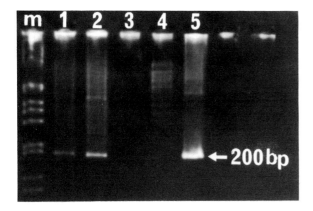

Figure. Amplifications from aqueous humor samples from patients: 4% agarose gels stained with ethidium bromide. Lane m: a size marker. Lane1: sample DNA from case 1. Lane 2: sample DNA from case 2. Lane 3 and 4: samples from patients with cataract. Lane 5: a positive control. Number 200 in gel indicates the expected size of the amplified product.

Discussion

Tuberculosis is not a disease of a past. It is worth noting that occurrence of extrapulmonary tuberculosis is increasing among patients with human immunodeficiency virus type I infection . Early diagnosis from small samples and early medical intervention can contribute not only to therapeutic improvement of affected individuals, but also to prevent of the disease and protection of medical staff. For this purpose, polymerase chain reaction is very helpful in clinical laboratory.

REFERENCES

1 Yamaguchi R, Matsuo K, Yamazaki A, Abe C, et al. Infect Immun 1989; 57: 283-288
2 Narita M, Matsuzono Y, Shibata M, and Togashi T. Acta Paediatr 1992; 81: 997-1001.

Advances in Ocular Immunology
R.B. Nussenblatt, S.M. Whitcup, R.R. Caspi and I. Gery, eds.   449

ACQUIRED OCULAR TOXOPLASMOSIS - LATE ONSET

J.Melamed

Dept.of Ophthalmology, Medical School, Federal University
of Rio Grande do Sul, Porto Alegre - RS, Brazil.

INTRODUCTION

Recently it was demonstrated that Acquired Ocular Toxoplasmosis
(**AOT**) occurs often in Brazil, specially in the southermost state
of Rio Grande do Sul (1,2,3,4,5,6). We have also observed several
cases in which **AOT** appears years after acute systemic infection.
We report here a case of 13-year latency between infection and
the onset of ocular signs.

CASE REPORTS

A woman,39, consulted on July 27,1992,complaining of "floaters"
and blurred vision in her left eye. She had scarce muttonfat
KPs, flare+, vitritis++,and a focal lesion of exudative retinochoroiditis close to the optic nerve (fig.1). After ruling out
other causes, toxoplasmosis was diagnosed,based on the presence
of antitoxoplasmic antibodies, plus clinical picture and previous
history, and treated successfuly with the usual therapy(fig.2).

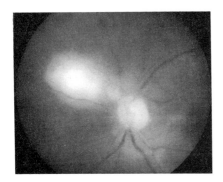
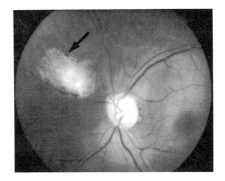

Figure 1. Mother's left eye.
An active lesion can be seen
supranasally to the optic
nerve.

Figure 2. The same lesion
after treatment showing
pigment clusters at edges
(arrow).

The patient had presented toxoplasmic infection 13 years earlier, when she was in the last trimester of pregnancy. Her daughter, born prematurely at 34 weeks, with hepatosplenomegaly and jaundice, was diagnosed as presenting congenital toxoplasmosis and treated with trimetropin + sulphametoxazole. The antitoxoplasmic antibody titers at the time were 1:32,000, both for mother and daughter. The daughter consulted on September 24,1990, presenting numerous retinochoroidal scars in both eyes (figs.3 & 4).

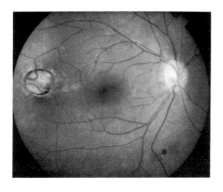

Figure 3. Daughter. Right eye presenting a typical para-macular punched-out scar with a retinochoroidal vascular shunt.

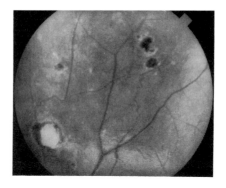

Figure 4. Daughter, left eye. Several darkly pigmented scars are scattered on the fundus.

At the time, a CT scan of the brain showed hydrocephalus, with marked enlargement of the third and lateral ventricles and calcifications in the brain (figs.5 & 6).

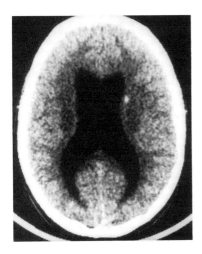

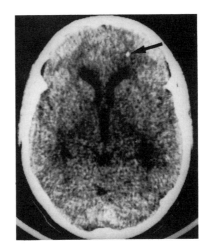

Figure 5. Daughter, CT scan
showing marked dilatation
of the ventricular system.

Figure 6. CT scan exhibiting
an intracerebral calcification
(arrow).

On June 15,1993, the daughter presented an active lesion in the
right eye (fig.7). Another exudative lesion was found in the left
eye on February 21,1994 (fig.8).

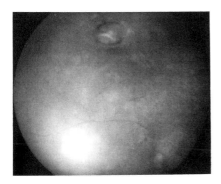

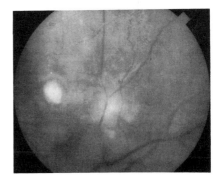

Figure 7. Daughter, right eye.
Active exudative lesion with
severe vitritis.

Figure 8. Daughter, eight
months later.Other recurrent
lesion with accompanying
vasculitis appearing in the
left eye.

452

COMMENT

Most authors have described ocular lesions of **AOT** accompanying acute systemic infection(7,8,9,10,11,12,13,14,15).We concluded, on the contrary,that,specially in adult patients,the possibility of late appearing **AOT** should be considered (2,4,16).

REFERENCES

1 Melamed J., Round Table on Ocular Toxoplasmosis, I South-Brazilian Meeting on Uveites, Gramado, 1984.
2 Melamed J., Peculiaridades da toxoplasmose ocular no Rio Grande do Sul, Arq.Bras.Oftal. 51, 197, 1988.
3 Silveira C., Belfort R.Jr., Burnier M.Jr., Nussenblatt R., Acquired toxoplasmic infection as the cause of toxoplasmic retinochoroiditis in families. Am.J.Ophthalmol.106:362,1988.
4 Melamed J., Peculiarities of ocular toxoplasmosis in Rio Grande do Sul, Brazil, In: Belfort R.Jr., Petrilli A.M.N. , Nussenblatt R.(eds), World Uveitis Symposium, São Paulo,Roca, 1989.
5 Melamed J., Clinical Appearance of Toxoplasmic Retino-choroiditis, Recent Advances in Uveitis, Proceedings of the Third International Symposium on Uveitis, Brussels, Kugler Publications, Amsterdam/New York, 1993.
6 Beniz J., Toxoplasmose ocular adquirida. Arq.Bras.Oft., 56, 134, 1993.
7 Hogan M.J., Kimura S.G., O'Connor G.R.,Ocular toxoplasmosis, Arch.Ophthal. 72:592, 1965.
8 Baron H.G., Zuccarini J., Consideraciones acerca de un caso de ocriorretinitis toxoplasmica con diagnostico parasitolo-gico de certeza, Arch.Oftal. B.Aires, 41:67, 1966.
9 Perkins E.S., Ocular toxoplasmosis, Brit.J.Ophthal. 57,1, 1973.
10 Saari M., Vuorre I., Neiminen H., Räisänen S., Acquired Toxoplasmic Chorioretinitis, Arc.Ophthalmol. 94:485, 1976.
11 Gump D.W., Holden R.A., Acquired Chorioretinitis Due to Toxoplasmosis, Ann.Int.Med., 90:58, 1979.
12 Reese L.T., Shafer D.M., Zweifech P., Acute Acquired Toxo-plasmosis, Ann.Ophthalmol., 13:467, 1981.
13 Sacks J.J., Roberto R.R., Brooks N.F., Toxoplasmosis In-fection Associated With Raw Goat's Milk, JAMA 248:1728, 1982.
14 Asbell P.A., Vermund S.H., Hofeldt A.J., Presumed Toxo-plasmic Retinochoroiditis in Four Siblings, Am.Ophthalmol., 94:656, 1982.
15 Alezzandrini A.A., Toxoplasmosis ocular aguda adquirida(nue va forma de inoculación), Arch.Oftalmol., B.Aires, 59:135, 1984.
16 Melamed J., Toxoplasmic Retinochoroiditis, Ph.D. Thesis - Medical School, Federal University of Minas Gerais, Belo Ho rizonte, 1991.

Advances in Ocular Immunology
R.B. Nussenblatt, S.M. Whitcup, R.R. Caspi and I. Gery, eds.

Immunohistopathology of the lacrimal gland in AIDS-related sicca syndrome

R. A. Neves,[ab] J. E. Dutt,[a] A. Rodriguez,[a] J. Merayo-Lloves,[a] R. Belfort Jr,[b] and C.S. Foster[a]

[a] Immunology and Uveitis Service, Massachusetts Eye and Ear Infirmary, Harvard Medical School, 243 Charles St., Boston, MA 02114 USA

[b] Ocular AIDS Service, Paulista School of Medicine, Sao Paulo Hospital, Rua Botucatu 822, Sao Paulo 04023, Brazil

INTRODUCTION

Keratoconjunctivitis sicca was first observed in three HIV infected patients by Ulirsch and Jaffe in 1987 [1]. Since its initial description, an increasing number of reports have been published showing the incidence of a Sjögren's-like syndrome in positive individuals. The clinical manifestations present in such patients have included xerophthalmia, xerostomia and salivary gland enlargement [2-4].

Reports of the immunohistopathologic characteristics of salivary gland biopsies performed in patients with AIDS have demonstrated the presence of a diffuse lymphocytic infiltration mainly composed of CD8[+] T-cells [5,6]. We analyzed lacrimal gland biopsies performed immediately post-mortem in five individuals with AIDS who had suffered from severe dry eye symptoms.

PATIENTS AND METHODS

Palpebral lobe biopsy of the right lacrimal gland was performed immediately post-mortem in five male patients with AIDS class IV. The patients' mean age was 32.4 years. Sicca syndrome was previously diagnosed on clinical basis, with a Schirmer test values ≤ 5 mm (range 0 - 5 mm) and Rose Bengal staining scores ≥ 7 according to the classification of van Bijsterveld [7].

Biopsy specimens were snap-frozen in OCT-compound, 4μ cryosections were mounted on gelatin-coated slides and stained with a panel of monoclonal antibodies directed against different immune cell surface markers using an immunoperoxidase technique [7]. Briefly, the sections were air-dried and acetone-fixed prior to blocking with 5% normal donkey serum in PBS-BSA. This was followed by a 45 minute incubation with the primary antibodies (Table 1). After three PBS washes, endogenous peroxidase activity was blocked using 0.3% H_2O_2. The sections were then incubated for a further 45 minutes with biotinylated donkey anti-mouse IgG. Following three PBS washes, a final 45 minute incubation was done using peroxidase-conjugated streptavidin. The color reactions were developed using 3-amino-9-ethylcarbazole and hydrogen peroxide in acetate buffer. Experimental controls included sections without the addition of primary antibodies. Cell counts were obtained from 5 high-power fields (x400) using a 10 x 10 mm^2 grid.

RESULTS

A moderate stromal and acinar destruction was observed in all specimens. There was a marked lymphocytic infiltrate. The infiltrate was mainly composed of $CD3^+$ T-cells, most of which were of the $CD8^+$ phenotype. The CD4:CD8 ratio was 1:4. The HLA-DR expression was also prominent. (Table 1)

Table 1
Immunohistopathology characteristics of the lacrimal glands in AIDS-related sicca syndrome.

Monoclonal antibody specificity	Cell counts* (Mean ± SD)
Pan-T cells ($CD3^+$)	42.5 ± 4.3
T helper/inducer ($CD4^+$)	9.42 ± 1.2
T suppressor/cytotoxic cells ($CD8^+$)	35.6 ± 3.9
Monocytes ($CD14^+$)	24.0 ± 5.4
B lymphocytes ($CD22^+$)	19.5 ± 3.3
HLA-DR	44.3 ± 2.9
Control	Negative

* Obtained from 5 high-power fields (x400) using a 10 x 10 mm^2 grid.

DISCUSSION

Keratoconjunctivitis sicca occurs in less than 1% of the general population. In AIDS patients, the reported incidence may vary from 21% to 56% [2, 4] in adults or children. The association of xerostomia, salivary gland enlargement and a lymphocytic interstitial pneumonitis (LIP) in these patients suggests that a unique clinical entity is responsible for the sicca syndrome, and this is called "diffuse infiltrative lymphocytosis syndrome" (DILS). Studying salivary gland and lung biopsies in AIDS patients, Itescu [5] found a diffuse CD8+ lymphocytic infiltration of the parenchyma. The same infiltrative pattern has been observed in other organs causing gastrointestinal, renal and neurologic complications [6].

Although isolated dry eye syndrome has been described in some HIV-infected patients [2], to the best of our knowledge, no reports regarding the histologic and immunohistopathologic characteristics of the lacrimal gland in AIDS patients suffering from sicca syndrome have been published. This is probably due to the difficulty in obtaining such specimens. We observed moderate disorganization of the glandular structure, atrophic duct epithelium and some degree of interstitial fibrosis in all specimens. The lymphocytic infiltrate with CD8+ predominance and the inversion of the CD4:CD8 ratio (1:4) found in these specimens are very similar to those features described in salivary gland of patients with DILS.

The histopathology of the salivary gland in patients with Sjögren's syndrome is also characterized by a lymphocytic infiltrate with a predominance of CD8+ T-cells and with a high expression of HLA-DR2 and DR3 [8,9]. By contrast DILS is strongly associated with both HLA-DR5 and DRw6 [5]. Our results showed also an increased expression of class II MHC molecules.

These results suggest that the lacrimal gland disease in these patients with AIDS-related sicca syndrome may be a part of the "diffuse infiltrative lymphocytosis syndrome", although an isolated ocular involvement may be present.

The therapy for DILS with AZT has successfully controlled the inflammatory process of limited glandular disease, but requires the addition of prednisone in cases of extraglandular disease. In severe cases of dry eye syndrome, the former monotherapy can represent a successful approach [6].

REFERENCES

1. Ulirsch RC, Jaffe ES. Sjogren's syndrome-like illness associated with the acquired immunodeficiency syndrome related complex. Hum Pathol 1987; 18:1063-8.
2. Lucca JA, Farris RL, Bielory L, Caputo AR. Keratoconjunctivitis sicca in male patients infected with human immunodeficiency virus type 1. Ophthalmol 1990; 97:1008-1010.
3. Couderc LJ, D'Agay MF, Danon F et al. Sicca complex and infection with human immunodeficiency virus. Arch intern Med 1987;147:898-901.
4. Neves RA, Sato EH, Freitas D, Oliveira CF, Belfort Jr R. Lacrimal dysfunction in pediatric AIDS. In The Lacrimal Gland. Eds Sullivan D 1994(in press).
5. Itescu S. Diffuse infiltrative lymphocytosis syndrome in human immunodeficiency virus infection - A Sjogren-like disease. Rheum Dis Clin North Am 17:99, 1991.
6. Itescu S, Winchester R. Diffuse infiltrative syndrome: A lymphocytosis disorder occurring in human immunodeficiency virus-1 infection that may present as a sicca syndrome. Rheum Dis Clin North Am 18:100, 1992.
7. van Bijsterveld OP. Diagnostic tests in the sicca syndrome. Arch Ophthalmol 1969; 82:10-14.
8. Chisholm DM, Mason DK. Labial salivary gland biopsy in Sjogren's disease. J Clin Pathol 1968; 21:656.
9. Harley JB, Reichlin M, Arnett FC et al. Gene Interaction at HLA DQ enhances autoantibody production in primary Sjogren's syndrome. Science 1986; 232:1145-1147.

Advances in Ocular Immunology
R.B. Nussenblatt, S.M. Whitcup, R.R. Caspi and I. Gery, eds.

Retinal and choroidal biopsy in AIDS patients with intraocular inflammation

G. Ortega-Larrocea, A.R. Rutzen, P.U. Dugel, L.P. Chong, P.F. Lopez and N.A. Rao

Doheny Eye Institute, University of Southern California School of Medicine,
1450 San Pablo Street, Los Angeles, California 90033, United States of America

INTRODUCTION

Although the etiologic diagnosis of intraocular inflammation is based usually upon the observation of characteristic clinical features combined with evidence from serologic and systemic evaluations, it is occasionally necessary to obtain an intraocular specimen in order to identify the specific etiologic agent and to determine the appropriate therapy. In some patients it is difficult to establish a specific diagnosis because the severe inflammation and resultant opacification of the ocular media preclude visualization of the ocular structures. In other patients, more than one diagnostic possibility must be considered. In as many as 33% of patients with intraocular inflammation, a specific etiologic diagnosis cannot be determined, [1] but in most patients, specific or empiric treatment results in a favorable clinical response. In those patients who do not respond to treatment, however, or who experience further clinical deterioration despite treatment, surgical diagnostic measures to confirm or revise the diagnosis may be required. In other patients, it may be necessary to exclude the possibility of malignancy or infection. In the present report, we describe the clinical and histopathologic features in 16 intraocular tissue biopsies from patients with AIDS and intraocular inflammation who underwent endoretinal, transscleral choroidal, or transscleral chorioretinal biopsy for etiologic diagnosis of intraocular inflammation.

PATIENTS AND METHODS

We performed a review of 16 consecutive intraocular tissue biopsies from 15 patients with AIDS and clinical signs of intraocular inflammation that were accessioned from 1984 to 1993. Inclusion criteria included: i) diagnosis of AIDS, ii) cells in the vitreous cavity, iii) retinal or choroidal lesions, and iv) the inability to determine an exact diagnosis through noninvasive means. The decision to biopsy was made by the operating surgeon and was based on the clinical circumstances of each case. Three patients have been included in previous reports [2,3].

Thirteen endoretinal, 2 chorioretinal, and 1 choroidal biopsy were performed in a manner similar to that previously described [4,5]; all patients in the endoretinal group had a retinal detachment and underwent biopsy at the time of retinal detachment repair. The preoperative diagnoses were in question in every case because of atypical clinical features or a lack of response to therapy. The differential diagnosis included possible cytomegalovirus retinitis (CMV) in 10 biopsies, progressive outer retinal necrosis (PORN) in 3, possible acute retinal necrosis (ARN) in 1, possible *Toxoplasma gondii* infection in 1, and a subretinal mass in 1 patient.

All 16 specimens were processed for light microscopy; 13 were processed for electron microscopy; 3 were studied using immunohistochemistry for CMV; 1 was tested using the polymerase chain reaction (PCR) for herpes virus group DNA and CMV DNA, and 1 was studied using in situ hybridization for CMV.

RESULTS

The results of histologic, electron microscopic, and additional studies are summarized in Table 1.

Table 1: Retinal, Choroidal, and Chorioretinal Biopsies in AIDS Patients

Biopsy no./age/sex	Preop dx	Rx	Histologic features	Electron microscopy	Pathologic diagnosis
1/NA/M*	Probable CMV	NA	Retinal disorganization, necrosis	Virus	Herpesvirus-group retinitis
2/34/M*	Probable CMV	G	Retinal disorganization, atrophy, gliosis	Virus	Herpesvirus-group retinitis
3/33/M*	Probable CMV	G	Retinal disorganization; immunohistochem negative CMV	Virus	Herpesvirus-group retinitis
4/30/M*	Probable CMV	G	Retinal necrosis, viral inclusions	Virus	Herpesvirus-group retinitis
5/41/M*	Probable CMV	NA	Retinal necrosis	Virus	Herpesvirus-group retinitis
6/52/M*	Probable CMV	G	Retinal disorganization; in situ negative CMV	Virus	Herpesvirus-group retinitis
7/44/M*	Probable CMV	F	Retinal atrophy, viral inclusions; immunohistochem positive CMV	-	CMV retinitis
8/38/M*	Probable CMV	NA	Retinal disorganization, necrosis	No virus	Retinal necrosis
9/36/M*	Probable CMV	G	Retinal atrophy, gliosis	No virus	Retinal gliosis
10/44/M*	Probable CMV	F	Retinal disorganization, gliosis; immunohistochem negative CMV	-	Retinal gliosis
11/29/M*	PORN	A	Retinal necrosis, vessels relatively preserved	Virus	Herpesvirus group retinitis
12/36/F#	PORN	A,G,F	Retinal necrosis	Virus	Herpesvirus-group retinitis
13/35/M*	PORN	A,F	Retinal atrophy, gliosis, vessels relatively preserved, PCR positive herpesgroup, PCR negative CMV	No virus	Herpesvirus group retinitis
14/26/M*	Probable ARN	A	Retinal disorganization, necrosis	No virus	Retinal necrosis
15/34/M†	Choroidal mass	-	Plasma cells, rare lymphocytes in choroid	-	Nonspecific choroiditis
16/43/M#	Toxo vs CMV, syphilis	G, PCN	Necrotic retina and RPE, Toxoplasma cysts	Toxoplasma	Toxoplasmic retinochoroiditis

*Endoretinal biopsy, #Chorioretinal biopsy, †Choroidal biopsy
NA=not available, CMV=cytomegalovirus, PORN=progressive outer retinal necrosis, ARN=acute retinal necrosis, G=ganciclovir, F=foscarnet, A=acyclovir, PCR=polymerase chain reaction, PCN=penicillin

Preoperative visual acuities ranged from 20/25 to light perception; preoperative visual acuities were limited by the presence of retinal detachment and, in some patients, by direct involvement of macular retinitis. Postoperative visual acuities ranged from 20/20 to no light perception with an average follow-up of 15 months. Postoperative visual acuities were improved from preoperative levels in 6 patients, the same in 1, and worse in 4. In the postoperative period, 1 patient had recurrent retinal detachment and 1 developed a cataract.

DISCUSSION

Among the patients with a clinical diagnosis of possible CMV, evidence for viral retinitis was detected in 7 of 10 biopsies, resulting in a diagnostic yield in establishing the diagnosis of viral retinitis of 70%; virus particles were observed with electron microscopy in 6 cases, and immunohistochemical staining for CMV was positive in 1 case. The patients whose specimens showed virus particles by electron microscopy usually demonstrated retinal necrosis. Those specimens that did not show virus particles by electron microscopy usually exhibited retinal atrophy and gliosis. When technically possible, it is advisable to obtain the biopsy specimen from the border of involved and uninvolved retina. Those specimens that clearly showed the zone of transition from normal to abnormal retina also demonstrated abundant virus particles when studied with electron microscopy.

The endoretinal biopsies in patients with probable CMV retinitis were performed relatively early in the AIDS epidemic, before the various clinical manifestations of CMV retinitis were well understood. In all cases, the preoperative diagnosis was in question, either because, a lack of response to treatment or atypical clinical features such as nonhemorrhagic retinitis, frosted branch vasculitis, or unusually severe vitreous inflammation. Endoretinal biopsies were undertaken because these clinical features were thought to overlap with the clinical manifestations of herpes zoster virus, herpes simplex virus, *Toxoplasma*, syphilis, and intraocular lymphoma [3]. As our understanding of the varied manifestations of cytomegalovirus has increased, however, our frequency of retinal biopsies in this group has diminished, as evidenced by the fact that a majority of biopsies in patients with possible CMV retinitis were performed between 1984 and 1986.

All 3 patients who had endoretinal biopsies with the preoperative diagnosis of the PORN syndrome, the diagnosis of viral retinitis was confirmed. Virus particles were detected by electron microscopy in two cases. In one case, PCR demonstrated DNA sequences of the herpesvirus-group, but was negative for the DNA of CMV. These findings are consistent with recent studies that conclude that this syndrome is probably caused by the herpes zoster virus. In contrast to the vaso-occlusive arteritis found in ARN, these specimens demonstrated remarkable preservation of the retinal vessels despite severe retinal necrosis and retinal atrophy (Figure 1). This finding correlated well with the clinical appearance of relative sparing of the inner retina and retinal vasculature until late in the course of the PORN syndrome (Figure 2) [2]. In the patient with the clinical diagnosis of ARN, the retina was gliotic and no virus particles could be detected. This specimen was obtained at the time of retinal detachment repair and exemplifies the observation that retinal detachments usually occur after the period of necrosis has passed, when the retina is thin and gliotic.

Electron microscopic features are sufficient to identify virus particles as members of the herpesvirus-group, but additional tests are required to determine the specific identity of the virus. Because antiviral medications have variable degrees of clinical effectiveness against various viruses, it is useful to know the specific identity of the pathogenic virus in order to rationally plan medical therapy. This can be achieved by techniques such as immunohistochemical staining, in situ hybridization, and the polymerase chain reaction to establish the specific identity of the offending virus. Only a few of our specimens were processed for immunohistochemistry, in situ hybridization, and PCR analysis because experience with these diagnostic techniques was limited during the early years of this study, and because the clinical significance of their results is still under investigation.

460

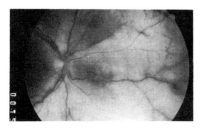

Figure 1. Fundus photograph, PORN syndrome.

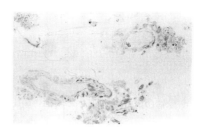

Figure 2. Histology, PORN syndrome (toluidine blue, x 100).

In most patients, vision was the same or better than the preoperative level. Unfortunately, most had visual acuities of counting fingers to no light perception, and only 4 patients had a final postoperative visual acuity of 20/400 or better. Two patients with 20/20 and 20/40 postoperative visual acuity, respectively, eventually suffered severe visual loss as a result of progression of retinitis. The predicted visual potential of these eyes was recognized as poor prior to the decision to perform the biopsy because of the severity of the intraocular pathology that prompted the biopsy. In most cases, the poor visual outcome of the operated eyes in these patients was due to either maculopathy from retinal detachment or progression of the disease to directly involve the macula, and not due to intraoperative or postoperative complications. Although the potential postoperative complications include retinal detachment, vitreous hemorrhage, proliferative vitreoretinopathy, cataract, and bacterial endophthalmitis, this study and previous studies have shown that with the use of modern microsurgical techniques, these complications occur relatively infrequently [4].

In difficult clinical situations in which the specific etiologic diagnosis cannot be determined through less invasive measures, intraocular tissue biopsies may be required. The risks of the procedure and the potential benefit from information obtained through the biopsy should be considered; intraocular tissue biopsy is indicated only when the results are expected to contribute to the patient's management. Intraocular tissue biopsies should be reserved for patients with the possible diagnosis of infection that is unresponsive to treatment, or patients with suspected malignancy (masquerade syndrome). In future cases, the use of new techniques such as the polymerase chain reaction and in situ hybridization may provide better understanding of the specific etiology of ocular inflammation in patients such as these, and guide therapy which may be eye-saving and, in some cases, life-saving.

REFERENCES

1   Henderly DE, Genstler AJ, Smith RE, Rao NA. Am J Ophthalmol 1987; 103: 131-136.
2   Forster DJ, Dugel PU, Frangieh GT, Liggett PE, Rao, NA. Am J Ophthalmol 1990; 110: 341-348.
3   Moorthy RS, Smith RE, Rao NA. Am J Ophthalmol 1993; 115: 742-747.
4   Freeman WR, Wiley CA, Gross JG, Thomas EL, Rao NA, Liggett PE. Ophthalmology 1989; 96: 1559-1565.
5   Peyman GA, Juarez CP, Raichand M. Br J Ophthalmol 1981;65: 723-726.

© 1994 Elsevier Science B.V. All rights reserved.
Advances in Ocular Immunology
R.B. Nussenblatt, S.M. Whitcup, R.R. Caspi and I. Gery, eds.   461

NOVEL APPROACH FOR THE TREATMENT OF ENDOGENOUS CANDIDA ENDOPHTHALMITIS

P. Pivetti-Pezzi, M. Accorinti, M.A. Abdulaziz, V. Ciapparoni, A.M. De Negri, F. Sadun

Institute of Ophthalmology, Ocular Immunovirology Service, University "La Sapienza", Rome - Italy

INTRODUCTION

The extensive use of immunosuppressive and antitumour agents, of prolonged antibiotic therapies and aggressive surgical procedures requiring post-surgical total parenteral nutrition may represent an increasing risk for the development of endogenous fungal endophthalmitis (1). The therapeutical approach to endogenous fungal endophthalmitis may be conditioned by the clinical status of the patients which may not allow the use of either highly toxic drugs or ocular surgical procedures. Amphotericin B has long been the mainstay therapy for deep-seated fungal infections as well as for fungal endophthalmitis but its use is often complicated by the onset of severe side-effects (2). Fluocitosine may also be effective but the risk of haematological toxicity and the resistance to this drug by candida organism often suggest a limited use, mostly in association with other drugs. On the contrary intravitreal injections of amphotericin B seem to be a useful help to systemic drugs in controlling intraocular fungal infections (3). More recently fluconazole, a new azole compound, has become available for the treatment of deep-seated fungal infections having shown a long half-life in the blood and a good penetration into the eye either administered orally or intravenously . Fluconazole may represent a new interesting drug for the treatment of endogenous fungal endophthalmitis (4,5).
We report our experience in the treatment of endogenous candida endophthalmitis related to post-surgical total parenteral nutrition with fluconazole alone or in combination with intravitreal amphotericin B.

PATIENTS AND METHODS

At the Ocular Immunovirology Service of the University of Rome "La Sapienza", from 1988 to 1993 we observed seven patients with endogenous fungal endophthalmitis related to post-surgical total parenteral nutrition. The patients, 6 males and 1 female, mean age 49.5 years (range: 22 - 66 years) were submitted to a complete ophthalmological evaluation at the onset of the ocular disease, weekly for the first month and according to the clinical evolution therafter. In all the patients, after a clinical diagnosis of bilateral fungal endophthalmitis, a research for the isolation of fungi from the blood or on the catheter tips were performed.

Table 1
Endogenous candida endophthalmitis: clinical features at onset

	Vitreous reaction	Posterior pole exudates	Peripheral exudates	V.A.	Fluconazole (mg/day)	Intravitreal Amphotericin B
1 RE	+	+	+	10/10	600	no
LE	++	++	++	2/10		7.5µg x1
2 RE	++	+++	+	6/10	400	no
LE	+++	+++	++	c.f.		no
3 RE	++++	+	+++	h.m.	600	no
LE	------	-----	-----	10/10		--
4 RE	++	++	++	5/10	600	no
LE	++	++	++	2/10		no
5 RE	++	++	++	6/10	600	5 µg x1
LE	++++	n.e.	n.e.	h.m.		no
6 RE	+++	++	+	c.f.	400	5 µg x2
LE	++	-----	+	10/10		no
7 RE	+++	++	++	2/10	400	5 µg x2
LE	++++	n.e.	n.e.	h.m.		5 µg x2

V.A.= visual acuity, RE=right eye; LE=left eye; n.e.= not evaluable;c.f.=counting fingers; h.m.= hand motion

Table 2
Endogenous candida endophthalmitis: clinical features at the end of follow-up

	Vitreous fibrosis	Retinal fibrosis	Retinal detachment	V.A.	Resolution time (days)	Follow-up (months)
1 RE	-----	-----	-----	10/10	120	30
LE	-----	-----	-----	10/10		
2 RE	-----	-----	-----	10/10	130	22
LE	++	-----	-----	1/50		
3 RE	+	-----	-----	10/10	90	9
LE	-----	-----	-----	10/10		
4 RE	+	-----	-----	5/10	65	3
LE	+	-----	-----	5/10		
5 RE	++	+	-----	7/10	110	8
LE	n.e.	n.e.	-----	h.m.		
6 RE	++	++	+	2/50	72	48
LE	-----	-----	-----	10/10		
7 RE	++	+	-----	3/10	153	6
LE	++	+	+	5/10		

V.A.= visual acuity, RE=right eye; LE=left eye; n.e.= not evaluable;c.f.=counting fingers; h.m.= hand motion

Once obtained the confirmation of the clinical diagnosis of fungal infection all the patients were administered fluconazole therapy. The initial dose, according to the clinical status, ranged from 400 to 600 mg daily, administered intravenously.

In 4 patients (5 eyes) because of the poor ocular conditions intravitreal amphotericin B was added : one patient received one single dose of 7.5 µg/0.1 ml in one eye; another patient one single dose of 5 µg/0.1 ml in one eye while the remaining two subjects received two doses of 5 µg/ 0.1 ml in one and in both eyes, respectively. The mean follow-up was 18 months (range : 3 - 48 months).

RESULTS

Table 1 shows the clinical features of our patients at the onset of the disease. All the patients experienced a sudden decrease in visual acuity in at least one eye; a severe anterior chamber and vitreous reaction was observed in 69.2% and 92.3% of the patients, respectively. White infiltrates located at the posterior pole were detected in 6 patients (92.3%) while all of the cases showed an exudation in the midperiphery. Intravenous fluconazole therapy was administered to all the patients at the initial dose of 400-600 mg according to the systemic status. In 3 patients we obtained a real improvement of vitreo-retinal exudates after 1 month of therapy. In the other four cases, after the same therapeutic course, the endophthalmitis did not show a regression or an halt in progression. Therefore we decided to administer amphotericin B 5-7.5 µg/0.1 ml intravitreally as reported in table 1. A second dose of intravitreal amphotericin B (5 µg) was given because of an unsatisfactory response in 2 patients (3 eyes) 7-10 days after the first injection. After noting an ophthalmoscopic evidence of the regression of vitreo-retinal infiltrates, the doses of fluconazole were reduced to 200-450 mg and administered orally until no more signs of intraocular inflammation were observed. A complete resolution of endogenous candida endophthalmitis was therefore detected after a mean time of 106 days (range: 65-153 days).

The clinical features of the patients at the end of follow-up are reported in table 2. All the patients showed an improvement in visual acuity and no reaction in the anterior chamber. Vitreous and retinal fibrosis developed in 9 (69,23%) and 5 eyes (38,16%) respectively and lead to a peripheral tractive retinal detachment in 2 eyes, both treated successfully with standard surgical procedures. No side-effects related to intravenous/oral fluconazole or intravitreal amphotericin B were observed.

One patient died of adenocarcinoma methastasis, we lost track of another patient after he had stopped treatment for one month and one is still in treatment. Four patients have been out of therapy for a mean time of 24 months (range: 6 - 44 months) without any evidence of ocular recurrences.

DISCUSSION

Disseminated candidiasis is being recognized with increasing frequency in patients with a variety of underlying diseases and in those submitted to aggressive surgical procedures requiring total parenteral nutrition. Candida endophthalmitis in particular occurs in nearly 30% of patients with candidemia and it may also be found in those without documented candidemia (6). Candida endophthalmitis has a poor visual prognosis in most cases if left untreated, consequently adequate therapy is always required. For many years amphotericin B was the only drug available, but it usually has many toxic effects (2) when administered systemically so it cannot be used in patients in poor systemic conditions. Intravitreal amphotericin B has also been used with good results and no side-effects but, as a sole therapy, it does not prevent the onset of a candida infection in other organs. Recent reports in the literature have shown the efficacy of fluconazole in the treatment of deep-seated fungal infections (7). This drug has been found to penetrate the blood-ocular barrier and to be effective in the treatment of endogenous candida endophthalmitis (4,8,9,10), and does not seem to be toxic. Our results confirm that the intravenous administration of 400-600 mg of fluconazole may be effective in the treatment of parenteral nutrition-related candida endophthalmitis. Furthermore, even if the mean duration of the therapy in order to achieve a complete resolution of the intraocular inflammation was 106 days, no side-effects appeared during fluconazole administration. In 5 eyes of 4 our patients we also used amphotericin B intravitreally at the recommended dosage (3,10) without retinal toxicity to intensify the systemic therapy because of the poor response achieved. The final outcome of our cases, which may be considered unsatisfactory, has to be mainly due to the primary localization of the retinal exudates involving the macula and the optic nerve rather than to a partial therapeutic success. In conclusion our experience is similar to that reported by other Authors (8,9) in demonstrating the efficacy and safety of fluconazole, systemically administered, in the treatment of mild cases of endogenous candida endophthalmitis. More severe cases may require a combination of intravenous fluconazole and intravitreal amphotericin B and this association seems to be less toxic than most other antifungal agents available.

REFERENCES

1) Brod R.D., Flynn H.W. Jr. Curr. Opin. Ophthalmol. 1991; 2:306-309
2) Goodman L.S., Gilman A. : The farmacological basis of therapeutics. Macmillan Publ. Comp., New York, USA, 1985.
3) Adenis J.P.. J. Fr. Ophthalmol. 1986; 9,5 : 403-410.
4) O'Day D.M., Foulds G., Williams T.E., Robinson R.D., et al. Arch. Ophthalmol. 1990; 108: 1006-1008.
5) Savani D.V., Perfect J.R., Cobo L.M., Durak D.T. Antimicrob. Agents Chemother. 1987; 31: 6-10.
6) Brooks R.G. Arch. Intern. Med. 1989; 149: 2226-2228.
7) Van't Wout J.W., Mattie H., van Furth R. J. Antimicrob. Chem. 1988; 21: 665-672.
8) Laatkainen L., Tuominen M., Von Dickhoff K. Am. J. Ophthalmol. 1992; 113: 205-207.
9) Urbak S.F., and Degn T. Acta Ophthalmol. 1992; 70: 528-529.
10) Pivetti-Pezzi P., Tamburi S., Bozzoni F., Da Dalt S., et al. Boll. Ocul. 1992; 2: 255-264.

Advances in Ocular Immunology
R.B. Nussenblatt, S.M. Whitcup, R.R. Caspi and I. Gery, eds.

Long-term systemic acyclovir in the management of recurrent herpes simplex keratouveitis.

A. Rodriguez, W.J. Power, R.A. Neves, and C.S. Foster

Immunology & Uveitis Service, Massachusetts Eye & Ear Infirmary, Harvard Medical School, Boston, Massachusetts, U.S.A.

INTRODUCTION

Herpes simplex virus is one of the most frequently encountered infectious agents in patients with iridocyclitis secondary to viral infection, accounting for 1-9% of the cases [1]. The intraocular inflammation may precede or occur in conjunction with herpetic keratitis [2]. In most instances, the onset of uveitis is abrupt, and its clinical course is recurrent [1,2]. It is the recurrence of the inflammation which is responsible for the high rate of severe ocular complications leading to permanent visual loss [2,3].

Although the pathogenesis of the disease is unknown, virologic and immunologic mechanisms seem to be implicated [4,5]. Severe intraocular inflammation might be triggered by active viral replication accompanied by the release of "live" viral particles into the anterior chamber, and sustained by the action of the immune system in its attempt to clear out free virus and infected cells [2,5]. Prevention of latent virus reactivation and replication in the intraocular tissues would reduce recurrence complications. Acyclovir, is a potent and selective inhibitor of herpes simplex virus replication, and has been shown to have good intraocular penetration when administered systemically [3,4].

We report herein, our experience in the management of patients with presumed herpetic keratouveitis using long-term oral acyclovir in order to prevent recurrence of inflammation and hence limit its severe, sight-threatening ocular complications.

PATIENTS AND METHODS

A total of 20 patients with presumed herpetic keratouveitis were included in this study. The diagnosis of herpetic keratouveitis was based on a previous or concomitant history of dendritic, geographic epithelial and interstitial or disciform stromal keratitis accompanied by endothelial keratic precipitates, anterior chamber inflammatory reaction, iris stromal atrophy and posterior synechiae.

During active inflammation (at presentation or during a recurrence), all patients were managed with aggressive topical steroids. Systemic corticosteroids were only administered concomitantly with antivirals in those uveitis cases in which topical steroids were ineffective in controlling inflammation. The initial prednisone dose employed was 1 mg/kg/day which was tapered rapidly and stopped within a period of 4 to 6 weeks. These patients were then maintained on topical steroids until complete resolution of all inflammation. Cycloplegics and glaucoma medications were given as necessary.

Oral acyclovir was administered at a dose range of 1 to 2 g/day during acute recurrent attacks of iridocyclitis, and then adjusted to a long-term prophylactic dose of 600-800 mg/day according to body weight, once the intraocular inflammation had subsided. Only those patients followed for a minimum of 8 months under that antiviral prophylactic therapeutic regimen were included in the study. The rate of recurrence of intraocular inflammation was recorded for each patient throughout their follow-up.

Fisher's exact test was used to compare the recurrence rate of uveitis between patients who continued on long-term prophylactic oral acyclovir and those who discontinued the treatment. A p value < 0.05 was considered significant.

RESULTS

Twelve men and 8 women with a mean age at onset of keratouveitis of 52.9 years (range 19 - 78 years) were included in the study. All patients had a previous history of severe and prolonged recurrent herpetic keratitis.

At initial presentation to our Service, most patients (75%) presented with stromal keratitis; 11 of these patients (55%) had a disciform keratitis and 4 patients (20%) presented with an interstitial keratitis. The remaining 5 patients (25%) presented with epithelial herpetic keratitis. The anterior chamber inflammatory reaction was graded as moderate (1.5 - 3+ cells) in 11 patients (55%), and severe (>3+ cells) in 9 patients (45%). Moderate to extensive posterior iris synechiae were observed in 11 patients (55%), and stromal iris atrophy was present in 8 patients (40%).

Thirteen patients (65%) continued on long-term oral acyclovir therapy throughout their follow-up time, and 7 patients (35%) discontinued the medication at different time points during the follow-up. The mean follow-up time for those patients who continued on oral acyclovir therapy was 2.2 years (range 10 - 60 months). Three patients developed a single recurrent episode of iritis while under this therapeutic regimen. Two of these patients experienced a recurrent episode within a mean period of 16.2 months after the oral acyclovir was tapered below 600 mg/day (p <0.05). The other patient had a breakthrough episode of uveitis while on prophylactic acyclovir (800 mg/day), requiring aggressive topical and systemic corticosteroid therapy. In striking contrast, 16 recurrent episodes occurred in the 7 patients in whom acyclovir was stopped (p<0.05). Of these patients, the initial recurrent episode occurred within an average of 4.3 months following cessation of therapy.

The most common ocular complication in our study population was cataract, which developed in 65% of the patients. Cystoid macular edema occurred in 7 patients (35%), most of whom (71.4%) had experienced recurrence of inflammation secondary to discontinuation of prophylactic acyclovir therapy. Secondary glaucoma developed in 4 patients (20%), 3 of whom (75%) had experienced at least one attack of intraocular inflammation while off prophylactic acyclovir therapy.

DISCUSSION

The intraocular inflammation secondary to herpes simplex infection may present as a mild transient form secondary to an irritative or reactive iritis associated with epithelial keratitis resulting from a self-limited neurological reflex mechanism [1,2]. However, it is the more severe form of uveitis, resulting from the presence of HSV antigens and probable replication of "live" viral particles in the anterior chamber, which is responsible for the severe ocular complications and profound visual impairment attendant to recurrent herpetic keratouveitis [4,6]. All of our patients suffered from moderate to severe recurrent anterior uveitis significant enough to be referred to our Service for further management.

The intraocular inflammation is mostly a nongranulomatous iridocyclitis with a mild to severe anterior chamber inflammatory reaction composed of fibrin, and white and red blood cells with small to medium size KPs [1,2]. The KPs interference with endothelial cell function, along with the transient rise in the intraocular pressure during the peak of the inflammation may give rise to stromal and epithelial edema as well as Descemet's folds [7]. Eleven of our patients (55%) presented with epithelial and/or stromal edema secondary to herpetic stromal keratitis and/or a transient elevation in the intraocular pressure during recurrent episodes of inflammation. The iris may show congestion, edema, and after multiple recurrent episodes of inflammation, extensive posterior synechiae; and a characteristic iris stromal atrophy may occur [6]. In our series, 40% of the patients were found to have atrophic changes within the iris stroma as noted by transillumination.

The pathogenesis of herpetic iridocyclitis remains unknown. Viral replication can occur in the anterior chamber and uveal tissue. Electron microscopy studies have shown evidence of herpes virus particles in iris biopsies [8], and virus antigen has been detected by immunofluorescence inside inflammatory cells within the anterior chamber of patients with severe herpetic uveitis [9]. Viral reactivation and replication within the anterior segment of the eye might initiate an immune response against the virus in which humoral as well as cell-mediated immune mechanisms may be involved [8,9].

Treatment of herpetic keratouveitis is based on the use of topical and/or systemic corticosteroids along with antiviral therapy. Long-term oral acyclovir reduces recurrent inflammation by preventing viral reactivation and replication; thereby reducing ocular complications that can lead to blindness [3]. In our series, this prophylactic therapeutic strategy resulted in a significant reduction in the rate of recurrence of inflammation. Although the optimal therapeutic regimen with long-term systemic acyclovir is still controversial, in our experience, the maintenance prophylactic dose (600 - 800 mg/day) should depend on the body weight of the individual patient [3]. Side effects from long-term systemic acyclovir are very rare [10]; none developed in our patients.

In conclusion, herpes simplex virus keratouveitis is a serious ocular infectious disease in which recurrence of inflammation results in extensive corneal scarring, iris atrophy, cataract formation, secondary glaucoma, and inflammatory macular edema, all of which may lead to severe visual impairment. Our results suggest that the long-term prophylactic use of systemic acyclovir may be of great benefit in the prevention of recurrences, and hence may prevent the blinding complications of this disease.

REFERENCES

1. Wilhelmus KR, Falcon MG, Jones BR. Herpetic iridocyclitis. Intl Ophthalmol 1981;4:143-150.
2. O'Connor GR. Recurrent Herpes simplex uveitis in humans. Surv Ophthalmol 1976;21:165-170.
3. Foster, CS, Barney NP. Systemic acyclovir and penetrating keratoplasty for herpes simplex keratitis. Doc Ophthalmol 1992;80:363-369.
4. Liesegang T. Ocular herpes simplex infection: pathogenesis and current therapy. Mayo Clin Proc 1988;63:1092-1096.
5. Pepose JS. Herpes simplex keratitis: role of viral infection versus immune response. Surv Ophthalmol 1991;35:345-352.
6. Hogan MJ, Kimura SJ, Thygeson P. Pathology of herpes simplex keratoiritis. Am J Ophthalmol 1964;57:551-564.
7. Vannas A, Ahonen R, Makitie J. Corneal endothelium in herpetic keratouveitis. Arch Ophthalmol 1983;101:913-915.
8. Witmer R, Inomato T. Electron microscopic observation of the iris in herpes uveitis. Arch Ophthalmol 1968;79:331-337.
9. Kaufman HE, Kanai A, Ellison ED. Herpetic iritis: demonstration of virus in the anterior chamber by fluorescent antibody techniques and electron microscopy. Am J Ophthalmol 1971;71:465-469.
10. Colin J, Malet F, Chastel C. Acyclovir in herpetic anterior uveitis. Ann Ophthalmol 1991;23:28-30.

© 1994 Elsevier Science B.V. All rights reserved.
Advances in Ocular Immunology
R.B. Nussenblatt, S.M. Whitcup, R.R. Caspi and I. Gery, eds.

THE MODE OF HIV ACQUISITION AND THE PREVALENCE OF RETINAL FINDINGS

Richard F. Spaide, M.D.
Anton Gaissinger, Diploma Medical Engineering
Joseph R. Podhorzer, M.D.
From the Department of Ophthalmology, St. Vincent's Hospital and Medical
Center of New York, Suite 506 O'Toole Building, 36 Seventh Ave., New York,
NY 10011. Mr. Gaissinger is currently at the Technical University of München,
Germany.

ABSTRACT

To investigate the relationship between the mode of HIV acquisition and
retinal findings a cross-sectional study was performed on 323 consecutive male
patients with a positive serodiagnosis for HIV. The patients were stratified into
two groups according to their predominant risk factors for HIV acquisition, and
these were designated Sexual and Intravenous. Patients in the Sexual group
were more likely to have cotton-wool spots (odds ratio = 2.96, p=0.0065) and
cytomegalovirus retinitis (odds ratio = 5.13, p=0.0076), than were patients in
the Intravenous group after adjustment for their CD4+ T-lymphocyte counts by
logistic regression. This study suggests that the ocular manifestations of HIV
infection are associated with the mode of HIV acquisition.

INTRODUCTION

In patients with AIDS, the frequency and severity of medical problems
escalate with declining CD4+ T-lymphocyte counts. Other factors, such as mode
of HIV acquisition, are associated with increased prevalence of specific
opportunistic infections and manifestations of AIDS, as well. Sexually
transmitted diseases, Kaposi's sarcoma,[1] enterocolitis,[2] amebiasis,[3] and certain
gastrointestinal carcinomas are more common in patients with homosexually
acquired HIV infection. Active tuberculosis occurs more frequently among
patients with HIV acquired through intravenous drug use.[4] The aim of the
present study is to evaluate the prevalence of retinal findings in a group of 323
consecutive male patients with HIV infection in reference to their mode of HIV
acquisition.

PATIENTS AND METHODS

The cohort of patients in this study were examined in the HIV-
Retinopathy Clinic at St. Vincent's Hospital during a ten month period ending
October, 1993. The eligibility criteria for inclusion in the study were: 1) male

sex, 2) positive Western blot analysis for HIV, 3) T-lymphocyte assay within 3 months of the ocular examination, 4) knowledge of risk factors for HIV acquisition, 5) the risk factor being either intravenous drug use or homosexual or bisexual activity. During the time period of the study 368 consecutive male HIV patients were examined in the HIV-Retinopathy Clinic, but 45 did not meet the eligibility criteria for the study. The study design was approved by the Institutional Review Board of St. Vincent's Hospital and Medical Center of New York.

To aid in analysis, patients were classified into 2 groups according to their predominant risk factors for HIV acquisition, and these groups were designated Sexual and Intravenous. The Sexual group was comprised of patients with the risk factor for HIV acquisition being homosexual or bisexual activity. The Intravenous group was comprised of patients with the risk factor for HIV acquisition being intravenous drug use. (These two groups have the highest risk for HIV acquisition in the United States.[5])

RESULTS

Of the 323 patients meeting the eligibility criteria for this study, the risk for HIV acquisition was identified as intravenous drug use in 68 (21.1%), and sexual in 255 (78.9%), with homosexual acquisition implicated in 241 and bisexual in 14. (Table 1). The mean CD4+ counts of the Sexual and Intravenous groups were compared and the difference between the two groups was not significant (p=.12, independent sample t-test). The mean CD4+/CD8+ ratios of the two groups were not significantly different in the two groups either (p=.20).

The mean CD4+ T-lymphocyte counts of patients with no retinopathy was 253.7 (standard deviation 231). The mean CD4+ T-lymphocyte counts of patients with cotton-wool spots only was 93.2, cotton-wool spots with cytomegalovirus retinitis was 44.4, and cytomegalovirus retinitis only was 22.5. The mean CD4+ counts of the patients with retinopathies were compared using one-way ANOVA, and a significant difference was found. Post hoc analysis using the Student-Newman-Keuls test showed a significant difference in the mean CD4+ T-lymphocyte counts of the cotton-wool spots only and cytomegalovirus retinitis only groups.

Cotton-wool spots, found with or without associated cytomegalovirus retinitis, were present in 76 (23.5%) patients. The prevalence of cotton-wool spots was higher in the Sexual group than in the Intravenous group (p=0.0038, chi-square test). Among patients with cotton-wool spots, 57.1% of the Intravenous group and 91.3% of the Sexual group had CD4+ counts less that 200, which is one of the diagnostic criteria for AIDS. Cytomegalovirus retinitis was found in 40 patients (12.4%) patients. The prevalence of cytomegalovirus retinitis was higher in the Sexual group than in the Intravenous group (p=0.0078, chi-square test).

Logistic regression was performed to evaluate sexual acquisition of HIV infection and CD4+ T-lymphocyte counts as risk factors for the development of cotton-wool spots and cytomegalovirus. The odds ratios, with the corresponding 95% confidence intervals and associated p-values are shown in Table 3. CD4+ T-lymphocyte counts less than or equal to 100 were strongly associated with the development of HIV-related retinopathies. Sexual, as opposed to intravenous acquisition of HIV infection, independently conferred an odds ratio of 2.97 for the development of cotton-wool spots and 5.23 for cytomegalovirus retinitis.

Table 1
Logistic Regression of Predictors for HIV-Related Retinopathies

Variable	Odds Ratio	95% Confidence Interval	p-value*
Cotton-Wool Spots			
Sexual Acquisition	2.97	1.92 - 4.6	0.0065
CD4 ≤ 100	5.23	2.8 - 9.76	<0.0001

Model chi-square = 41.9, 2 df, p<.0001

Cytomegalovirus Retinitis			
Sexual Acquisition	5.12	2.41 - 10.87	0.0076
CD4 ≤ 100	13.86	4.17 - 46.12	<0.0001

Model chi-square = 42.8, 2 df, p<.0001

DISCUSSION

This study of 323 consecutive male HIV patients confirmed past findings that cotton-wool spots and cytomegalovirus retinitis were associated with low CD4+ T-lymphocyte counts.[6] This study found that cotton-wool spots and cytomegalovirus retinitis were significantly more common in patients with sexual acquisition of HIV.
In the present study, the two groups had similar CD4+ counts, making the extent of HIV disease, as measured by the CD4+ count an unlikely explanation for the different prevalence of the retinopathies detected. Indeed, even after using logistic regression to control for the CD4+ count, the associations were still found.

In the present study, cotton-wool spots were more common in patients with low CD4+ counts, particularly for patients in the Sexual group. The exact cause of cotton-wool spots in HIV patients is not known. It has been suggested that cotton-wool spots may be related to HIV infection of the retinal capillary endothelium.[7,8] In the present study, patients in the Sexual group were more likely to have cotton-wool spots than patients in the Intravenous group. Since both groups had HIV infection, and similar CD4+ counts, it appears unlikely that HIV infection of the capillary endothelium alone can explain the development of cotton-wool spots.

We found that cytomegalovirus retinitis occurred more frequently in patients of the Sexual group. The exact reason for the increased prevalence is not known with certainty, but suppositions, based on the epidemiology of cytomegalovirus, can be made. Although cytomegalovirus infection may be contracted early in life under conditions of crowding or poor hygiene, in industrialized countries, infections after childhood are commonly contracted through sexual activity. In various studies the risk factors for seropositivity for cytomegalovirus in patients with or without concurrent HIV infection have been identified to include: a recent sexual partner, more than 2 lifetime sexual partners,[9] frequent sexual partners,[10,11] early age of intercourse,[11] a past history of sexually transmitted diseases,[10,12] and anal-receptive intercourse.[10]

Blood transfusion is also a possible vector for the transmission of cytomegalovirus. Intravenous drug users, through needle sharing, may inadvertently transfer blood that has refluxed into the syringe. The risk for seroconversion for cytomegalovirus after the transfer of the small amount of blood associated with needle sharing is not known. The risk for seroconversion after receiving a unit of blood, a much larger amount, is estimated to be 2-3%.[13] In one study of HIV infected patients, 100% of homosexual men, but only 57% of hemophiliacs, were seropositive for cytomegalovirus.[14] An implication of these findings is that exchange of blood, although a possible vector, may not be an efficient mechanism for transferring cytomegalovirus infection.

HIV-related retinopathies have been associated with low CD4+ counts in previous studies. The present study also identified sexual, as opposed to intravenous, acquisition of HIV as a risk factor associated with both cotton-wool spots and cytomegalovirus retinitis. There may be factors, inherent in the differing life styles of these two high risk groups, that may be associated with the retinal manifestations of HIV infection. It is possible, though, that repeated exposure to cytomegalovirus, spread through high risk sexual practices, may put the recipient at increased risk for cytomegalovirus retinitis. If this were true, it is possible that safer sexual practices could limit the spread of cytomegalovirus infection and its ocular sequelae.

REFERENCES

1.   Beral V., Peterman T.A., Berkelman R.L., Jaffe H.W.: Kaposi's sarcoma among persons with AIDS: a sexually transmitted infection? Lancet 335(8682):123, 1990.

2.   Quinn T.C.: The polymicrobial etiology of intestinal infections in homosexual men. N Engl J Med 309:576, 1983.

3.   Schmerin M.J., Gelston A., Jones T.C.: Amebiasis: An increasing problem among homosexuals in New York City. JAMA 238: 1386, 1977.

4.   Selwyn P.A., Hartel D., Lewis V.A.,Schoenbaum E.E, Vermund S.H., Klein R.S., Walker A.T., Friedland G.H.: A prospective study of the risk of tuberculosis among intravenous drug users with human immunodeficiency virus infection. N Eng J Med 320: 545, 1989.

5.   Centers for Disease Control: HIV/AIDS Surveillance Report, March 1991, pp 1-22.

6   Kuppermann, B.D., Petty J.G., Richman M.D., Mathews W.C., Fullerton S.C., Rickman L.S., Freeman W.R.: Correlation between CD4+ counts and prevalence of cytomegalovirus retinitis and human immunodeficiency virus-related noninfectious retinal vasculopathy in patients with acquired immunodeficiency syndrome. Am J Ophthalmol 115: 575, 1993.

7   Pomerantz R.J., Kuritzkes D.R., de la Monte S.M., Rota T.R., Baker A.S., Albert D., Bor D.H. Feldman E.L., Schooley R.T. Hirsh M.S.:Infection of the retina by human immunodeficiency virus type 1. N Engl J Med 317: 1643, 1987.

8.   Jabs D.A., Green W.R., Fox R., Polk B.F., Bartlett J.G.: Ocular manifestations of the acquired immune deficiency syndrome. Ophthalmology 96:1092 1989.

9.   Sohn Y.M. Oh M.K., Balcarek K.B., Cloud G.A., Pass R.F.: Cytomegalovirus infection in sexually active adolescents. J Infect Dis 163: 460, 1991.

10.   Collier A.C., Meyers J.D., Corey L., Murphy V.L., Roberts P.L., Handsfield H.H.: Cytomegalovirus infection in homosexual men. Relationship to sexual practices, antibody to human immunodeficiency virus, and cell-mediated immunity. Am J Med 82:593, 1987.

11.   Chandler S.H., Holmes K.K., Wentworth B.B., Gutman L.T., Wiesner P.J., Alexander E.R., Handsfield H.H.: The epidemiology of cytomegalovirus infection in women attending a sexually transmitted disease clinic. J. Infect Dis 151:344, 1985.

12.   Hyams K.C., Krogwold R.A., Brock S., Wignall S., Cross E., Hayes C.: Heterosexual transmission of viral hepatitis and cytomegalovirus infection among United States military personnel stationed in the western Pacific. Sexually Transmitted Diseases 20:36, 1993.

13.   Ho, M: Epidemiology of cytomegalovirus infections. Reviews of Infectious Diseases 12:S701, 1990.

14.   Jackson M.A., Erice A., Englund J.A., Edson J.R., Balfour H.H.: Prevalence of cytomegalovirus antibody in hemophiliacs and homosexuals infected with the human immunodeficiency virus type 1. Transfusion 28: 187, 1988.

Index of authors